A History of Forensic Science in 10 Publications

How They Established Current Practice

Sean Doyle

Linked Forensic Consultants Ltd
Wellington, New Zealand

WILEY

This edition first published 2026

Registered Office(s)
John Wiley & Sons, Inc., 111 River Street, Hoboken, NJ 07030, USA
John Wiley & Sons Ltd. New Era House, 8 Oldlands Way, Bognor Regis, West Sussex, PO22 0NO, UK

Wiley-VCH GmbH, Boschstr. 12, 69469 Weinheim, Germany

John Wiley & Sons Singapore Pte Ltd, 134 Jurong Gateway Road, #04-307H, Singapore 600134

For details of our global editorial offices, customer services, and more information about Wiley products visit us at www.wiley.com.

The manufacturer's authorized representative according to the EU General Product Safety Regulation is Wiley-VCH GmbH, Boschstr. 12, 69469 Weinheim, Germany, e-mail: Product_Safety@wiley.com.

Wiley also publishes its books in a variety of electronic formats and by print-on-demand. Some content that appears in standard print versions of this book may not be available in other formats.

Library of Congress Cataloging-in-Publication Data:
Names: Doyle, Sean, 1955- author
Title: A history of forensic science in 10 publications : how they established current practice / Sean Doyle, Linked Forensic Consultants Ltd, Wellington, New Zealand.
Description: Hoboken, NJ : Wiley, [2026] | Includes bibliographical references and index.
Identifiers: LCCN 2025034108 | ISBN 9781394170760 hardback | ISBN 9781394170777 pdf | ISBN 9781394170784 epub
Subjects: LCSH: Forensic sciences—History
Classification: LCC HV8073 .D688 2026
LC record available at https://lccn.loc.gov/2025034108

Cover Design: Wiley
Cover Image: © Stuart McCall/Getty Images

Contents

About the Author

Sean Doyle is a consultant forensic scientist and a director at Linked Forensic Consultants Ltd, a New Zealand-based company specialising in critically reviewing scientific evidence. He cofounded the consultancy in 2010, having spent decades as a forensic scientist working with UK law enforcement agencies and prosecution authorities. He completed his government career as the Principal Scientist at the Forensic Explosives Laboratory, now part of Dstl.

Sean is also a cofounder, a director and Director of Quality at The Forensic Isotope Ratio Mass Spectrometry (FIRMS) Network Ltd, an English-based company with an international board of governors that promotes the forensic application of stable isotope analysis.

For many years, he lectured at universities in NZ and England on various aspects of forensic science at undergraduate and postgraduate levels. Over his career, he has partnered with universities in many joint projects.

Sean is a Chartered Chemist and a Fellow of both the Royal Society of Chemistry and the Chartered Society of Forensic Science. In 2025, he celebrates his fiftieth year as a forensic scientist.

He is the author of many publications, book chapters and a standard text, Quality Management in Forensic Science.

Sean is still active in case work and has recently been involved in the trial of Mark Lundy and the appeal of Scott Watson in New Zealand. Historically, he has had some exposure to many actual and potential miscarriages of justice, from Sally Clark and the Birmingham 6 in England to Shandee Blackburn in Queensland, Australia.

Acknowledgements

Like all authors, I owe a huge debt of gratitude to many people for their help in writing this book, especially to the living authors of the publications selected, whose helpful suggestions and insights have significantly improved the book.

Sir Alec Jeffreys
William C Thompson
Edward L Schumann
D Michael Risinger
Michael J Saks
Claude Roux

I am especially grateful to Pierre Margot, whose correspondence proved to be an education.

I am also grateful to those who helped in various ways, including reviewing, offering helpful advice and providing information and general guidance.

Christian Bachhiels
Stefan Köchel
Heather Wolfram
Jeffrey Teitelbaum
Matthew and Gerald Doyle
Rosemary Marryat

As ever, any errors in the text are mine alone.

I also wish to express my gratitude to the following: the patient editors at Wiley; Tom Holland and Dominic Sandbrook, whose podcast 'The Rest is History' was the initial inspiration for this book. Last but certainly not least, I want to thank my beloved wife, Dianne, for her patience and encouragement.

List of Abbreviations

REGION	ABBR	
USA	A2LA	Assessment Accreditation Services
A&NZ	A&NZ	Australia and New Zealand
USA	AAFS	American Academy of Forensic Sciences
USA	ABC	American Board of Criminalistics
	ACE V	Analysis Comparison Evaluation & Verification [of fingerprints]
INTL	AFTE	Association of Firearm and Toolmark Examiners
	AI	Artificial Intelligence
A&NZ	ANZPAA	Australia New Zealand Police Advisory Agency
USA	ANAB	ANSI American National Accreditation Board
USA	ANSI	American National Standards Institute
USA	ASB	AAFS Standards Board
USA	ASCLD/LAB	Association of Crime Laboratory Directors/Laboratory Accreditation Board
INTL	ASTM	American Society for Testing and Materials [SDO]
USA	ATF	Bureau of Alcohol Tobacco, Firearms and Explosives
USA	BJA	Bureau of Justice Assistance
	BPA	Bloodstain Pattern Analysis
USA	CAC	California Association of Criminalists
	CAI	Case Assessment and Interpretation
UK	CBE	Commander of the Order of the British Empire
	CCTV	Closed-circuit TV
USA	CEBR	DNA Capacity Enhancement for Backlog Reduction
UK	CH	Order of the Companions of Honour
CHE	CHE	Helvetic Confederation [Switzerland]
E&W	CID	Criminal Investigation Department [Police]
UK	CRFP	Council for the Registration of Forensic Practitioners
USA	DEA	Drugs Enforcement Agency

REGION	ABBR	
	DNA	Deoxyribonucleic acid
USA	DOJ	Department of Justice
	E&W	England and Wales
EUR	EAFS	European Academy of Forensic Sciences
EUR	ENFSI	European Network of Forensic Science Institutes
CHE	ESC	École des sciences criminelles [School of Criminal Sciences, University of Lausanne]
USA	FBI	Federal Bureau of Investigation
UK	FRS	Fellow of the Royal Society
USA	FSAB	Forensic Specialties Accreditation Board
E&W	FSR	Forensic Science Regulator
E&W	FSS	Forensic Science Service
USA	FSSB	Forensic Science Standards Board
UK	HMG	His Majesty's Government
INTL	IAI	International Association of Identification
INTL	IEC	International Electrotechnical Commission [SDO]
INTL	ILAC	International Laboratory Accreditation Cooperation
USA	IOM	Institute of Medicine
INTL	ISO	International Organization for Standardization [SDO]
	LCN DNA	Low copy number DNA
	LR	Likelihood ratio
	LT DNA	Low template DNA
EUR	MAE	Member of the Academia Europaea
	mtDNA	mitochondrial DNA
	NAA	Neutron Activation Analysis
USA	NAE	National Academy of Engineering
USA	NAS	National Academy of Sciences
USA	NCFS	National Commission of Forensic Science [DoJ]
	nDNA	Nuclear DNA
	NGS	Next Generation Sequencing
A&NZ	NIFS	National Institute of Forensic Science
USA	NIJ	National Institute of Justice
USA	NIST	National Institute of Standards and Technology
USA	NRC	National Research Council
USA	NSTC	National Science and Technology Council

REGION	ABBR	
E&W	NSY	New Scotland Yard, Headquarters of the London Metropolitan Police
UK	OBE	Officer of the Order of the British Empire
UK	OM	British Order of Merit
USA	OSAC	Organisation of Scientific Area Committees
USA	PCAST	President's Council of Advisors on Science and Technology
	PCR	Polymerase Chain Reaction
	PGS	Probabilistic Genotyping Software
	QA	Quality Assurance
	QC	Quality Control
	QMS	Quality Management System
UK	RARDE	Royal Armament Research and Development Establishment
	RFLP	Restriction Fragment Length Polymorphism
	RFU	Relative Fluorescent Unit
	RNA	Ribonucleic Acid
	SDO	Standards Development Organisation
	SGM	Single Gamete Multiplex
USA	SoFS	Subcommittee on Forensic Science
	STR	Short Tandem Repeat
USA	SWGDAM	Scientific Working Group on DNA Analysis Methods
USA	SWGFAST	Scientific Working Group on Friction Ridge Analysis, Study and Technology
USA	SWGGUN	Scientific Working Group on Firearms and Toolmarks
	TOR	Terms of Reference
USA	UCB	University of California, Berkley
USA	UCI	University of California, Irvine
USA	UCR	University of California, Riverside
UK	UK	United Kingdom of Great Britain and Northern Ireland
UK	UKAS	United Kingdom Accreditation Service
USA	USA	United States of America
	VNTR	Variable Nucleotide Tandem Repeats
	WW	World War

Terms, Definitions and Explanations

Introduction

In addition to the specialist, this work is also aimed at the general reader interested in the history of forensic science, so some technical terms are defined and explained in alphabetical order with some context to aid understanding.

Many of these explanations, or parts thereof, are repeated in the main text, but this section will enable the reader to quickly check meanings when necessary.

Bias – Cognitive Bias – Tunnel Vision – Observer Effects

Cognitive bias is an error in thinking. The fundamental premise is that human beings are not independent and objective observers. We tend to come with preconceived ideas, are receptive to information confirming those ideas, and reject information that does not. There is a whole raft of different cognitive biases that contribute to poor decision-making. Tunnel vision and confirmation bias are two (of many) that particularly affect crime investigation and, in turn, forensic science.

Tunnel vision is the tendency to select evidence to build a case to secure a conviction. Confirmation bias tends to favour information that confirms preconceptions independently of the information's accuracy while ignoring conflicting or contradictory evidence.

The main remedy is for all involved, including forensic scientists, to keep an open mind.

Case Assessment and Interpretation

Case assessment and interpretation (CAI) is an approach to decision-making in an operational forensic science organisation based on the principles of Bayesian inference. In practice, it involves assigning likelihood ratios (LR) to candidate evidence types to determine which might deliver the most probative value, saving time and money. CAI engages the forensic scientist at an early stage of a criminal investigation and at the crime scene. The steps are as follows.

1. Define customer requirement
2. Assess how forensic science can help by assigning LRs to evidence types
3. Agree on a forensic examination strategy
4. Carry out examinations
5. Interpret the results using an LR approach
6. Communicate the test results and opinion

CAI is not a rigidly defined process, but it can guide workflow so that time and energy are spent on the issues and items expected to produce the most valuable information.

References to CAI occur throughout the book, with a detailed discussion in Chapter 8.

Chromosome

A chromosome is a package of DNA. The DNA molecule is about two meters long. Getting it to fit into the nucleus of a cell, which is between 5 and 20 millionths of a meter, is a challenge. To achieve that aim, the DNA is coiled and folded to form chromosomes, which compact and organise the DNA molecule within the cell nucleus.

It is important to think of chromosomes as packets or units of DNA. In the nucleus of a human cell, there are 46 chromosomes in 23 pairs, one of which determines sex. One of each pair is either from Mum or Dad.

Common Law and Civil Law

Strictly speaking, science should be the same everywhere. In contrast, legal systems differ and vary by jurisdiction. The major difference is between Common Law and Civil Law.

Common Law relies on an adversarial approach, where two opposing sides present their cases to uncover the truth. In contrast, civil law is inquisitorial or non-adversarial, considering any evidence that might be relevant and gathering all the facts. It is often conducted by a judge. Both systems aim to uncover the truth, and each has its strengths and weaknesses.

Common law is derived from the law of medieval England. In addition to operating in England and Wales, it also operates in former colonies of what was the British Empire, such as Australia, and parts of the United States.

Common law is based on precedent and judicial decisions, i.e. case law, rather than being documented or codified; it is evolutionary and adopts an adversarial approach to weighing evidence, uncovering the truth and delivering justice. In this system, lawyers act for the prosecution. Their role is to present the facts to prove the crime with which a defendant is charged. The prosecutor represents the state, whereas the defence lawyer, or attorney, acts primarily as the protector of the defendant's rights and interests. The evidence is placed before a neutral judge and/or jury, which determines the truth. Perhaps the most important right is to a presumption of innocence, which applies in most jurisdictions. It is important to note in passing that these role differences produce divergent ethical responsibilities.

In the adversarial system, because of the presumption of innocence, the burden of proof usually lies with the prosecution. The defence is not required to prove anything, and the defendant is not required to give or present evidence.

The strength of evidence presented is tested by cross-examination of witnesses of both fact and opinion, and plea bargaining is common.

In the common law/adversarial system, for evidence to be admitted, it must be relevant and probative. Many rules exclude relevant evidence that might not be probative and vice versa. These rules aim to focus the court on the most cogent evidence. In simple terms, the adversarial system excludes evidence that might be considered in the civil law/inquisitorial system.

Despite the lofty claims made for the adversarial system, that it will uncover the truth, it is, in reality, a gladiatorial contest in which both sides want to win, and winning is more important than the truth. In addition, the prosecution often has all the resources of the state at its disposal, creating an uneven contest and far from an 'equality of arms'. These factors can and do contribute to miscarriages of justice.

Civil law is codified, i.e. written down, and has its roots in Roman law and, more recently, the Napoleonic Code of 1804. This system applies in continental Europe, such as the Penal Code in France, and the former colonies of non-British European powers. Civil law has an inquisitorial approach. In contrast with the adversarial system, which has many rules that exclude certain types of evidence, an inquisitorial system is inclusive and considers all evidence that might be relevant. The inquiry is often led by a judge who establishes the facts based on the evidence. Experts are usually appointed by the court and are expected to act impartially, assisting the court to understand complex issues. As such, they are usually not subject to cross-examination, a key element in the adversarial system. In addition, Plea bargaining is rare.

Criminology and Criminalistics

Providing concise and simple definitions or explanations of these terms acceptable to all academics and practitioners, even today, would be a challenge. The distinctions have been and remain quite fluid. There is a section of Chapter 10 devoted to a discussion of these terms and their history.

While inconsistencies in meaning in the same language add to the confusion, translations have not helped. The German 'kriminalistik' and the French 'criminalistique' are often translated into English as 'criminology'.

When this story starts back in the nineteenth century, those who considered themselves criminologists were mostly engaged in trying to identify the criminal type through physical characteristics (criminal anthropology) so that, once identified, measures could be taken to protect society from crime.

Today, criminology is a broad interdisciplinary field encompassing all aspects of crime: its causes, criminal behaviour and its punishment (penology), legislation, law enforcement, the criminal justice system and society's response to crime. It is a subject founded on the social sciences rather than the natural and life sciences such as chemistry, physics and biology.

Criminalistics might be defined as the recognition, examination and interpretation of physical evidence utilising the natural and life sciences. However, for Edmond Locard, 'criminalistique' seems to have meant, more broadly, the scientific investigation of crime.

Applying the term criminalistics to a discipline somewhat akin to what is generally understood to be forensic science began in California in the 1940s. It was borrowed from European sources, where in some quarters it had the same meaning as criminology. It was used to distinguish those applying the natural and life sciences to the investigation of crime, criminalists, from criminologists. The term criminalistics, having been 'born' in California, has largely remained there.

Fallacy

A fallacy is an error in reasoning that results in poor decision-making. Two fallacies relevant to forensic science are the prosecutor's and defender's fallacies, which are the subject of Chapter 5. Respectively, these fallacies risk unfairly strengthening the prosecution or defence case.

Forensic Science and Terminological Ambiguity

Ambiguity extends to the meaning of 'forensic science' itself, which remains contested. Some seem to think it cannot be defined, only described (Fraser 2020). Others consider forensic science to be the science of the trace or 'traceology' (Margot 2011; Roux et al. 2021), and some more prosaically consider forensic science as science in the service of the law and justice (Doyle 2019). Many others take the far more utilitarian view that forensic science is any science that might be applied to the resolution of legal disputes. This understanding aligns with the broad view expressed in the international standard ISO 21043:2018 'Forensic sciences – Part 1: Terms and definitions'. The meaning of the term 'forensic science' is a major topic in this book.

Paul Kirk, in his Ontogeny paper, the subject of Chapter 3, characterises forensic science as '*synthetic*', by which he probably meant prepared or made artificially – an odd word – and '*conglomerate*', a mixture, combination and/or mingling of things. However, it is more syncretic than eclectic.

Whatever the definition, forensic science is at the service of the law and justice; it aims to reconstruct past events, help solve the crime and deliver justice.

Gene

A gene is a sequence of three of the four bases (A, T, C, G) on the DNA molecule (see Nucleic acids in the following text) that codes – carries instructions for – a particular amino acid. There is a series of these three base codes. RNA then assembles the amino acids into proteins to form cells, and cells get together to form tissues, which go on to form organs such as a pair of lungs.

Genome

Another term to be familiar with is genome. The human genome is a complete set of genetic information in human cells, encoded as DNA within the 23 chromosome pairs in cell nuclei and in a small DNA molecule found within individual mitochondria. These are usually treated separately as the nuclear genome and the mitochondrial genome.

Hierarchy of Propositions

In arriving at an evaluative opinion (see 'Opinions' later in the text), consideration must be given to the level of the propositions evaluated. Offence-level propositions are for the fact-finder or jury. Provided the forensic scientist has sufficient information, activity-level propositions might be evaluated. This is the ideal. However, in practice, it is not often that the forensic scientist can evaluate activity-level propositions.

With DNA evidence, there is also a sub-source category. Modern DNA analysis methods are so sensitive that even a few cells or parts thereof are enough to give useful profiles. In those cases, the identity of a contributor might be known, but not the cellular source, that is, what type of cell the DNA came from. Hence, the sub-source category. The following table (Table Terms.1) uses the example of an alleged sexual assault to demonstrate the levels in the hierarchy.

Table Terms.1 Hierarchy of propositions.

Level	Proposition – Yes/No	Evaluator
Offence	Sexual assault	Jury/factfinder
Activity	Sexual contact	Forensic scientist
Source	Semen	Ditto
Sub-source	DNA contributor	Ditto

Inference – Methods of Reasoning: Deduction, Induction and Abduction

Inference may be thought of as reaching a logical conclusion based on evidence and reasoning or, more simply, explaining observations and findings.

Human beings use inferential reasoning to make decisions all the time. For example, whether to take an umbrella on a walk.

Whenever it is cloudy and overcast, it is likely to rain. It is cloudy and overcast today, so an umbrella is taken. This is deduction: the application of a general rule (if it's cloudy and overcast, it's likely to rain) to a specific case (today's weather).

The Met Office has forecast rain every day this week and, so far, it has rained. Today's forecast is for rain, so an umbrella is taken. This is induction and is based on past events, but it might not always be true. Even though rain is forecast, it might not rain.

The lawn is wet; it either rained, or maybe I left the sprinkler on. I can't see the sprinkler, so it probably rained. An umbrella is taken just in case it rains again. This is abduction, suggesting the most plausible explanation based on available evidence.

Fundamental activities in forensic science are making observations, for example, bloodstain patterns at the scene of a suspicious death, analysing the patterns and then providing an explanation of how that pattern was produced. There is often more than one possible explanation, in which case the forensic scientist must assess the relative likelihoods of those explanations by some rational and logical process and report which is the most likely. Ideally, this should be by formulating an evaluative opinion (see 'Opinions' in the following text). However, there is more than one route from observation to explanation, and these include the three inferential methods of deduction, induction and abduction.

Deduction

Deduction is the classical process of reasoning from general principles to specific instances.

1. All swans are white.
2. The bird is a swan.
3. The bird is white.

Another example

1. All beans in the bag are black.
2. The beans in my hand are from the bag.
3. The beans in my hand are black.

If premises 1 and 2 are true, then the conclusion or explanation 3 must also be true. Some argue that this is just a statement of the obvious and is not a productive means of producing new knowledge.

In deduction, the explanation is inferred or predicted.

The weakness is that you cannot know that premise 1 is true until, for example, all swans have been observed. We now know that there are black swans. This is part of the logical weakness of fingerprint evidence. It is impossible to conclude with certainty that a person's fingerprints are unique until the fingerprints of all persons, living and dead, have been observed, which is impossible.

In forensic science, deduction is used when applying known scientific principles, laws or facts to a particular case to reach a conclusion. Examples include applying the physics of ballistics to a shooting, or the molecular biology of the DNA molecule to DNA profiling.

Induction

Induction involves reaching a conclusion based on a series of observations. This is a common process in science and is the basis of the scientific method. Experiments are conducted to test a theory or an explanation. If the theory passes the test, then it is accepted with the understanding that further experiments may show the explanation to be false.

In contrast with deduction, which predicts the explanation, induction predicts or infers a rule.

Using the bag of beans example, a handful of beans are taken from the bag on several occasions, and each time, it is found that all the beans are black. The conclusion is that all the beans in the bag are black. The weakness is that there might be a white (say) bean in the bag, but it was missed in the sampling.

In forensic science, induction is used in pattern analysis and profiling. In comparison, discipline examiners will establish over time which features are less common than others. The relative rarity of features will assist in attributing a source.

Inductive inference is the basis of the scientific method, which includes the elements of theorising, experiment and observation. In forensic science, there must be a theory to test, and that is where abduction comes in.

Abduction

Abduction can be thought of as simply providing rational and reasonable explanations for observations and findings.

In forensic science, abduction is crucial in generating possible explanations (propositions or hypotheses) that might be subjected to inductive and/or deductive reasoning and evaluation.

Summary

All three inferential processes contribute to the scientific investigation of a crime. Observations are made at the scene, and possible explanations are generated (abduction), based on knowledge gleaned from similar scenes, for example, where to look for particular evidence types (induction), the scene is processed, and the crime is reconstructed partly by applying the laws of physics (deduction).

Inference – Bayes and The Likelihood Ratio

In addition to the inferential processes of deduction, induction, and abduction used in forensic science is Bayesian inference. The Reverand Thomas Bayes (1702–1761) was an English statistician and polymath who is credited with formulating an equation that bears his name. It is beyond the scope of this book, but Bayes' theorem is probably one of the most important equations in human history. It helps us to explain everything![1]

In the simplest of terms, Bayesian inference involves updating existing beliefs when new information becomes available.

In the case of forensic science, once the previous inferential methods have played their part and are left with some plausible explanations for the observations and findings, the question then arises: which is the most likely explanation? Determining which is the more likely is achieved by employing part of Bayes' equation called the likelihood ratio, which will be encountered many times in this book and is a major subject of Chapter 6 on interpretation.

In technical terms, it is a ratio of two conditional likelihoods or probabilities, in criminal matters, one relating to the prosecution case and the other, an alternative, relating to the defence case. The likelihood ratio (LR) is expressed mathematically as follows.

$$LR = \frac{p(E|H_p)}{P(E|H_d)}$$

In words, this can be read as the likelihood of the evidence (observation or finding) if the explanation that supports the prosecution case is true, i.e. guilt, divided by the likelihood of the evidence if the explanation that supports the defence case is true.

Essentially, the LR can take one of three values. If the value is greater than one, then an explanation that supports the prosecution case is more likely to be true. If the value is less than one, then the explanation that supports the defence case is more likely. If the value is close to zero, then neither explanation is favoured. Essentially, the scientific evidence is of no help to either party.

Guilt and Not-Guilt

In discussions around Bayesian reasoning, the word 'innocence' is not used. In many jurisdictions, the law is based on a presumption of innocence. The outcome of a criminal trial is either guilt or not-guilt, conviction or acquittal. In addition, when considering alternative propositions in a Bayesian framework, the propositions essentially support either guilt or not-guilt.

Law Enforcement and Justice

It is important to recognise that law enforcement is just part of the (criminal) justice system. Law enforcement refers to the agencies and individuals that enforce laws and regulations. In many jurisdictions, that will be a police force but may also include, for example, immigration officers and, in the United States, agents of the FBI, ATF and DEA. Law enforcement officers are responsible for investigating crimes, making arrests, and maintaining public order and safety.

---

1 Readers wishing to know more should read *Everything is Predictable: How Bayes' Remarkable Theorem Explains the World* By Tom Chivers

In common law jurisdictions, such as those of the United States and Australia, law enforcement agencies will investigate a crime and, in most cases, then turn over their findings to prosecutors, who will decide whether to charge the suspect with a crime and proceed with a prosecution. In civil law jurisdictions, a justice will lead the investigation and direct law enforcement agents.

Criminal justice is the system by which crimes are investigated, prosecuted and punished. The criminal justice system is the network of agencies intended to manage accused and convicted criminals. In addition to law enforcement, it includes courts, prosecutors, defence lawyers, and prisons. The treatment of victims of crime should also be considered part of the system. Criminal justice professionals are responsible for ensuring that individuals accused of crimes are treated fairly and that criminal offences are punished appropriately.

For a criminal case to go to trial before a tribunal of fact, often a judge and jury, some conditions usually need to be met. The law enforcement agency needs to have sufficient evidence to support the charge. The prosecuting agency considers whether there is a reasonable chance of conviction and that the prosecution is in the public interest.

Therefore, there is a clear distinction between law enforcement and justice. If forensic science sees itself as solely the servant of law enforcement, then it risks abusing its role. It needs to see itself as the servant of the law, helping to deliver justice. However, the early development of forensic science as 'police science', a title which still has resonance today, and the continuing close relationship between forensic science and law enforcement agencies, sometimes effectively being part of the same agency, puts justice at risk and has contributed to numerous miscarriages of justice. These issues are explored in Chapters 9 and 10.

A failure to recognise or at least give due consideration to the fact that law enforcement is just part of the justice system, and the resultant risk to justice is a topic discussed in this book.

Miscarriage of Justice

A miscarriage of justice occurs when someone is convicted of a crime they did not commit or acquitted of a crime they did commit. The consequences of either outcome are wide-ranging.

The wrongful conviction of the innocent impacts the individual by denying freedom and causing reputational and psychological damage. It impacts the family, causing emotional and perhaps financial distress, together with damaging relationships. The crime is not 'solved', and the victims of the crime are denied justice.

If the wrong person is convicted, the guilty party remains at large, risking further crimes, and if the crime was violent, public safety is at risk. In addition, public trust is eroded, and appeals can be very costly.

Similarly, in the case of a wrongful acquittal, the victims are denied justice. In addition, the criminal remains at large and may re-offend. If the crime was violent, the safety of the victims and the public is at risk. Such acquittals may also demoralise law enforcement agents. Given the finality of a not-guilty verdict, the acquittal of the truly guilty is hard to rectify.

Therefore, miscarriages of justice have profound consequences for the parties involved, society and the justice system's integrity. All criminal justice stakeholders, particularly lawmakers, law enforcers, lawyers and judges, should do all in their power to reduce the risk.

It could be argued that one of the principal aims of forensic science should be to reduce the risk of a miscarriage of justice.

Nucleic Acids (DNA & RNA)

Deoxyribonucleic Acid (DNA)

DNA carries the genetic code as a series of bases: adenine, thymine, cytosine and guanine (A, T, C, G). Pairs of these bases form the rungs of the twisted ladder that is the double helix of DNA; A can only pair with T, and C can only pair with G.

nDNA is DNA in the nucleus of cells
mtDNA is DNA in the mitochondria of cells; the mitochondria are the engine rooms of cells

Ribonucleic Acid (RNA)

RNA assembles the amino acids coded for by the DNA molecule into proteins. Proteins are the building blocks of life.

Science and the Scientific Method

While philosophers of science argue over the meaning of these terms, a simple explanation is that the word science generally has one of two meanings: a body of knowledge, such as chemistry, and a means of gaining new knowledge by theory, observation and/or experiment followed by peer review, also known as the scientific method. Any of the three initial processes can begin the journey to new knowledge, e.g. a new theory may suggest itself to a researcher, experiments are then conducted to test the theory, and the results of those experiments either support the theory or not, resulting in the confirmation, rejection or modification of that theory. Alternatively, an observation may suggest a new theory to be tested by experiment. In drawing conclusions, the scientific method relies mostly on induction. A theory is proposed and tested by experience, experiment and observation, and a conclusion is drawn. However, all the inferential methods play a part in obtaining new knowledge.

Every scientific theory is considered a 'working hypothesis' in the almost certain knowledge that the hypothesis will one day be overturned, overtaken or at least modified. Indeed, this is the most powerful aspect of the scientific method: the assumption that current knowledge is incomplete or even wrong and that theories must continually be questioned and tested.

This lack of certainty at the heart of science and the need for certainty and finality when resolving legal disputes gives rise to a continuing tension between the law and science.

Short Tandem Repeat

As the name implies, these are short lengths of DNA with a sequence of bases that repeats, e.g. a 2-base pair 4x repeat sequence; (C, A) (C, A) (C, A) (C, A). Short tandem repeats (STRs) are highly variable among the population and can, therefore, be used to distinguish between individuals. In modern DNA analysis, it is these STRs that are targeted, removed and their relative quantities measured to produce the profiles for comparison.

Social Darwinism

Social Darwinism is a term used to describe the practice of misapplying the biological evolutionary language of Charles Darwin to politics, the economy, and society.

Social Darwinists tend to believe in *'the survival of the fittest'*—the idea that certain people become powerful in society because they are innately better. Social Darwinism has been used to justify imperialism, racism, eugenics and social inequality.

As explained in Chapter 1, according to Charles Darwin, evolution requires a multitude of generations to determine the *'fittest'*, whereas social Darwinists start by identifying who they believe are the fittest and then engineer their survival and advancement at the expense of those deemed unfit.

Opinions

When a forensic scientist is called to give expert evidence, it is often in the form of an opinion. That opinion may be expressed in one of three ways: categorical, probabilistic and evaluative.

Categorical Opinion

A categorical opinion falls into one of some predefined categories, such as 'match', 'no match' or 'inconclusive'.

Sometimes, they are expressed as a likelihood or probability, e.g. 'the writings are most probably of common authorship', but still fall into defined categories. The difficulty with categorical opinions is that they are in the form of a Bayesian posterior probability, and therefore, some unreported prior must have been assumed.

One form of Bayes' Theorem is as follows.

$$\text{Posterior} = \text{LR} \times \text{Prior}$$

The current belief, the Prior, is updated by the LR to give a new belief, the Posterior.

The posterior and prior probabilities are the province of the fact finder and off limits to the forensic scientist. The likelihood ratio is provided by the forensic scientist, enabling the fact-finder to update the prior to give a new posterior probability.

By reporting a posterior probability, the role of the fact-finder or jury is usurped. In addition, the same unreported assumed prior might also be relied upon by the fact-finder, and so it might be double-counted and given unwarranted weight. These issues are more fully explored in Chapter 6.

Probabilistic Opinions

Probabilistic opinions are expressed on a continuous scale of certainty and are usually expressed evaluatively as a likelihood ratio with a narrative explanation such as 'the DNA is more likely to have come from person A than person B'. Probabilistic opinions can also be expressed as a random match probability, that the DNA is more likely to have come from person A than from some random individual in the population. Probabilistic opinions are to be preferred to categorical opinions.

Evaluative Opinion – What Does the Evidence Mean?

An evaluative opinion is one of evidential weight, assigning a likelihood ratio based upon case-specific propositions and a clear framework of circumstances that is provided for use as evidence in court.

In cases where the assigned LR is greater than one, that would lead to opinions of the following general type.

> *'The findings are far more likely if the questioned and reference materials have the same source rather than different sources'.*

In simpler terms, an evaluative opinion provides an assessment of the strength of evidence to be attached to the findings in the context of the alleged circumstances.

An evaluative opinion is to be distinguished from an investigative opinion. The following table (Table Terms.2) may help highlight the differences.

Table Terms.2 Differences between investigative and evaluative roles.

Investigative Role	Evaluative Role
Tends to be crime-focused.	Tends to be suspect-focused.
Tends to be at the beginning of the criminal justice process.	Tends to be at the culmination of the criminal justice process.
Helps the investigator make decisions.	Helps the court take decisions.
Type of questions: What happened? What is this? Who could be involved?	Type of questions: Is Mr Smith the source of the DNA or is it someone else? Did Mr Smith drive the car or was he a passenger?
Suggests explanations for the observations and gives guidance.	Evaluates the observations (i.e. results) given at least two mutually exclusive propositions.
Open-ended process.	More formal and structured.
Explanations need to encompass all realistic possibilities to avoid bias and avoid potentially misleading the inquiry.	Assigned probabilities should be calibrated; rates of misleading opinions should be low and documented.

Differences between investigative and evaluative roles (Hicks, et al. 2022). The investigative role relies on abduction.

Quality

Quality is the degree to which a product or service is fit for its intended purpose. In the case of a forensic science provider, it is the extent to which the results it generates can be relied upon by a tribunal of fact, such as a court of law, to reach a safe decision or verdict by a fair process, i.e. the extent to which it helps to deliver justice.

Organisational and technical competence is usually demonstrated by conformance with international standards such as ISO/IEC 17025 for laboratory activities and ISO/IEC 17020 for crime scene activities. Individual competence can be demonstrated through certification by a body conforming to ISO/IEC 17024. Conformance is independently assessed and assured by an accreditation body.

These and other standards provide a framework that reduces the risk of unreliable and misleading evidence contributing to a miscarriage of justice (Doyle 2019).

Introduction

Forensic science and its practitioners have entered the public imagination mainly through television series and film media. Brilliant minds, often employing state-of-the-art science and technology, solve the most intractable crimes in under six hours if it is a television series and under three hours for a film. Sadly and, I suspect, unsurprisingly, the reality is somewhat different from the dramatic portrayal in popular fiction. Forensic scientists do not interrogate suspects; those who examine the crime scene and recover evidence are often not those who process samples at the laboratory. The interpretation and reporting of the results obtained are often undertaken by a further group of specialists (specialised scientists). Even so, the reality of forensic science is no less an exciting and interesting story than its fictional counterpart.

Forensic science's journey from its earliest gestation to where it is today is full of drama and interest. This book charts the development of forensic science from its earliest beginnings to the powerful role it has today in solving crime and delivering justice. It does so by the selection and review of publications that had a major impact on the practice of forensic science at the time and contributed to the development of current practice, management and delivery.

But what is forensic science? You will find it often explained that the term 'forensic' is derived from 'of the (Roman) forum', pointing to the use of forensic science to help settle (legal) disputes. All well and good, but the meaning of 'science' in 'forensic science' is a little harder to pin down. Ordinarily, 'science' has one of two meanings: a body of knowledge, as in the science of chemistry, or as a way of finding out about the universe through observation, experiment and theorising (proposing explanations), key elements of what is known as the scientific method.

Jointly, the individual meanings do not easily apply to 'forensic science'. It is an eclectic and syncretic science. Forensic science, in its practice and for its success, draws on a whole raft of sciences, all the major ones: biology, physics and chemistry and their numerous subcategories, e.g. molecular biology, biochemistry, analytical chemistry, geology, etc. Mathematics, particularly statistics, also has a major role, as do psychology and logic. So, the narrow 'body of knowledge' idea does not apply to this scientific magpie. Generating new knowledge by observation, experiment, and theory does not easily apply to forensic

A History of Forensic Science in 10 Publications: How They Established Current Practice, First Edition.
Sean Doyle.

science. It is retrodictive; forensic science aims to reconstruct past events and determine their causes by analysing evidence collected in the present.

Forensic science disciplines are many and varied. Their classification depends on the purpose of the classification and who is classifying. Nevertheless, two broad classifications are as follows.

1. The comparison of features which rely solely on the knowledge and experience of the examiner, such as fingerprints, footwear, handwriting and tool marks, etc.
2. The making of measurements which rely, at least in part, on analytical science, such as DNA analysis and forensic chemistry – the analysis of drugs, ignitable liquids, poisons, explosives, etc.

In either case, the findings need to be interpreted and communicated, and again, there are two broad approaches as follows.

1. Reporting restricted to certain categories, categorical reporting: 'yes, no, or maybe'.
2. Reporting a likelihood or probabilistic reporting; the blood is likely to be that of the victim.

So, it begins to become clear why forensic science is so hard to define other than simply something like 'science in support of the law and justice'.

Science – A Historical Perspective

In charting the history of forensic science, albeit by a personal route, it is important to have some appreciation of the history of 'science'. The term, as we understand it today, had its origins in the sixteenth century; before that, the 'queen of sciences' was theology. Before that time, most, if not all, of the knowledge *Homo sapiens* (our species) needed could be gleaned from oral tradition, religious texts and philosophy. The Scientific Revolution dawned with what the historian Yuval Noah Harari calls '*the discovery of ignorance*' (Harari 2011). *Homo sapiens* realised that they did not know the answers to some of the most important questions, and by attempting to answer them, new knowledge was created by which power, influence and wealth could be accrued, thus promoting further research. This acceptance of ignorance is one of the defining characteristics of science. The lack of certainty of being 'right' creates tension between science and legal processes, which aim to end in certainty and bring finality.

Based on this potted history, any suggestion that forensic science, as commonly understood, can find origins earlier than the sixteenth century is on shaky ground.

Why This Book?

Few, If Any, Books on the History of Forensic Science

There haven't been many, if any, histories of forensic science published. A comprehensive treatise, although of undoubted benefit to specialist scholars, would not be of great interest to the broader readership that this book aims to reach. The central aim of this book is to chart the course by which current practice in forensic science was established, by seeking out the publications that have shifted forensic science in the direction that has led to today's practice. In doing so, it aims to highlight to students and academics some of the most important works establishing current practice, at least in the author's opinion, and to present that journey in a way that hopefully will attract the non-specialist reader interested in knowing a little more about the science behind 'CSI'. The steps along the way are science, philosophy, logic, statistics, psychology and regulation. This book is also a celebration of the pioneers of forensic science.

The History of Forensic Science Is Not Taught

Unfortunately, few forensic science courses cover the historical development of forensic science, with some notable exceptions, and, as a result, earlier knowledge and wisdom are lost, either for good or need to be re-learned. The time and energy of many forensic scientists are focused on identifying and applying the latest technological developments. Therefore, if lessons are not to be forgotten or relearned, then a historical perspective should be acquired by students.

The first of the publications, the Handbook of the Austrian lawyer Hans Gross (1847–1915), written at the end of the nineteenth century, is a good example. Among other things, the Handbook is a comprehensive guide to crime scene investigation (CSI) and is as applicable today as it was when it was written over a century ago. Some modern CSI textbooks record the same principles as the Handbook but make no mention of either the Handbook or Hans Gross.

Target Readership

This book is intended for undergraduates studying forensic science and related subjects, as well as their teachers. It also caters to users of forensic science, such as lawyers and police officers. Additionally, anyone with a general interest in the history and development of forensic science, crime investigation, or true crime stories will find this book valuable. Furthermore, members of the public who may be called to jury service in a trial involving scientific evidence will find this a useful resource.

Anglophone Bias

The book has an Anglophone/English-speaking bias. Apart from a short chapter on Edmond Locard's 'Criminal Investigation and Scientific Methods', only works published in English or for which an English translation is available have been considered.

Therefore, there is less discussion than there should be of Rudolphe Archibald Reiss (1875–1929) and Edmond Locard (1877–1966). As we shall learn, in 1909, Reiss established a school of forensic science (Institut de Police Scientifique) at the University of Lausanne, Switzerland, which today, under a different title, is a world-leading forensic science research and teaching institute. In 1910, Locard, after a visit to the Lausanne school, established the first police forensic science laboratory in Lyon, France.

However, the roles of these pioneers in the development of forensic science are discussed and given the impact of the publications selected, the Book is not significantly weakened by the absence of detailed chapters on their works.

An Overview of the Publications

The book charts the history and development of forensic science as it is practised today and provides a look at what the future may hold. Several publications have been selected, the subjects of which have significantly contributed to that development.

Those publications are as follows.

Title in English	Author(s)	Year
A Handbook for Examining Magistrates, Police Officers, Gendarmes, etc.	Hans Gross	1893
Criminal Investigation and Scientific Methods	Edmond Locard	1920
The Ontogeny of Criminalistics	Paul Kirk	1963
Hypervariable 'minisatellite' regions in human DNA	Alec Jeffreys et al.	1985
Interpretation of statistical evidence in criminal trials: The Prosecutor's Fallacy and the Defense Attorney's Fallacy	William Thompson & Edward Schumann	1987
Interpreting Evidence: Evaluating Forensic Science in the Courtroom	Bernard Robertson & Tony Vignaux	1995
ISO/IEC 17025:1999 General requirements for the competence of testing and calibration laboratories	ISO	1999
The Daubert/Kumho Implications of Observer Effects in Forensic Science: Hidden Problems of Expectation and Suggestion	Michael Risinger et al.	2002
Strengthening forensic science in the United States: a path forward	NAS/NRC	2009
The Sydney Declaration – Revisiting the essence of forensic through its fundamental principles	Claude Roux et al.	2022

1893/1 The Handbook – Gross

The story these publications tell begins in the late nineteenth century in continental Europe, where several criminologists, those who study crime in its broadest sense, struggle to find a physical characteristic that will identify the 'criminal type'. It is their mistaken belief that there is a criminal type whose identification might enable society to be better protected from crime. During that time, an Austrian lawyer, an examining magistrate, Hans Gross, decided to turn to science and the scientific method to identify the criminal.

Gross was frustrated by the lack of relevant knowledge acquired during his university education. In response and over a 30-year career, he amassed a near-encyclopaedic body of knowledge to aid him in the pursuit of the truth.

Gross had little faith in human witnesses and was arguably the first to look to science and the scientific method of detailed observation, suggesting explanations for findings and testing those explanations, a search for objective evidence untainted by human weaknesses. The Handbook is a detailed treatise on the investigation of crime using the scientific method and, in particular, crime scene investigation.

Gross exercises the role of the investigating officer, directing matters and resources and calling on experts as and when needed.

1920 Criminal Investigation – Locard

Locard's seminal work, 'L'enquete criminelle et les methodes scientifique' has not been translated into English. It is listed and discussed in recognition of its importance and that of the author. Locard's contribution to the development of forensic science is recognised and discussed in several other chapters in this book. His most famous contribution is the so-called exchange principle, usually paraphrased as *'as every contact leaves a trace'*. Or more precisely, as follows.

> *It is impossible for a criminal to act, especially considering the intensity of a crime, without leaving traces of this presence.*
>
> *(encyclopedia.com 2019)*

Locard's view was that the violent nature and intensity of a criminal act were such that multiple signs of the criminal's presence would be left at the scene. This focus on Locard's signs, the 'trace', is a theme in this book.

The works of both Gross and Locard are aimed at maximising the forensic exploitation of the crime scene, ensuring that every ounce of evidence is recognised, recovered, and its probative value assessed.

It is also important to note that both Gross and Locard considered themselves criminologists and not forensic scientists, however defined. They would have considered their scientific endeavours to be part of the broader field of criminology, the study of all aspects of crime.

Many authors argue, and this point is developed in the book, that the contribution made by Gross and Locard to the development of forensic science could only have occurred in jurisdictions in which the inquisitorial or civil law system of justice operates, i.e. continental Europe. In this system, the mindset is to gather and process all potentially relevant evidence. In contrast, in the adversarial or common law system, which operates in, for example, the US and Australia, the mindset is to gather and process just sufficient evidence to identify and successfully prosecute the criminal. This difference in approach affects all justice system stakeholders and should be given due consideration in suggesting paths forward for forensic science.

1963 The Development of Forensic Science – Kirk

The next publication selected raises the question: What is forensic science? Readers may be surprised to learn that this fundamental question is far from settled. Some accept that it is a disparate and disconnected set of disciplines, with fingerprint examiners doing it one way and DNA analysts doing it another way. Others would wish to see forensic science as a single science and promote it as the science of the trace, as might have been understood by Gross and Locard, with current clues enabling the reconstruction of past events.

While some authors argue that although the law may differ by jurisdiction, the science shouldn't. However, forensic science is to a significant extent a servant of the law and must bend to its demands. What might be considered relevant and admissible scientific evidence in one jurisdiction may be considered irrelevant or inadmissible in another. Scientific evidence deemed to be of sufficient quality in one jurisdiction may be judged to be insufficient in another. Other factors that work against the concept of forensic science as a single science will be explored in this book.

Kirk calls his science criminalistics, which is broadly equivalent to forensic science. Another recurring theme in the book is the terminological ambiguity in forensic science; trying to pin down exactly what terms mean is often a challenge.

In his paper, Kirk also raises the issue of the profession of forensic science and asks what its fundamental principles are. A question he does not attempt to answer, but a later publication does.

He controversially defined forensic science as the science of individualisation, a phrase that will be encountered often in this book. Individualisation may be thought of as attributing evidence to a particular source to the exclusion of all others. For example, the bullet was fired from a particular gun and no other. Such categorical assertions are wrong in logic, and more probabilistic interpretations are suggested, such as the bullet was more likely than not to have been fired from a particular gun.

Thus, this paper sets a developmental agenda and begins a discussion of the nature of forensic science, which, as will become clear, continues to this day.

1985 DNA Fingerprinting – Jeffreys

It is argued in the book that this work put the 'science' in 'forensic science'. DNA fingerprinting provided a scientific means of identifying the criminal, a role that had become exclusive to fingerprinting. Jeffreys' method was highly discriminatory, providing powerful evidence of identity. As such, in its early days, it was subjected to intense scrutiny, particularly in criminal trials. In time, DNA evidence overcame those initial challenges and, in so doing, held a mirror up to other evidence types, mostly so-called feature comparison methods such as fingerprint examination. The question arose: If DNA was subject to such scrutiny, why wasn't fingerprint evidence? Fingerprint evidence had been accepted for decades. When an examiner identified the source of the questioned print, to the exclusion of all others, that evidence was accepted without question. However, in contrast with DNA evidence, there was no scientific basis for such a claim, which was essentially founded on the assumption that no two people had matching fingerprints. An assumption that had never been questioned or tested. As will be explored further in this book, fingerprint examination remains controversial to this day, both in its methods and conclusions.

1987 Logical Fallacies – Thompson and Schumann

The contribution of this work to the development and current practice of forensic science was essentially philosophical. This publication drew the attention of forensic scientists to two related errors in thinking, or logical fallacies, which they call the prosecution and defence fallacy. The publication includes experimental data that demonstrates how these fallacies can unfairly strengthen the evidence in favour of the prosecution and defence. By far, the most common and the one with the highest risk is the prosecutor's fallacy. This fallacy is the logical equivalent of arguing that because my cat has four legs, it must be a cow. The details of these fallacies will be discussed in the chapter.

1995 Interpreting Evidence – Robertson and Vignaux

This is included as it represents the introduction and impact of Bayesian reasoning on forensic science. Thomas Bayes (1702–1761) is credited with this approach to dealing with uncertainty. In essence, Bayesian reasoning is updating existing beliefs as new information becomes available. Seems like common sense? Yes, we are all Bayesians! While not a consequence of Bayesian reasoning, at the heart of the approach to interpretation in this publication is the likelihood ratio. The likelihood ratio will be mentioned often in this book. In technical terms, it is a ratio of two conditional probabilities, in criminal matters, one relating to the prosecution case, and the other, an alternative, relating to the defence case. The likelihood ratio (LR) is expressed mathematically as follows.

$$\mathrm{LR} = \frac{p(E|\,H_p)}{P(E|\,H_d)}$$

In words and using a real-world example, it is the probability of the degree of resemblance found between questioned and reference handwriting if they are of common authorship, divided by the probability of that degree of resemblance if they are not of common authorship. The vertical line symbolises 'if', which signals the condition. If the LR is greater than one, the evidence favours the prosecution's assertion of common authorship and if less than one, the evidence favours the defence case that the writings are by different people. There are many other examples in this book, as this is an important concept to understand. The likelihood ratio is also discussed in the section on Terms, Definitions and Explanation.

This publication makes clear that scientific evidence must conform to four principles.

- Logic – which essentially is to avoid the fallacies identified by Thompson and Schumann by considering the probability of the evidence and not that of the prosecution or defence hypotheses
- Balance – to consider only two mutually exclusive explanations for the evidence
- Transparency – to report the basis for conclusions reached and highlight any weaknesses
- Robustness – conclusions/opinions must be based on valid data and relevant research.

These principles will be encountered often in the book.

1999 Standards to Improve Quality – ISO/IEC 17025

This publication has been selected because quality systems have become a major tool for ensuring the quality and reliability of scientific evidence. This is an international standard, conformance to which demonstrates technical competence and the ability to produce valid results. Following several miscarriages of justice, quality systems were seen as a means of restoring confidence in forensic science and in those providers found to be contributors to those miscarriages of justice.

Some understanding of quality systems and their impact on forensic science as it is practised today is essential.

2002 Cognitive Bias – Risinger et al.

After logic and statistics contributed to the development of forensic science, along came psychology. This erudite publication provided a detailed account with examples of how long-known cognitive biases (errors in thinking) could affect forensic science and, unless recognised and effectively managed, might contribute to a miscarriage of justice.

After a period of gestation, Itiel Dror and colleagues in 2006 picked up the baton and conducted research at University College London to demonstrate the detrimental effects of bias. After an initial denial of the issue with claims that forensic scientists were so independent of mind that they were immune to bias, and in time, forensic science recognised the danger and adopted systems to minimise the risk. However, some forensic practitioners remain unconvinced of the danger.

2009 Strengthening Forensic Science – National Academies of Science (NAS)

This was a major report preceded by a huge amount of work completed by a multitude of contributors. It is a publication that is still being cited today, 16 years later. The initiative was prompted by continuing miscarriages of justice. The report records in detail the problems and challenges and makes several recommendations. As with initiatives of this type, few of those recommendations have been implemented. However, as a snapshot of the state of US forensic science at the time and a record of possible paths forward, it is an excellent report and essential reading for forensic scientists.

Among the recommendations that have been implemented is the need for standardisation, to be delivered in part by the accreditation of organisations and the certification of individuals. The need to standardise procedures was met, in due course, by the US National Institute of Standards and Technology/Organisation of Scientific Area Committees (NIST/OSAC) and its register of standard methods and procedures and its lexicon of terms.

2022 One Science – The Sydney Declaration – Roux et al.

In a sense, we come full circle with this publication, as it harks back to the criminology of Gross, Locard and other contemporaneous pioneers in continental Europe. It promotes forensic science as the unified science of the trace, traceology, i.e. clues present at the crime scene enabling the reconstruction of past events. On that basis, it argues for a greater role for forensic scientists in the criminal justice system. For example, being at the scene to direct the scientific investigation as a matter of course and using information gained as forensic intelligence to aid more effective policing, public safety and security.

The challenge to the vision is the deeply entrenched status quo. At present, forensic science is an eclectic mix of unconnected disciplines and other parties, police investigators and examining justices, unwilling to cede a leading role to a scientist at the scene, the preference for experts to be on tap and not on top.

1

The Handbook

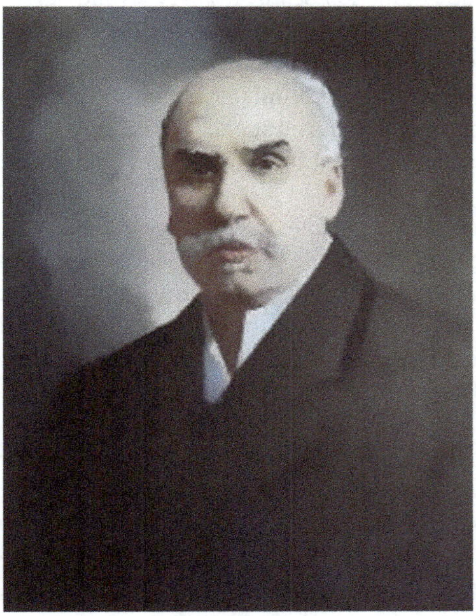

Image 1.1 Hans Gross. BP48Fadhillah/Wikimedia Commons/CC0 1.0.

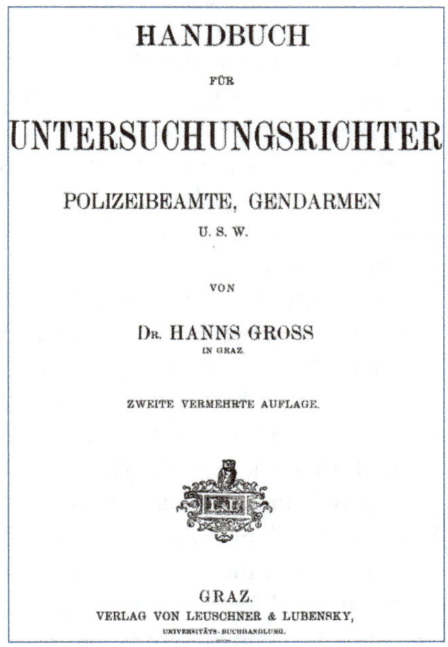

HANDBUCH

FÜR

UNTERSUCHUNGSRICHTER

POLIZEIBEAMTE, GENDARMEN

U. S. W.

VON

DR. HANNS GROSS

IN GRAZ.

ZWEITE VERMEHRTE AUFLAGE.

GRAZ.

VERLAG VON LEUSCHNER & LUBENSKY,

UNIVERSITÄTS-BUCHHANDLUNG.

Image 1.2 Title page of the handbook. Gross (1894)/Leuschner & Lubensky/Public Domain.

Name of the Publication

Title, *Handbuch für Untersuchungsrichter, Polizeibeamte, Gendarmen u.s.w.* which can be translated as ‘A Handbook for Examining Magistrates, Police Officers, Gendarmes, etc.’. The subtitle ‘als System der Kriminalistik’ (as a system of criminalistics) was added to the third German Edition published in 1899.

A History of Forensic Science in 10 Publications: How They Established Current Practice, First Edition.
Sean Doyle.

Introduction

The first edition of the Handbook (as the publication will be referred to in this book) was published in 1893.[1] Its author was Hans Gross, then an examining magistrate and public prosecutor, and later Professor of Criminal Law at the Karl-Franzens University of Graz, Austria. His Handbook is by far the largest publication discussed in this book and is certainly one that, both directly and indirectly, has had a major impact on the development of forensic science and its current practice, hence its inclusion in this work.

The Handbook treats crime investigation as a scientific endeavour requiring all the skills of a research scientist for its success. It reveals that Gross was very much a member of the trace- or clue-driven school of forensic investigation, with forensic science defined as the 'science of the trace'. Fellow members of that school include Edmond Locard (1877–1966) and others, as discussed in later chapters of this book, particularly Chapter 10 on the Sydney Declaration.

Most importantly, the publication demonstrates that Gross attached more weight to physical evidence than human testimony. He considered humans better interpreters than recorders and prone to numerous potentially biasing influences. The unreliability of human testimony is explored in greater depth in another of Gross' publications, 'Criminalpsychologie' (Gross 1898).

The Handbook, among other things, sets out the principles of effective crime scene management and investigation, i.e. protecting the integrity of physical evidence, including preservation, chain-of-custody and contamination avoidance. These are principles that continue to apply to this day. It also highlights the dangers of cognitive biases such as tunnel vision, i.e. focusing on one theory or explanation to the exclusion of others. Furthermore, and presciently, the Handbook foreshadows offender profiling and the use of facial recognition as a means of identifying criminals.

The Handbook, particularly in later editions, also describes operational procedures for the recovery and examination of numerous evidence types including firearms, fingerprints, blood splatter, hair, poisons, handwriting and so on.

A measure of the importance and significance of the publication, and its impact on the development of forensic science and its current practice, is its longevity. For example, it was first translated into English by two English lawyers, a father and son, based in Madras, India. That first English edition, published in 1906, adapted and augmented the 1904 fourth German edition of the Handbook for the investigation and prosecution of crime in India at the time of the British Raj. Following that first edition in English, another five followed, the last published in 1962. In addition, there were 10 editions published in German, the last in 1978. There are accounts of the Handbook being used by police investigators at New Scotland Yard (NSY), London, up until the 1970s. Although those later English editions probably bore little resemblance to Gross's Handbook (Wilson 1952; Adam 2016).

The decline in interest in the Handbook in the German-speaking world was, in part, a symptom of its subject matter becoming less relevant in the developing academic field of criminology. Criminology is the study of crime and society's response to crime, drawing on the law and the behavioural and social sciences. The continuing use of the Handbook in the English-speaking world was partly the result of its adoption and adaptation by law enforcement agencies, particularly New Scotland Yard in London, as an instructional and operational manual.

The Handbook was also translated into several other languages including French thereby influencing Edmond Locard (1877–1966) to whom the adage 'every contact leaves a trace' is falsely attributed – the so-called 'exchange principle' – and possibly even Rudolphe Archibald Reiss (1875–1929) who in 1909 founded the Institut de police Scientifique at the University of Lausanne, Switzerland. Locard and Reiss, in addition to Gross, are pioneers in the development of forensic science. Both feature a little later in its history and are discussed in this book. Locard specifically acknowledges the debt he owes to Gross. Locard, at the time Director of the Laboratory of Police Technique Lyon in France and vice president of the International Academy of Criminology[2], wrote.

> *However, the first author who clearly described cases where this research* [studying dust for the purpose of discovering *'criminological evidence'*] *has been made is Hans Gross. One can hardly speak highly enough of the worth of this magistrate; he was one of the initiators of criminology; and he envisaged not merely a particular phase of the science, but its broadest aspects.*
>
> *(Locard 1929).*

Biography of the Publication

The Handbook was first published in 1893 with the title in German 'Handbuch für Untersuchungsrichter, Polizeibeamte, Gendarmen u.s.w.', which can be translated as 'A Handbook for Examining Magistrates, Police Officers, Gendarmes, etc.'. The contents of the Handbook were drawn from Gross's near encyclopaedic knowledge and experience gained in over two decades of structured learning and practice as an examining magistrate and public prosecutor, all poured into one extensive publication.

In Austria, as in most of continental Europe, the system of civil law applies, which is based on the inquisitorial approach of gathering facts. In this system, an examining magistrate, or justice, directs the investigation of crime and not the police or other law enforcement agents. A judicial officer may also prosecute the case, act as the fact-finder, reach a verdict and hand down a sentence; all roles exercised by Gross, but of course not simultaneously. Therefore, the civil law system was ideal for facilitating the acquisition of the knowledge and experience recorded in the Handbook. This process would have been far more difficult, if not impossible, in a common law jurisdiction such as those of England and Wales or the United States, where the role of an examining magistrate does not exist, and the police, or other law enforcement agencies, take the lead in the investigation of crime.

The distinction between the inquisitorial approach of civil law, which emphasises gathering information, and the adversarial approach of the common law system, which has many rules to exclude potentially relevant information, is crucial in charting the history of forensic science.

A consequence of the difference between the continental system of civil law and the system of common law, derived from English law, and the lack of an examining magistrate in common law jurisdictions was the slower development of forensic science in such jurisdictions, particularly in England (Adam 2016; Burney and Pemberton 2016a,b). This resulted in what was initially described as 'police science' in the United Kingdom and United States, a blurring of the role of the forensic scientist and what is and is not forensic science. This lack of clarity continues to this day. These points are developed further in Chapter 10 on the Sydney Declaration section, as is the 'science of the trace'.

The Handbook had 10 editions in German, the seventh onwards being edited by others and the final edition published in 1978. As mentioned earlier, it was to the third German edition published in 1899 that Gross added the subtitle 'als System der Kriminalistik' (as a system of criminalistics). This was the first recorded use of the term 'criminalistics', and this is the basis for the claim that Gross is the 'founder' or 'father' of criminalistics (Block 1979a; Dillon 1977), among other offspring. However, as discussed later, Gross's meaning of the term criminalistics was closer to criminology than today's 'forensic science'.[3] Nevertheless, the Handbook is replete with scientific procedures and a reliance on scientific expertise to investigate crime successfully; today, collectively termed 'forensic science'.

The 1893 first German edition was published in two parts, part 1 in 11 sections and part 2 in 10 sections, 21 sections overall. From the fourth German Edition (1904) onwards, the Handbook was published in two volumes. The sixth German Edition (1914) was the last one edited by Gross himself. From the eighth German Edition (1941) onwards, the title was simply 'Handbuch für Kriminalistik'.

As recorded in the introduction, the Handbook was first translated into English in 1906 by the father and son barristers John Adam and J. Collyer Adam, practising in Madras, India, at the time of the British Raj. The translators adapted the text for 'India and the Colonies' (p. 13 of the Kindle Edition), and it is based on the 1904 German fourth edition, which the translators updated and modified for their jurisdictions. For practical reasons, they rejected the two-volume model; their edition is divided into five parts.

There followed a series of later editions in English edited by members of New Scotland Yard (NSY), London, and the fifth and final English edition was published in 1962, edited by Sir Richard Leofric (aka Levfric) Jackson CBE[4] (1902–1975), barrister-at-law and a member of the Criminal Investigation Department (CID) at NSY. Sir Richard was at the time Assistant Commissioner of the CID and also President of Interpol, the International Police Criminal Organisation, then headquartered in Paris, France.

The 1962 edition in English retains the basic structure of the original English edition but omits the sections on 'Wandering Tribes' and 'Superstitions'. It also updates the text to reflect the time and its use by police officers and includes new sections on Road Accidents and the Criminal Records Office, a source of intelligence, recording crimes and their perpetrators. This edition also highlights the role of Interpol in the cross-border prevention and suppression of crime.

According to Turner (Turner 1952–1953), and as recorded earlier, the later English editions included significantly less of Gross's text, with more additions by the 'editor'. This is certainly borne out by the comparative brevity and additional sections of the 1962 edition, edited by Jackson. In the opinion of Turner, what is required for an English speaker to hear the authentic voice of Gross is a translation of the 1914 edition, being the last which was the sole responsibility of Hans Gross. Sadly, no such translation has been made, so the 1906 Adams' translation is the best source on offer in English, and it is the Kindle edition that is the basis for this chapter. The English and German editions are listed in Table 1.1.

Table 1.1 List of German and English editions.

Edition	German	Editor	English	Editor
First	1893	Hans Gross	1906[a]	Adams and Adams
Second	1894	Hans Gross	1924	Adams (Jnr)
Third	1899[b]	Hans Gross	1934	Norman Kendal
Fourth	1904	Hans Gross	1949	Robert Howe[c]
Fifth	1908/6	Hans Gross	1962	Richard Jackson
Sixth	1914	Hans Gross		
Seventh	1922	Erwein Höpler		
Eighth	1942	Ernst Seelig		
Nineth	1954	Ernst Seelig		
Tenth	1977/78	Friedrich Geerds		

a. Based on the 1904 fourth German edition.
b. It was to this edition that 'as a system of criminalistics' was added.
c. A contemporary reviewer considers this edition to have little in common with Gross' Handbook, which underwent a major revision by Gross for the sixth Edition in 1914 (Wilson 1952).

Professional Biography of the Author

Hans (Johannes) Gustav Adolf Gross was born on the Feast of Stephen, December 26th, in the year 1847 in the city of Graz, the capital of the then Duchy of Styria, part of the Austro-Hungarian Empire. Part of the Duchy is now in Slovenia, but Graz remains Austrian.

Graz is Austria's second-largest city, with a population of over a quarter of a million and remains the capital of the state of Styria. By car, Graz is about 200 kilometres south of Vienna and is surrounded by green hills. It remains a picturesque location in the eastern Alps and is now a World Heritage Site with a museum dedicated to Hans Gross (University of Graz n.d.).

Gross studied law at the University of Graz and, after graduating in 1870, became an examining magistrate in the then-industrial area of Upper Styria and later a public prosecutor in Graz. He spent 30 years as a judge, a career culminating in being appointed the presiding judge of a senate (panel of judges) of the Court of Appeal[5] in Graz. It was during these three decades that Gross acquired the wide-ranging knowledge and experience that was the source material for the Handbook.

His frustration with the lack of knowledge he had acquired at university, which would enable him to uncover the truth when investigating crime, led him to engage in a period of structured self-education studying the natural sciences (biology, physics and chemistry), medicine and psychology and scientific procedures such as microscopy. These efforts eventually bore fruit in the publication in 1893 of his seminal work, the Handbook 'Handbuch für Untersuchungsrichter, Polizeibeamte, Gendarmen u.s.w.' (Grassberger 1956).

As discussed later, the natural sciences developed rapidly in the nineteenth century. The power of science and the scientific method may have encouraged or inspired Gross to look to science as a useful ally in the investigation of crime and uncovering the truth, which Gross felt was often obscured by the unreliability of human witnesses.

In 1898, while remaining a justice and having never taught in a university before, he was appointed a Professor in Ordinary for Criminal Law and Justice Administration at the University of Czernowitz, which, at that time, was also part of the Austro-Hungarian Empire. It is now part of Ukraine, close to the border with Romania and named Chernivtsi. Czernowitz has had a rich and fascinating history in the nineteenth and early twentieth centuries, but that history lies beyond the scope of this book. It is, however, a stunningly beautiful city full of nineteenth-century Habsburg architecture.

Another major achievement and of long-lasting influence was the publication in 1898 of the journal 'Archives for Criminal Anthropology and Criminalistics', in German 'Archiv für Kriminal-Anthropologie und Kriminalistik'. In addition to founding the journal, Gross was its first editor. According to Gross, the journal aimed to make criminology a practical scientific aid to criminal law (Gross 1899), echoing Gross's overall aim of providing practical guidance. In 1916, the year after his death, the journal changed its name to 'Archives of Criminology' and is still published today with the full title 'Archiv für Kriminologie unter besonderer Berücksichtigung der gerichtlichen Physik, Chemie und Medizin', making it the oldest existing criminological journal.

In 1902, Gross was appointed Professor of Law at the German University of Prague, then also part of the Austro-Hungarian Empire, and finally, in 1905, Professor of Criminal Law at the Karl-Franzens-University, his *alma mater*, in his home city of Graz.

In 1912, Gross achieved one of his life's ambitions and founded The Criminological Institute at the Graz University in the face of opposition from legal academics who felt that criminology, including what is now termed forensic science, was too narrow a field to merit even a separate area of study, let alone an institute. However, the success of the Institute can be measured by the fact that it only closed its doors in 1978, the cause being that it had failed to adapt to the broadening scope of criminology, remaining too narrow in its focus (Bachhiesl 2014).

In 1915, Hans Gross fell ill with pneumonia, his criminological institute being located in the unheated basement of the main building of the University (Bachhiesl 2014). He died on the 9th of December 1915.

As already indicated, Gross's legacy and impact on forensic science are immense.

In addition to the Handbook and the Journal 'Archives of Criminology', he also wrote a major work on criminal psychology (Gross 1905), which is now mostly of historical interest. As an indication of his legacy and impact, he has variously been called the father or founder of scientific criminology (Bachhiesl 2020), criminal research and modern police technique (Dillon 1977), scientific techniques in crime detection (Block 1979b) and criminalistics (Block 1979a; Dillon 1977), and some general biographies have included offender profiling. In addition, one of New York's most famous private detective agencies is named after him, 'The Gross Investigation Bureau'.

In introducing the French translation of the Handbook, M Gardiel, Professor of Criminal Law at Nancy, France, described Hans Gross as follows.

> *... an indefatigable observer; a far-seeing psychologist; a magistrate full of ardour to unearth the truth, whether in favour of the accused or against him; a clever craftsman; in turn, a draftsman, photographer, modeller, armourer; having acquired by long experience a profound knowledge of the practices of criminals, robbers, tramps, gypsies, [and] cheats ...*
>
> *(Adam 1924).*

Contexts

Science

As is clear from the Handbook, Gross relied heavily on science in his approach to investigating crime. The word 'science' with its modern meaning was first coined in 1833 by the Church of England priest, polymath and master of Trinity College, Cambridge, England, William Whewell (1794–1866), replacing the term 'natural philosophy'. The word has its origins in the Latin word '*sciens*', meaning knowing. As pointed out in the section on Terms, Definitions and Explanations, in its modern usage, science has two basic meanings: a body of knowledge, such as the science of chemistry and a way of finding out about the universe using what is commonly termed the scientific method. The scientific method derives new knowledge through any combination of observation, theory and experiment and then subjecting the results to peer review. It is important to note that at the heart of the scientific method is the principle that every theory is, in effect, a working hypothesis which must be tested until it is overturned or augmented by new knowledge; science accepts no certainties.

The absence of certainty in science is often a frustration in a judicial process; the Law seeks certainty to support the requirement for finality.

To understand how much the meaning of the word 'science' has changed, it is important to note that historically, the 'queen' of sciences was theology[6]!

Notable nineteenth-century scientific advances included Louis Pasteur's (1822–1895) vaccine against rabies and his advances in the understanding of disease; Dimitri Mendeleev's (1834–1907) creation of the periodic table of elements which enabled scientists to predict the characteristics of as yet undiscovered elements; the creation of electromagnetism (electricity) as a new branch of science and a better understanding of energy in thermodynamics and its conversion from one form to another. Electromagnetism and thermodynamics drove technological advances such as increasing the efficiency of steam engines and the generation of electricity.

However, by far the most important advance with an almost seismic impact on science and, more importantly, on society at large was the publication in 1859 of '*On the Origin of Species by Means of Natural Selection*' by Charles Darwin (1809–1882). The publication spawned a whole new branch of knowledge: evolutionary biology or Darwinism. It is widely considered to be one of the most important advances in knowledge in human history. Its consequences and impacts are still being felt today; for example, there is no longer a need for a creator God to explain the diversity of nature.

Unfortunately, Darwin's theory gave rise to the notion of 'survival of the fittest', which is not a consequence of Darwin's evolutionary model but an erroneous distortion. This notion led to the (false) idea, among others, that some 'races' are superior.[7] The notions of 'survival of the fittest' and racial superiority are among the defining principles of so-called social Darwinism.

This misunderstanding of Darwinism at the time also had a significant impact on late nineteenth-century criminology. As demonstrated, not even Hans Gross, with his focus on facts, rationality and logic, was immune to the influence of the Darwinian swirl of ideas around at the time. His belief in science as a means of uncovering the truth may have led Gross to the belief, in good faith, that science supported the idea of the inferiority of wandering tribes or gypsies – which of course it does not.

Hans Gross considered himself a criminologist. As mentioned earlier, towards the end of his career, he was Professor of Criminal Law at the Karl-Franzens University in his home city of Graz and established an Institute of Criminology at that University. Therefore, it is important to get some understanding of the intellectual environment into which Hans Gross emerged, i.e. criminology in the late nineteenth century. Among the beliefs of criminologists at that time, derived from their (mis)understanding of Darwinism, was that human beings had the potential to revert to an earlier stage of evolution; the process was termed 'atavism'. Therefore, one aim of criminology was to identify the atavistic criminal type and protect society by permanently imprisoning the individual so identified. Accepting the existence of these atavistic criminal types led to the notion that the punishment or sanction should fit the criminal and not the crime (Bergman 2005).

Identifying the 'criminal type' so that such types could be 'removed' from society was a major effort in late nineteenth-century criminology. In addition to the idea of an evolutionary backwards step, there was the idea that criminals had certain physical characteristics. The aim was to find those physical characteristics. This idea was exploited by Sir Francis Galton[8] (1822–1911, English) in fingerprints and by Cesare Lombroso (1835–1909, Italian) in medical physiology, all technically called anthropological criminology and tainted by social Darwinism with the notions of 'survival of the fittest' and racial superiority, which was essentially racism.

Anthropological criminology at the time attached credence to the idea that inferior 'races' are less evolved, more prone to crime and therefore more likely to be 'criminal types'. Galton stands out by being credited as the 'father' of eugenics[9] (Aubert-Maison 2009). Eugenics was based on the idea that undesirable human characteristics should be removed by selective breeding; unfortunately, a step towards the 'racial health' policies of the Nazis and the genocide of the holocaust. These ideas lead to the conclusion that criminals are born, the product of nature and not nurture, and once identified, should in some way be removed from society.

While a discussion of the *Origin of the Species* in late nineteenth century western Europe, its impact on late-nineteenth and early-twentieth-century criminology and indeed on world history is beyond the scope of this book, it is important for the reader to correctly understand the notion of 'survival of the fittest', first coined by the English philosopher Herbert Spenser (1820–1903). As stated earlier, the notion is not a consequence of Darwin's theory of evolution but is the basis of social Darwinism, which influenced many criminologists at the time. The outcome of evolution by natural selection is that the fittest survive and not the survival of the fittest. Nature requires thousands of generations in a stable ecosystem to determine the fittest. Social Darwinists start from the position of identifying the 'fittest' in society, who then need to be protected so that they can flourish. In essence, social Darwinists misused or misunderstood the *Origin of the Species* in an attempt to provide scientific support for their bogus theories, which have been thoroughly discredited, but sadly, even today, find echoes.

In conclusion, then, there is no scientific support for the concept of a criminal type, and the racial theories and ideas of these 'fathers' of criminology – Galton and Lombroso – have been thoroughly discredited. Today's criminologists are increasingly of the view that the causes of crime lie in a combination of predisposing biological traits together with social circumstances, which lead to criminal behaviour. Neither traits nor circumstances alone inevitably lead to crime. Criminal behaviour is the product of both nature and nurture, and probably more of the latter.

Gross is on record as rejecting the work of Lombroso as statistically flawed and concluding that.

> *The truth is that there is neither criminal born nor a type of criminal.*
>
> *(Block 1979c)*

However, Gross does believe that.

> *... persons of feeble intelligence, full of hereditary defects and morally shipwrecked, fall into crime more readily than others ...* Section iii, - Examination of the accused, end of Chap II.

This reveals that Gross was not entirely untainted by social Darwinism. According to Stefan Köchel, the current curator of the Hans Gross Kriminalmuseum at the University of Graz, Gross and his successors at the Institute of Criminology often criticised Cesare Lombroso and the idea of anthropological criminology, but in fact had serious problems with distancing themselves from their own criminological ideas. After the death of Gross, so-called 'Kriminalbiologie' (biological criminology) was invented at the Institute, which later turned out to be very attractive in support of the ideology of the National Socialists in the late 1930s and early 1940s.

The adoption of science in support of the investigation of crime in the late nineteenth and early twentieth century was all part of a general trend recognising the importance of science, the realisation that knowledge was power and that many unknowns remained. The nineteenth century saw science institutionalised, the establishment of schools of science and institutions of learning.

The drive of the late nineteenth century criminologists to observe, measure and theorise is reflective of the perceived power of science and the scientific method.

History

So, having set the scientific, criminological, and, to some extent, societal scene in which the Handbook was born, the picture is completed with a word or two about the historical backdrop. The history of the German-speaking peoples in the nineteenth century is complex.

However, the following may be of relevance to the genesis of the Handbook. Victory in the Franco-Prussian War (1870–1871) led to the unification of Germany in 1871 and the creation of the German Empire under the Kaiser, Wilhelm 1 (1797–1888), administered by Otto von Bismarck (1812–1898). Although Austrians were among the German-speaking peoples and both what constituted the new German empire and Austria shared a common history as part of the Holy Roman Empire[10], of which Vienna was a recent capital, Austria remained part of the Austro-Hungarian Empire. Again, the reasons are complex, but essentially, such a union may have destabilised Europe, a risk recognised by those holding the levers of power at the time.

Because of its history, the Austro-Hungarian Empire was far more ethnically diverse than newly established Germany, and the presence of many 'wandering' tribes within that empire, together with social Darwinian ideas may partly explain Gross' intense dislike of gipsies expressed in the Handbook.

The Structure of the Handbook and Relevant Content

Introduction

The subject and aim of the Handbook are succinctly stated in the introduction to the 1906 English edition.

> *It is a Manual of Instruction for all engaged in investigating crime, its aim being, not only to deal in detail with subjects coming directly within the province of the criminal investigator, but to also inform that official in what cases and in what manner specialists may or must be resorted to.*

The Handbook is, of course, specifically aimed at an examining magistrate or the person leading or directing a criminal investigation; the 'Investigating Officer' in English translations. The Handbook contains an almost encyclopaedic knowledge of every element of crime and its investigation as understood in the late nineteenth and early twentieth century, much of which remains relevant today, hence the Handbook's longevity. It assumes the investigator has at his/her disposal, police and the necessary experts. Forensic science and the role of the forensic scientist are woven into the text as Gross recognises that science and scientific investigators are essential contributors to a successful outcome, uncovering the truth.

The Handbook is based on and gives expression to Gross's fundamental beliefs.

- The unreliability of human testimony.
- The power of science and the scientific method to uncover the truth.
- Properly managed and exploited, the crime scene will enable past events to be accurately reconstructed.

As mentioned earlier, the first German Edition of the Handbook (1893) was in two parts, the first one subdivided into 11 sections, the second one into 10 sections. However, it is important to note that the basis for this commentary is the first English edition of the Handbook (1906), which is based on the fourth German Edition (1904). This English edition is a single volume in four parts and has 1436[11] pages.

Part 1 – with the title 'General', pages 31–484 (453 pages),
Part 2 – 'Knowledge special to the investigating officer', pages 485–727 (242 pages),
Part 3 – 'Crafts special to the investigating officer', pages 728–988 (260 pages), and
Part 4 – 'Particular offences', pages 989–1390 (401 pages).

Each part covers a series of topics and subtopics. For example, Part 1 discusses the following topics.

- The Investigating Officer,
- Examination of Witnesses and Accused,
- Inspection of Localities,
- Equipment of the Investigating Officer,
- The Expert and How to Make Use of Him, and
- The Legitimate Sphere of the Public Press

The final topic in Part 1 demonstrates a remarkably modern understanding of the benefits of a good relationship between the investigator and journalists.

Part 1 'General' is perhaps the most relevant to the current practice, management and delivery of forensic science and is therefore explored in greater detail below. Briefly, Part 1 describes the duties and responsibilities of the investigator, and the knowledge and skills required to successfully manage and progress an investigation, including crime scene management and the use of experts such as microscopists, chemists, biologists and physicists. Part 1 refers to forensic disciplines which would be recognised today, including firearms, document examination, photography and fingerprints.

Part 1 also details operational procedures at the crime scene and includes warnings to keep an open mind. It includes the requirements to accurately and comprehensively record the scene and ensure that everything that might advance an investigation is recovered and its integrity maintained. Of particular relevance is the avoidance of what is termed 'Preconceived Theories', today termed confirmational bias or tunnel vision, i.e. only recognising evidence that supports a particular theory and ignoring that which doesn't. Tunnel vision can result in a miscarriage of justice, and indeed, often has. Bias is the subject of Chapter 8.

Part 2 'Knowledge Special to the Investigating Officer' describes strategies employed by criminals, such as disguises and false identities, which the investigator needs to be aware of. This part also sets out the required knowledge for the examination of firearms and other weapons, such as knives and swords.

Part 2 also includes a major section on 'Wandering Tribes', which gives expression to the social Darwinism discussed earlier. Gross was of the view that wandering tribes, also called gypsies, were a separate class of people and by their nature were possessed of criminal tendencies, tendencies not possessed by '... *the civilised man* ...' (page 579). Those who first translated the Handbook into English, the father and son barristers John Adam and J Collyer Adam, '*adapted* the Handbook "... *to Indian and Colonial practice* ..."'. The influence of social Darwinism, essentially racism, in 'Western' societies in the late nineteenth and early twentieth centuries is reflected in this 1906 edition. This edition finds the same class with 'criminal tendencies' among the nomadic tribes of the Indian subcontinent. This seems remarkable given the clear cultural and societal distinction between say Bohemian gypsies and the Bediyas of Bengal!

Part 3 'Crafts Special to the Investigating Officer' details the skills required by an investigator, which in the nineteenth century included drawing and modelling skills, and the detection and deciphering of secret writings.

Part 4 'Particular Offences' includes offences against the person; theft, fraud and arson. This part provides information on the methods used by criminals in committing the specified offences, including the use of weapons to inflict wounds, for example, by stabbing, bludgeoning and shooting. Poisoning and poisons are included, as are burglary/breaking and entering. The Handbook describes the 'tools of the trade' such as skeleton keys, metal files, drills and crowbars. Also included are the falsification of documents, such as passports, and the use of ignitable liquids, means of ignition and improvised timers for use in arson attacks.

Many of the topics covered in the Handbook are of their time and place, and some, such as 'Wandering Tribes' and 'Superstitions', are omitted from later English editions. Those topics, which to a certain extent reflect the racist and misogynistic views of the time, are of no significance in terms of pointing towards or contributing to current forensic science practice. However, they remain of considerable historical interest to criminologists as is Gross' other major work 'Criminal Psychology' (Gross 1918) and these two volumes, together with the journal 'Archiv für Kriminal-Anthropologie und Kriminalistik' (Archives of Criminal-Anthropology and Criminalistics), published up until 1916 under that title, are significant works contributing to the development of criminology.

Part 1 'General'

As this is the part of the Handbook that most directly links to current practice, selected sections are examined and discussed in a little more detail.

Part 1 is intended to detail the essential principles and qualities required by an investigator (p. 12) and to inform the investigator of what science has to offer. Advice is also given on the examination of witnesses and the accused, and the effective management and exploitation of crime scenes.

The Investigating Officer

Section i General Considerations, p31

Listed here is the very broad range of knowledge, skills and attributes required to be a competent investigator of crime. This includes the '*vigour of youth*' an '*acquaintance with all branches of the law*', '*languages*' and bookkeeping. In addition, '*to understand slang, read ciphers and be familiar with the processes and tools of all classes of workmen.*' The actual list is far wider and amounts to the need for a polymath or some kind of super person, which Gross seems to have been.

Section ii The Duties of the Investigating Officer p35

This text might be summarised as: investigators need to be prepared to 'go the extra mile', as the '... *culprit must be discovered at any price.*'

Section iii The Procedure of the Investigating Officer p36

Here, the Handbook includes a requirement to approach the investigation with an open mind and guard against premature conclusions which might lead the investigation in the wrong direction. It emphasises the importance of working effectively with the police and the risks and opportunities presented by that relationship. It identifies types of persons who might provide important eyewitness evidence. It then goes on to describe the *modus operandi* for certain types of crime and expresses a somewhat misogynistic view of the role of women as a potential cause of crime. A view that remains in later English editions, unfortunately.

Section iv Preconceived Theories p51

This section deals with the risk of a type of cognitive bias (error in thinking) known as tunnel vision (latching onto an erroneous theory and ignoring contradictory evidence) and how to reduce that risk. This is extremely prescient in that a recognition of the potential impact of cognitive bias did not emerge in mainstream forensic science until the early 2000s (Risinger et al. 2002). Cognitive bias is the subject of Chapter 8.

At this juncture, it is important to emphasise that, despite the warnings clearly stated in the Handbook, tunnel vision still plagues the investigation of crime, contributing to miscarriages of justice. There are far too many examples to mention everyone. A common pattern is as follows: the conviction of the 'prime suspect' based on a firm belief in the guilt of the accused by law enforcement and prosecuting authorities, supported by weak, non-existent or even fabricated evidence and later, often decades later, exoneration based on DNA evidence. Two recent examples are Andrew Malkinson in England (Dugan 2023) and Archie Williams in the United States (Bastian 2021), and for an idea of the scale of the issue, see the report of Gould (Gould et al. 2013). One of the most powerful examples of tunnel vision leading to miscarriages of justice – well, actually just wrongful convictions – at an industrial scale is the so-called Post Office Scandal in the United Kingdom (Willis 2021).

The Handbook draws attention to behaviours that result in tunnel vision. '... *an opinion is formed which cannot be got rid of* ...' and therefore, '... *the details of the case are no longer studied with entire freedom of mind* ...' (p52)

Gross's insights into the dangers of cognitive bias and tunnel vision as recorded in the Handbook are, with hindsight, extraordinary. Although the potential for cognitive bias to distort scientific conclusions had been recognised since the writings of Francis Bacon in the seventeenth century (Bacon 1620) it seems clear that the risk of such bias had not been fully recognised in the late nineteenth century, and, as mentioned above, not until the late twentieth in mainstream forensic science, as discussed in Chapter 8. It should be noted in passing that Francis Bacon is considered by some to be a major contributor to the concept of the scientific method as it is currently understood (Stanford Encyclopedia of Philosophy 2012).

It is also interesting to note that Gross unknowingly recognises the power of the prior probability[12] in Bayesian inference, which is defined in the section on Terms, Definitions and Explanations and discussed in Chapter 6.

> *... where the problem is whether a violent death is caused by suicide or by unknown causes. ... It is safe to affirm with certainty that an enormous proportion of such cases is due to the hand of another.* (p56)

Section v Certain Qualities Essential to an Investigating Officer p60
Here, the Handbook specifies the requirement for accurate record-keeping.

> *... he* [the Investigating Officer] *must set out details in the official records exactly as they have been seen or said, for it goes without saying that this will be so done.* (p62)
> *Since 'exactness', or accuracy of work, is of so much importance in all branches of research, this accuracy must also be applied to the work of the Investigating Officer.* (p63)

Here, Gross emphasises his point that investigating crime is akin to conducting scientific research, and the same rigour must be applied.

Inspection of Localities

Section i Preparation p213
This section highlights the importance of effective crime scene recording; any errors made at the scene could well render any further progress redundant.

> *His report of an inspection of localities is a real touchstone for the Investigating Officer. In no other duty are address, power of observation, logical reasoning, methodised energy, and keeping the end ever in view, so clearly revealed; ...* (p213)

To properly and thoroughly manage and exploit a crime scene, a competent assistant is considered essential.

Section ii What to Do at the Scene of Offence p217
The potential for cognitive bias and tunnel vision is emphasised again, this time in the examination of the crime scene. Any mistakes made at the crime scene must be recognised and immediately corrected.

> [Preconceived theories] ... *frequently causes him* [the crime scene examiner] *to go wrong in his reckonings. For this reason, the faults of his first impression must be corrected on the spot and his plans and intentions modified accordingly.* (p219)

In the Handbook, Gross, in a demonstration of the breadth of his scholarship, quotes the Catholic theologian and Doctor of the Church, Saint Thomas Aquinas (1255–1274) in Summa Theologica, who, following Aristotle, teaches that the circumstances affecting a human act are comprised under these seven heads.

> *Quis, quid, ubi, quibus auxiliis, cur, quomodo, quando?*
> *Who, what, where, with what, why, how, and when?* (p219)

These heads are interpreted as follows.

> *What was the crime, who did it, when was it done, and where, how done, and with what motive, who in the deed did share?*

The Handbook recommends committing these words to memory, '... *to prevent many a grave mistake.*' (p220)

In acquiring, critically assessing and interpreting eyewitness accounts, the Handbook recommends keeping eyewitnesses separate from each other to prevent them from exchanging information and potentially weakening the probative value of their testimony through collusion. With this measure in place, Gross attached significant weight to corroborative eyewitness accounts.

The Handbook emphasises the importance of excluding events, particularly the movement of items or persons, that occurred after the crime was thought to have been committed.

Section iii The Actual Description of the Scene of Offence p224

Here, the Handbook draws attention to the importance of accurately recording everything that might be of evidential value, however unlikely, before items are moved. The scene must be recorded in its undisturbed state.

The rule given regarding scene preservation is as follows.

> ' ... *never to change in any way the condition of the scene before it is described in the report.*' (p225)

Many modern crime dramas have the first responder moving items at the scene contrary to the Handbook's guidance and demonstrating the gap between fiction and the proper investigation of crime. Moving items or altering the scene in any way prior to recording may undermine the investigation and call into question the integrity of any evidential items recovered.

Guidance is then offered on the structure and general requirements of the description of the scene report. A detailed method of scene recording is documented, and the need to avoid inexact or ambiguous language is emphasised.

The importance and significance of, and how to record, bloodstain patterns are described in detail. Bloodstain pattern analysis following a violent crime is now a major activity within forensic science (Hanson 2004).

Many examples are given where what seemed trivial or unimportant at the time of the crime scene examination turns out to be the '... *pivot on which the whole case turned;...*' (p232)

The Handbook recommends that a sketch plan of the scene be made initially before writing and then annotated with written detail. Today, the scene would be sketched, photographed and, in some cases, a virtual scene created.

The need to distinguish clearly between subjective and objective evidence is stated.

Foreshadowing the use of cadaver dogs, the use of canines for the detection of corpses and tracking fugitives is recommended.

Equipment of the Investigating Officer p243

Listed here are items considered indispensable to the Investigating Officer. It being the early twentieth century, it consists mainly of appropriate stationery, but also lists, a tape measure and a pair of compasses. Interestingly also recommended is a pedometer placed in the investigator's boot for measuring distance. A cloth for collecting blood and Plaster of Paris for recording and preserving footprints and other impressions are also listed. All essentials to be carried in a '*Commissionstasche*' or field bag.

One very amusing passage has the following advice.

> *Smokers should always have a few cigars in reserve, for how often does not one in his haste forget his cigar case. A post mortem, for instance, is not a very pleasant thing for the mere lawyer, if he cannot smoke; even the brandy flask may be a very present help in such circumstances.* (p250)

The Expert and How to Make Use of Him

Section i General Considerations p252

In this section of the Handbook, Gross acknowledges the uncertainty at the heart of science, and he clearly understands the consequences that expert opinions often need to be qualified. Readers need to note that the lack of certainty in science is sometimes difficult to understand by non-scientists, including police, lawyers and judges.

The Handbook provides examples of experts beyond medicine and science who can advance an investigation but warns against pressuring them to offer opinions that won't withstand scrutiny. For instance, what was once considered impossible and led to unqualified certainty, such as the positive detection of an illicit substance, is now known to be possible in the form of a false positive result. Science evolves and progresses, uncovering new knowledge that challenges and may overturn earlier certainties.

Section ii Role of the Medical Jurisprudent p261

Regarding the certainty with which conclusions are offered, it may be helpful at this juncture to make a distinction between science and medicine. Medical practitioners are inclined to be very certain in their own minds of their opinions and present them with great confidence, even when erroneous; the story of Professor Sir Roy Meadow[13] and his evidence regarding sudden infant death syndrome (SIDS) is a good example (Dyer 2005). In addition, medical practitioners tend to rely heavily on abductive inference (Veen 2021), an educated guess based on knowledge and experience. In this type of reasoning, the simplest and most likely explanation for an observation or set of observations is sought. The risk is that the true explanation may lie beyond the knowledge and experience of the medical practitioner. Where the conclusion has a definite uncertainty associated with it, this uncertainty tends to be put to one side by the medical practitioner. There is rarely much evidence of the consideration of alternative explanations in the testimony of medical practitioners.

Scientists, on the other hand, are aware of the uncertainties associated with their opinions, or at least should be, and make use of the scientific method. This involves inductive and deductive reasoning to test explanations generated by abduction[14], as appropriate, and refining those explanations, including alternatives, in arriving at and offering opinions which are nearly always qualified and expressed in terms of a likelihood or probability. In addition, as discussed later in Chapter 6, forensic scientists tend to increasingly rely on Bayesian reasoning[15] when reasoning under uncertainty. So, while the Handbook offers a whole section of guidance on what is termed medical jurisprudence, it is not strictly science and as such it is beyond the scope of this book. However, it should be noted in passing that the topics include preserving parts of a corpse, tattooing, mental afflictions and hypnotism.

As an interesting aside, there is also much written in the Handbook about the relationship between an investigator and the medical jurisprudent known more recently as a forensic pathologist or medical examiner. That this relationship should be close and amicable (p261), such as to produce a '... *lively enthusiasm and active cooperation* ...' is recommended '... *as their collaboration will considerably aid the solution of the problem.*' (p262). It is of interest to consider how many successful fictional crime dramas, in books, plays and/or films, have been based on such a relationship between the medical examiner (however named!) and the investigator.

Section iii The Microscopist p310

A. Traces of Blood p312

In addition to being able to distinguish between blood and other stains, extraordinarily, the microscopist can measure 'blood globules' and by so doing distinguish between an animal or human source.

Bloodstain pattern analysis is also described and used to distinguish between arterial and venous blood splatter.

B. Excrement p319

This is not a common evidence type. However, the Handbook foreshadows the monitoring of wastewater to detect evidential substances (Hauser et al. 2019), so-called 'sewage forensics'. The Handbook claims that distinctions might be made between faecal matter, mainly of vegetable origin, and that of meat and linking types of seeds to a location. The earlier comments about medical practitioners and their reliance on abduction are supported by the following quotation.

> *The state of digestion of the figs exactly corresponded with the time which had elapsed between the eating of the figs and the murder of the girl.* (p320)

C. Hair p321

Hair is a more commonly encountered evidence type today, although weakened by scandals such as those at the FBI (FBI 2015). A standard work of the time is quoted.

> Dr Emile Pfaff's, '*The hair of man, its physiological, pathological and legal importance,*' (p321)

Regarding hair, the Handbook has.

> *We should in the first place not lose sight of the faculty of absorption possessed by human hair; it is capable of absorbing gases, odours, etc., with extreme facility and retains them for a relatively long time.* (p321)

Guidance is given on the recovery of hair, contamination avoidance and appropriate packaging. The Handbook emphasises, not for the first or last time, the need for precise and complete recording of those steps to prove the integrity of the evidential item.

Among other circumstances discussed and examples given is the potential for the exchange of pubic hair between a complainant and an alleged perpetrator in cases of alleged sexual connection.

In this section, there is an early example of offender profiling following the recovery of two hairs from a hat dropped by an assailant as he fled the scene. Based on the hair examination, it was '*concluded*' that the hairs belonged to a '*dark*' man, still fairly young but who was beginning to grow grey. He had recently had his hair cut, he was beginning to grow bald and '*inclined to stoutness*'. It was concluded that the assailant was ...

> *A man of middle age, of robust constitution, and inclined to obesity: black hair intermingled with grey hair, recently cut; commencing to grow bald.* (p329)

Interestingly, Gross in the Handbook claims that the approximate age of a person can be estimated by the rate of dissolution of a hair root in a solution of potassium hydroxide, of unspecified concentration. He claims that the hair root of children will dissolve immediately, but that of older people will dissolve in a matter of hours. No current scholarship can be found in support of this phenomenon.

There follows quite a treatise on hair examination, its morphology and evidence of treatments. In addition, the resistance of hair to post-mortem decay is noted.

Although stated in relation to hair, the Handbook draws attention to the fact that scientific evidence is most powerful in the negative, when it excludes, without doubt, a suspect from an investigation. This exculpatory power is most in evidence today in the work of the Innocence Project, (The Innocence Project 2023), in which current DNA profiling techniques are being used to exonerate those wrongfully convicted – ironically, many of those convictions were based on unreliable hair comparison evidence (FBI 2015).

As a warning against placing too much reliance on a particular evidence type and that evidence misdirecting the investigation and risking a wrongful conviction, the Handbook describes a case where two eminent hair examiners, finding a rare and unusual feature common in both the questioned and reference hair, identified a suspect who was later found to be innocent of the crime.

D. Other cases relating to Medicine p335
Here, the Handbook refers to toxicology and poisoning using plants.

E. Falsification of writing p339
The Handbook describes all the relevant elements, the pen, ink, paper, and seals, together with bleaching and other erasure techniques, in a reasonably comprehensive treatise.

F. Examination of Cloth, Woollens, Linen, & c. p340
The characteristics of cloths and paper are described together with the examination of fibres and the importance of fibre evidence.

G. Examination of stains p343

1. On Weapons and Tools p344
Here, and elsewhere in the Handbook, casework examples are given in which the instruction to the expert had been narrow or restricted and, as a result, has deprived the expert of relevant information, risking vital evidence being overlooked or missed. This is a lesson perhaps for jurisdictions that employ a market approach to forensic science, where forensic science provision is commoditised and compartmentalised, potentially denying experts relevant information, resulting in the production of misleading evidence. The point is also supportive of the model presented in the Sydney Declaration, the subject of Chapter 10.
Earth, dust, fibres and dried-up liquids are mentioned, as is dirt under fingernails.

2. Dust p348
The characteristics and composition of dust from various locations are described, e.g. the desert, a ballroom, and clothing from various persons.
The beating and shaking of garments and the collection of particulates obtained are described. This can shed light on the history of a person during the time the garment was worn.
Examining dust on other items, such as knives, might yield important evidence.
The examination of dust links Gross with Edmond Locard, and although not explicitly stated in the Handbook, Gross is clearly aware of the 'exchange principle' (every contact leaves a trace) and its probative value. In one of his publications, Locard duly acknowledges the debt owed to Gross (Locard 1928).

3. Stains on Clothes, etc. p352
This section focuses mainly on blood and spermatozoa.

4. Mud on Footwear p354
As evidence of location, types of soil and other evidence of location, e.g. flour attached to footwear.

Section iv The Chemical Analyst p355

The analytical chemist is considered to have the most value in cases of poisoning, to identify suspected toxic substances, which today is the discipline of toxicology.

Section v The Expert in Physics p359

According to the Handbook, the physicist can provide information on the flight or trajectory of projectiles, i.e. ballistics, the effects of light and the positions of the sun and moon in corroborating eyewitness testimony. The physicist might also shed light on the influence of weather and on the forces producing the effects observed, such as damage to items, breakages, tears and splits. While probably beyond the competence of a physicist, the Handbook also suggests that such an expert might provide useful insights into accident investigation and structural collapse.

In this section, the Handbook recommends that the investigator keep up to date with developments in the natural sciences (chemistry, physics, biology and geology) to ensure new developments that might be applied to the investigation of crime are identified and utilised.

Section vi Experts in Mineralogy, Zoology, and Botany p366

Mineralogists might determine the nature of a mineral to reveal the origin of the recovered dust, soil, or stains. Zoologists can measure the dimensions of '*blood globules*' and thereby suggest a source, and botanists can identify poisonous plants and types of wood which might be of probative value.

Section vii The Expert in Firearms p370

Much is written in the Handbook about the chemical analysis of bullet lead, from the projectile itself and residue in the barrel of the firearm, to link one to the other.

The Handbook includes an intriguing series of chemical tests used to determine the time elapsed since a firearm was discharged. (p375)

Section viii Handwriting p375

In the Handbook, by handwriting, Gross initially seems to mean graphology – the determination of personal traits based on handwriting features – a largely discredited practice which, even if it were successful, only reveals the personality of the author. While acknowledging that it might have utility in the future, Gross treats it sceptically. Graphology should be contrasted with Locard's graphometry discussed in the next chapter.

There follows a lengthy treatise and what is currently understood as the examination and comparison of handwriting, including forgery and traced forgery.

Section x Anthropometry – Bertillon System p439

The anthropometric system of identification involved the measurement and recording of certain physical characteristics, was developed by Alphonse Bertillon (1853–1914) in 1879 in the Paris Police Department and was for some time highly valued and utilised by many law enforcement agencies both in France and elsewhere. The system involved measuring certain dimensions of the body of criminals, e.g. the head and face. The 1906 English Edition of the Handbook describes the system in some detail. Bertillon's anthropometric method is discussed further in the next chapter.

Section xi Finger-Prints p445

While praising the anthropometric system of Bertillon for identification, this 1906 edition of the Handbook lists its disadvantages.

1. The instruments are expensive, easy to spoil, and can only be obtained from certain suppliers.
2. The persons who carry out the measurements must have had a special and complete course of instruction.
3. The measurements of the body can only be taken at appointed measuring stations, and by appointed measurers.

4. If the measurements are not properly taken, or being properly taken are then wrongly read or transcribed, the mistake cannot be discovered at the office where the records are kept, and thus all chance of a successful result is spoilt.
5. The taking of the measurements demands time, for to be reliable, they must be repeated three times.
6. It is necessary for the body to be partly exposed.
7. The measurements of young people alter as they arrive at maturity.
8. Double search is often rendered necessary.

The advantages of fingerprints are then listed for comparison.

1. The necessary accessories – a piece of tin, a bit of India rubber, and printing ink- are, above all, cheap and easy to procure.
2. Any person can, after half an hour's practice, take clear fingerprints.
3. The fingerprints can be taken by any policeman at any place.
4. To check a sequence of recorded fingerprints, the comparison of a single impression suffices.
5. The prints of the whole 10 fingers can be taken very much more quickly than body measurements.
6. It is not necessary for a person to remove his clothes.
7. The pattern of a fingerprint never alters during the life of an individual.
8. Mistakes being impossible, no second search is necessary.

Apart from 8, all other points are as valid today as they were when the then.

By highlighting the disadvantages of anthropometry and the advantages of fingerprints, Gross heralded the decline of anthropometry and the rise of fingerprints as a standard means of establishing the identity of criminals. The Handbook goes on to describe in some detail how to record fingerprints, their main features and their forensic utility (p448).

Even with the advent of facial recognition and DNA profiling, fingerprints currently remain an important tool in the investigation of crime and establishing the identity of criminals.

Section xii Geometrical Identification p471

This section refers to the proposal of a W Mathews (British Journal Almanac 2590 p412) using what we would now call facial recognition. Recognition was based on a comparison between photographic images of the face and making certain measurements/measuring certain distances, which were believed to change little over time, for example, the distance between pupils. Questioned and reference photographs are cut along either the horizontal axis of the pupils or through a vertical axis, being the central line intersecting the nose and lips. If the questioned and known photographs fit, then identity is confirmed.

Impact at the Time

The Handbook records the earliest use of the scientific method in the investigation of crime, a revolutionary approach at the time. It emphasises the rigours and benefits of that approach in uncovering the truth and solving crime. It is therefore the first major treatise on forensic science, certainly in Europe. It stresses the need to distinguish between objective and subjective evidence and the preference for the former, attaching more weight to physical evidence than to human testimony, which is considered less reliable.

The Handbook's impact is evident in its immediate translation into several languages and its adoption by investigators in both civil law jurisdictions, such as continental Europe, and common law jurisdictions, including the United Kingdom, as both an instructional and operational text. Later pioneers, such as Locard, acknowledged their debt to Gross and his Handbook.

In promoting fingerprints as a means of identification and highlighting the disadvantages of the anthropometric system of bodily measurements, later editions of the Handbook effectively sounded the death knell for anthropometry.

In terms of trace evidence, and principally regarding the examination of dust, the Handbook recognises the 'exchange principle' later attributed to Edmond Locard. Among the circumstances discussed and examples given is the potential for the exchange of pubic hair between complainant and suspect in cases of alleged sexual connection.

Impact Today

The Handbook documented operational procedures for the appropriate examination of numerous evidence types, including toxicology, hairs and fibres, body fluids, firearms and so on. This presaged the multi-disciplinary approach to the investigation of crime normally employed today.

As reported earlier, the fact that, in some form or other, the Handbook continued in service until the 1970s, certainly among the detectives at New Scotland Yard, London, United Kingdom, as an instructional and operational manual, bears witness to the lasting impact of the Handbook and the brilliance of its author.

It echoes the call by many authors in this book to beware of the 'preconceived ideas' resulting in tunnel vision.

Contribution to Current Practice

Perhaps the greatest contribution to the current practice of forensic science is in the scene principles elucidated by Gross, of control, preserve, record and recover, which remain fundamental to the forensic exploitation of a crime scene.

Control – restrict access to essential personnel and record all activities

Preserve – establish and maintain the integrity of the scene and all items at the scene

Record – record the scene in detail in its original state

Recover – recognise and recover items of potential evidential value according to a plan

In common law jurisdictions, the impact on current practice comes via police investigators. A detailed method of scene recording is documented, and the avoidance of inexact or ambiguous language is emphasised. The Handbook stresses that the scene must be recorded accurately in its undisturbed state. Guidance is given on the recovery and packaging of evidential items and avoiding contamination. The Handbook states the need to record precisely and completely the history of recovered items as a means of demonstrating integrity, i.e. every evidential item must have a record of its continuity or chain of custody.

The Handbook must be considered a foundational work in forensic science and has played a significant role in its development and in contributing to current practice.

Concluding Remarks

Having established several fundamental principles of crime investigation, particularly crime scene management and investigation, and extensively documented practice in support of those principles, of all the paternities assigned to Gross, the father of crime scene investigation is perhaps the most fitting.

The Handbook stresses the requirement for an open mind when investigating crime and guarding against hasty conclusions that might lead the investigation in the wrong direction. This is a recognition of the risk of latching onto an erroneous theory and ignoring contradictory information, a form of cognitive bias known as tunnel vision.

Among other things, the Handbook presages facial recognition, offender profiling and 'sewage' forensics.

Finally, the fundamental utility of the Handbook in the investigation of crime, its tactical and operational aspects, drawing on information from various sources and the early recording of forensic science practice can best be measured by its translation into many languages and its longevity from 'birth' in 1893 to the final German edition some 80 years later.

Later English editions of the Handbook were used by detectives at NSY, London, United Kingdom, as both an instructional and operational manual for crime investigation until the 1970s.

Key Takeaways

The Handbook was the first to:

- Employ the scientific method in the investigation of crime.
- Document the fundamental principles of crime scene management and investigation; control, preserve, record and recover.
- Identify the purpose of crime scene investigation as reconstructing past events.
- Recognise and give weight to the superiority of physical evidence over human testimony.
- Highlight the risk of cognitive bias and describe measures to reduce that risk; to avoid preconceived ideas and keep an open mind.
- Caution against the use of inexact or ambiguous terms.
- Coin the term 'criminalistics' but not as understood by later forensic scientists.[16]
- Document examination procedures for numerous evidence types.
- Detail the trace-driven model of forensic science repeated in the Sydney Declaration (Chapter 10).

Notes

1 Some sources have 1891. However, in this book, 1893 will be taken as the year of first publication.
2 In French the term 'Criminalistique' is used in the title of the Academy. The exact meaning of 'criminology' and 'criminalistics' in the late nineteenth and early twentieth century is unclear. See the section on Terms, Definitions and Explanations.
3 There is some suggestion that by adding the subtitle, Gross was merely emphasising the fact that it was a manual for the scientific investigation of crime, a marketing ploy.
4 Commander of the Order of the British Empire.
5 Courts of Appeal are often the highest courts in a jurisdiction unless there is a Supreme Court.
6 According to Thomas Aquinas (1255–1274).
7 There was a long-held popular view of 'Western superiority' that, for example, Africans (and later Jews) were in some way inferior. To some, Darwinism seemed to provide scientific support for these racist views: it did not.
8 A cousin of Charles Darwin.
9 It is beyond the scope of this book, but eugenics was remarkably popular even among so-called 'progressives' and retained the support of many, including some leading politicians and scientists until the 1940s. However, the atrocities of WW2 put paid to such racist notions for most right-thinking people.
10 Which, according to the French writer Voltaire (1694–1778) was neither holy nor Roman nor an empire!
11 All page numbers are from the Kindle edition of the 1906 first edition in English.
12 Also known as the base rate. In the case of suspected suicide, murder is the more likely explanation.
13 Meadow was also the author of the controversial Munchausen's syndrome by proxy.
14 The three methods of reasoning, abduction, induction and deduction, are described in the section on Terms, Definitions and Explanations. Abduction involves generating reasonable explanations, while induction involves testing those explanations or hypotheses, which are then refined by deduction.
15 Bayesian reasoning, a probabilistic approach, is discussed and described in the section on Terms, Definitions and Explanations and the chapter in interpretation Chapter 6
16 Criminalistics in the mind of Gross was closer to criminology, the study of crime in its broadest sense, while later forensic scientists meant the exploitation of physical evidence; see Terms, Definitions and Explanations and Chapter 10.

Bibliography

Adam, Alison. 2016. "Hans Gross and Criminalistics." In *A History of Forensic Science: British Beginnings in the Twentieth Century*, edited by Alison Adam, 63–66. Abingdon, Oxford: Routledge.

Adam, Alison. 2016. "The Influence of Scientific Criminology and Criminalistics." In *A History of Forensic Science: British Beginnings in the Twentieth Century*, edited by Alison Adam, 67. Abingdon, Oxford: Routledge.

Adam, John Collyer. 1924. "Introduction." In *Criminal Investigation*, x. Edizioni Savine.

Aubert-Maison, Dominique. 2009. "Sir Francis Galton: le fondateur de l'eugénisme [Sir Francis Galton: the father of eugenics]." *Medical Sciences (Paris)* 25: 641–45.

Bachhiesl, Christian. 2020. "Reading the Criminal in the Austrian School of Criminology: Unveiling the Deviant Character Through Measurement and Intuitive Introspection." In *Mind Reading as a Cultural Practice*, edited by Laurens Schlicht, Carla Seemann and Christian Kassung, 140. Palgrave Macmillan.

Bachhiesl, Christian. 2014. "The Graz School of Criminology – The criminological Institute at the Karl-Franzens-University of Graz (1912–1978)." *Studies in Law: Research Materials* 15: 5–20.

Bacon, Francis. 1620. *Novum Organum (New Tools)*. London: Joannem Billium.

Bastian, Casey. 2021. "After 36 Years in a Louisiana Prison for a Rape He Didn't Commit, Archie Williams Wins Freedom – and a TV Show Spotlight." *Prison Legal News*, 1 April. https://www.prisonlegalnews.org/news/2021/apr/1/after-36-years-louisiana-prison-rape-he-didnt-commit-archie-williams-wins-freedom-and-tv-show-spotlight/.

Bergman, Gerald. 2005. "Darwinian Criminality Theory: A Tragic Chapter in History." *Revista Di Biologia* 98: 47–69.

Block, Eugene B. 1979a. *Science vs Crime – The Evolution of the Police Lab*. San Francisco: Cragmont Publications.

Block, Eugene B. 1979b. *Science vs Crime: Scientific Crime Detection, the Inside Story*. First. Cragmont Publications.

Block, Eugene B. 1979c. "Time Brings Progress." In *Science vs. Crime: The Evolution of the Police Lab*, edited by Eugene B Block, 10. San Francisco: Cragmont Publications.

Burney, Ian, and Neil Pemberton. 2016a. "Gross Abroad: Early Debates on English CSI." In *Murder and the Making of English CSI*, edited by Ian Burney and Neil Pemberton, 77–85. Baltimore: Johns Hopkins University Press.

Burney, Ian, and Neil Pemberton. 2016b. "Teaching the Detectives." In *Murder and the Making of English CSI*, edited by Ian Burney and Neil Pemberton, 159–81. Baltimore: Johns Hopkins University Press.

Dillon, Duayne Joseph. 1977. *A History of Criminalistics in the United States 1850–1950*. D.Crim Dissertation, Berkeley: University of California, Berkeley.

Dugan, Emily. 2023. "Rape, DNA and Injustice: A Timeline of the Andrew Malkinson Case." *The Guardian*, 15 August. https://www.theguardian.com/law/2023/aug/15/dna-and-injustice-a-timeline-of-the-andrew-malkinson-case.

Dyer, Clare. 2005. "Professor Roy Meadow Struck Off." *British Medical Journal* 331: 177.

FBI. 2015. "FBI Testimony on Microscopic Hair Analysis Contained Errors in at Least 90 Percent of Cases in Ongoing Review." *FBI News Press Release*. 20 April. Accessed August 2023. https://www.fbi.gov/news/press-releases/fbi-testimony-on-microscopic-hair-analysis-contained-errors-in-at-least-90-percent-of-cases-in-ongoing-review#:~:text=%E2%80%9CThese%20findings%20confirm%20that%20FBI,Project%2C%20which%20is%20affiliated%20with.

Gould, Jon B., Julia Carrano, Richard Leo, and Joseph Young. 2013. "Predicting Erroneous Convictions: A Social Science Approach to Miscarriages of Justice." Research Report, US Department of Justice, National Institute of Justice.

Grassberger, Roland. 1956. "Pioneers in Criminology XIII–Hans Gross (1847–1915)." *Journal of Criminal Law, Criminology, and Police Science* 47: 397–405.

Gross, Hans. 1899. "Aufgabe und Ziel." *German 'Archiv für Kriminal-Anthropologie und Kriminalistik'* 1 (1): 1–34.

—. 1918. *Criminal Psychology – A Manual for Judges, Practitioners and Students*. First English. Translated by Horace M Kallen. Boston: Little, Brown, and Company.

—. 1898. *Criminalpsychologie*. Kessinger Publishing.

—. 1905. *Kriminal-Psychologie*. Leipzig: Vogel.

Hanson, Doug. 2004. "Bloodstain Pattern Analysis: Recreating the Scene of the Crime." *Law Enforcement Technology* 31 (2): 84–90.

Hauser, Frank M., Tim Metzner, Thorsten Rößler, Michael Pütz, and Steffan Krause. 2019. "Real-Time Wastewater Monitoring as Tool to Detect Clandestine Waste Discharges into the Sewage System." *Environmental Forensics* 20: 13–25.

Locard, Edmond. 1928. "Dust and its Analysis: An Aid to Criminal Investigation." *The Police Journal* 1: 177–92.

Locard, Edmond. 1929. "The Analysis of Dust Traces." *Revue Internationale de Criminalistique* 1 (Nos. 4–5): 176–249.

Risinger, Michael D., Michael J. Saks, William C. Thompson, and Robert Rosenthal. 2002. "The Daubert/Kumho Implications of Observer Effects in Forensic Science: Hidden Problems of Expectation and Suggestion." *California Law Review* 90: 1–56.

Stanford Encyclopedia of Philosophy. 2012. "Francis Bacon." *Stanford Encyclopedia of Philosophy*. 7 December. Accessed August 17, 2023. https://plato.stanford.edu/entries/francis-bacon/.

The Innocence Project. 2023. *Our Work. Restoring Freedom*. Accessed August 22, 2023. https://innocenceproject.org/restoring-freedom/.

Turner, Ralph T. 1952–1953. "Police Science Book Reviews." *Journal of Criminal Law, Criminology & Police Science* 43: 281.

University of Graz. n.d. *Hans Gross Kriminalmuseum*. Accessed August 7, 2023. https://universitaetsmuseen.uni-graz.at/de/unsere-sammlungen-und-ausstellungen/hans-gross-kriminalmuseum/.

Veen, Mario. 2021. "Creative Leaps in Theory: The Might of Abduction." *Advances in Health Sciences Education* 26: 1173–83.

Willis, Nick. 2021. *The Great Post Office Scandal: The Fight to Expose a Multimillion Pound IT Disaster Which Put Innocent People in Jail*. Bath: Bath Publishing.

Wilson, G. W. 1952. "Police Science Book Reviews." *Journal of Criminal Law and Criminology* 43 (2): 281–82.

2

The Exchange Principle

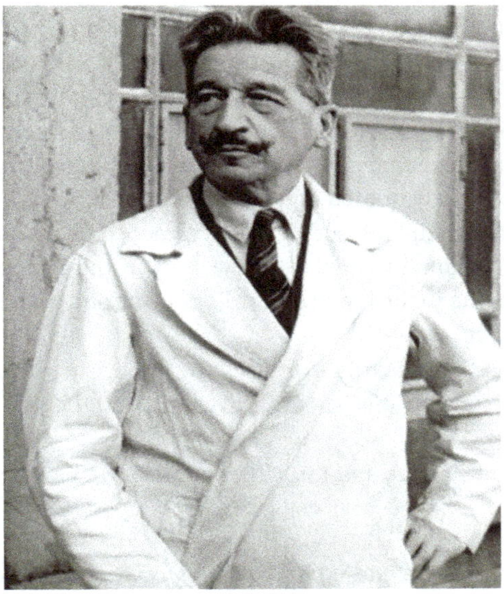

Image 2.1 Edmond Locard. ExploraLyon/ https://exploralyon.com/histoire-de-lyon-10-janvier-1910/last accessed on June 17, 2025/ Public Domain.

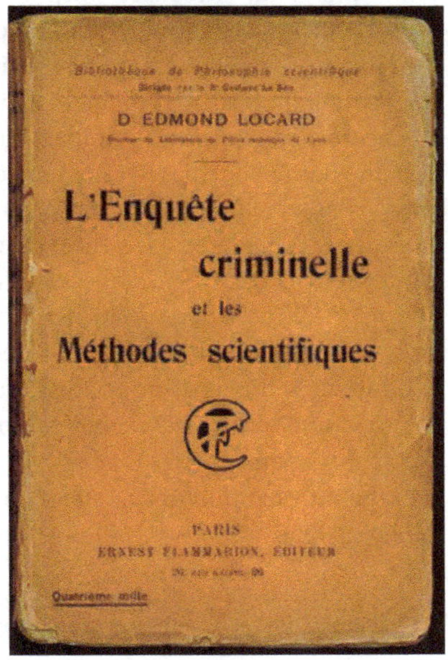

Image 2.2 Front cover. Criminocorpus/ Public Domain.

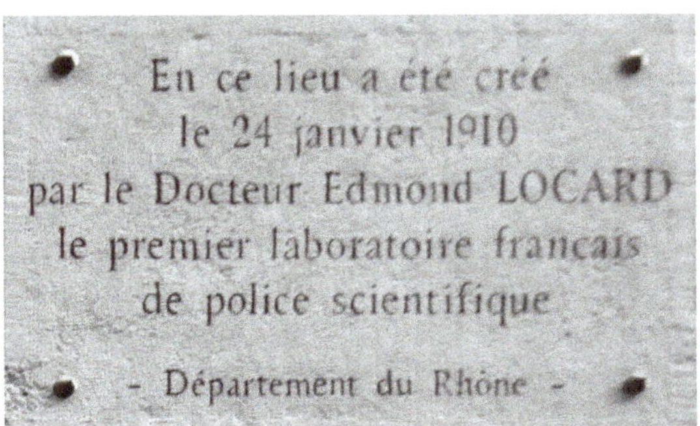

Image 2.3 Wall plaque in Lyon recognising the establishment of Locard's Laboratory. Otourly/Wikimedia Commons/CC BY-SA 3.0.

A History of Forensic Science in 10 Publications: How They Established Current Practice, First Edition.
Sean Doyle.

Name of the Publication

L'Enquête Criminelle et les Méthodes Scientifiques (Criminal Investigation and Scientific Methods) by Edmond Locard. The book was published in Paris, France, in 1920.

A digital copy of the publication may be found at https://criminocorpus.org/fr/bibliotheque/doc/2555/

This chapter uses an abbreviated English version of the title: 'Criminal Investigation'.

Introduction

While this book is focused on publications, no work on the history of forensic science would be complete without mention of Edmond Locard (1877–1966). Indeed, he is referred to in many of the other chapters of this book and is widely given the title 'Father of Forensic Science' (Frappa 2024). The inclusion of 'Criminal Investigation' permits some exploration of Locard's career and his impact on forensic science. However, to most forensic scientists, the name Locard will be associated with the 'exchange principle' often paraphrased as 'every contact leaves a trace', perhaps the most widely quoted aphorism in forensic science and widely considered as its most fundamental principle. Traces left at or removed from the crime scene act as silent witnesses, the interpretation of which tells the story of the crime. The status of the 'exchange principle' warrants the inclusion of Locard's book as one of the most influential in the history of forensic science.

However, it might come as a surprise to learn that Locard never used the aphorism. Still, its origin and that of the exchange principle do appear in 'Criminal Investigation', the subject of this chapter.

In the introduction to Chapter 4 on traces and stains, page 139 of the publication has the following text.

> *La vérité est que nui ne peut agir avec I'intensité que suppose I'action criminelle sans laisser des marques multiples de son passage ... tantot le malfaiteur a laissi sur les lieux des marques de son activité, tanto par une action inverse, il a emporti sur son corps ou sur ses vetements les indices de son sejour ou de son geste.*

This can be roughly translated as follows.

> *The truth is that no one can act with the intensity of criminal action without leaving multiple marks of its passage ... sometimes the criminal left on the scene the marks of his passage, sometimes, by a reverse action, he took away on his body or on his clothes the clues of his stay* [or his action].

The important point is that Locard never wrote 'every contact leaves a trace'. Nevertheless, the above quotation does record an exchange principle, and this is the source of the aphorism quoted in almost every undergraduate textbook on forensic science.

Of course, the exchange principle, as expressed as 'every contact leaves a trace', can never be proved, and one exception would render it false! Nevertheless, the principle is widely considered fundamental, and it remains Locard's most significant contribution to forensic science.

Unfortunately, 'Criminal Investigation' has not been translated into English, making a detailed review of this book very difficult, and it is the reason why this is a relatively short chapter. However, forensic science students and the general reader need to be aware of this publication, given Locard's reputation and influence in the English-speaking world and his significant impact on the development of forensic science in the French-speaking world.

In addition to the exchange principle, Locard is credited with establishing one of the world's first forensic science laboratories. At the time of publication in 1920, Locard was director of the technical police laboratory in Lyon, France, which he established a decade earlier in 1910.

During his career, Locard contributed significantly to the development of document examination, including handwriting, which he termed graphometry, and fingerprint examination.

Locard was also co-founder of the International Academy of Criminalistics (1929–1938), a collaboration between German, French and Dutch forensic scientists and criminologists.

Locard, like Gross, applied the scientific method to the investigation of crime, placing less reliance on human testimony.

Biography of the Publication

'Criminal Investigation' was published in Paris in 1920. In the front matter are listed other publications by Locard, which contributed to the publication. Their titles and details are translated as follows.

The Police. What it is. What it should be. 1 vol. in-12. Paris, Payot 1919.

Identification of repeat offenders. Library of Criminology. 1 vol. in-4 428 p. with 85 fig. Paris, Maloine 1909.

Instructions for technical research in criminal statements. (In collaboration with Gabriel Petisné.) 1 broch. in-12 with 8 fig. In Lyon, at the Laboratoire de police technique 1919.

Graphometry and identification of writings. Revue Scientifique.

Medical jurisprudence in the seventeenth century 1 vol. gr. in-8°. Lyon Storck 1902 (this is Locard's doctoral thesis).

Poroscopy, a new method of identifying criminals. 1 broch. with many figures. Lyon, Rey 1913.

For Locard, graphometry was the measurement of certain features of handwriting, which is a major section in 'Criminal Investigation'.

Poroscopy is the study of sweat pores and their use in identification. It is today considered the third level of fingerprint examination after overall pattern and minutiae. Locard is credited with pioneering poroscopy.

Fingerprint examination and document examination are major sections in the 'Criminal Investigation'.

The question arises as to why Locard's book did not have the wide impact of Gross's Handbook. A major contributing factor must be that it was not translated into other languages, particularly English. However, together with Gross, Locard can be considered one of the pioneers of forensic science and, in particular, traceology, which is discussed in Chapter 10 on the Sydney Declaration. The 'exchange principle' is perhaps Locard's greatest legacy.

Biography of the Author

According to most sources, Edmond Locard (1877–1966) was born on the 13th of November 1877 in Saint-Chamond in the Loire Department of the Auvergne-Rhône-Alpes region of France, about 50 km southwest of the city of Lyon.

Locard went on to study medical jurisprudence (legal medicine) at the University of Lyon and was a student of Alexandre Lacassagne (1843–1924), professor of legal medicine at the University and founder of the Lacassagne School of Criminology, a rival of Cesare Lombroso's Italian School. Lacassagne is worth a chapter in any history of forensic science, particularly in the field of toxicology. However, in this history of publications, it is his role as a teacher of Locard that is important. Lombroso is discussed in Chapter 1 of the Handbook.

After obtaining his doctoral degree in 1902, Locard undertook several internships in a variety of institutions, including the Paris Police under Alphonse Bertillon (1853–1914). There, Locard was introduced to Bertillon's anthropometric system of identification, employing physical measurements of an individual. Bertillon and anthropometry were discussed in Chapter 1 of the Handbook. However, anthropometry was an important stepping stone in the development of forensic science practice, and so a summary of its rise and fall is given in a following panel under Contexts.

Locard went on to study law and obtained his degree in 1905. He conducted further research on legal medicine and criminology.

In 1910, Locard acquired two attic rooms in Lyon's Palais de Justice and, together with two assistants, established the world's first forensic science laboratory. At that time, the focus was mainly on identifying criminals using Bertillon's anthropometry and fingerprints. Locard can be rightly considered the father of the forensic science laboratory. Image 2.3 is of a plaque in Lyon recognising the establishment of Locard's Laboratory.

During the First World War (1914–1918), Locard joined the cypher service of the French Secret Service, which probably accounts for the chapter on codebreaking in 'Criminal Investigation'.

In 1920, Locard published 'Criminal Investigation', introducing an exchange principle. He expanded his laboratory and developed fingerprint and handwriting examination and the microscopic examination of traces.

In 1921, Locard formalised his new method of handwriting examination by publishing it in Revue Scientifique. This method involved specified measurements of handwriting features, which he termed graphometry. The method is included in 'Criminal Investigation'.

In one of his few publications translated into English (Locard 1928), Locard acknowledges a debt owed to others. The idea of looking for traces, particularly dust, he recounts, was borrowed from Hans Gross and the fictional Sherlock Holmes. Incidentally, Locard himself was known as the 'Sherlock Holmes of France', one of many regional 'Sherlocks'.

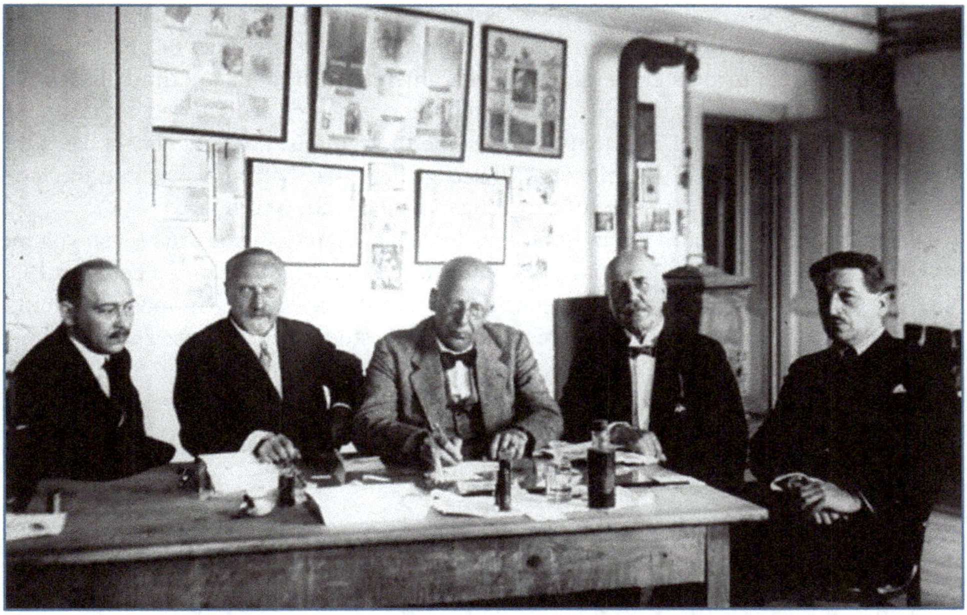

Image 2.4 Members of the Academy in Lausanne, 1929. Courtesy of Pierre Margot.

In 1929, at the University of Lausanne, Switzerland, Locard co-founded the International Academy of Criminalistics. Locard aimed to promote the field of forensic science on an international level, separating the scientific investigation of crime, which he called 'criminalistics', from the broader, more criminological aspects of the study of crime.

Image 2.4 shows members of the Academy meeting at the University of Lausanne. Edmond Locard is on the right. The other members are, from right to left, Marc Bischoff, professor of forensic science at the University of Lyon and successor to Archibald Riess, George Popp from Frankfurt, Germany, a chemist and microscopist; Christian Jacobus van Ledden Hülsebosch, a pharmacist from Amsterdam and in 1929 the president of the Academy. Sitting next to Locard is Siegfried Karl Türkel from Vienna, a lawyer turned criminologist.

The officers of the Academy in 1931 were as follows (Lonsea n.d.).

- Prof. Dr. Marc Bischoff. Vice President
- Dr. Robert Heindl. Vice President
- Dr. Edmond Locard. Vice President
- Prof. Dr. Georg Popp. Vice President
- Dr. Bruno Schultz. Vice President
- Dr. Siegfried Türkel. Secretary
- Dozent Christiaan Jacobus Van Ledden Hülsebosch. President.

In conjunction with co-founding the Academy, Locard also became editor-in-chief, then director of the Academy's publication Revue Internationale de Criminalistique, positions he held until the Academy broke up.

The Academy was wound up in 1938 as tensions between Nazi Germany and other European powers continued to mount. This event is discussed later under Contexts.

At this juncture, readers are reminded of the different definitions of criminalistics and criminology and the ambiguity surrounding those terms, which is discussed in the section on Terms, Definitions and Explanations. In some translations, the Academy is titled the 'International Academy of Criminology'. It seems clear that Locard considered the term 'criminalistique' to mean the scientific investigation and study of crime.

During his career, Locard wrote numerous works, including the famous seven-volume *Magnum Opus 'Treatise on Criminalistics'*, *'Traité de criminalistique'*, written between 1931 and 1941. In it, Locard provided a detailed study of the scientific methods of criminal investigation (fingerprints, traces, forgery, typographic studies, etc.). These seven volumes would become the 'bible' of French-speaking forensic science laboratories.

Locard retired as the director of the Lyon laboratory in 1951 to be succeeded by his son. Edmond Locard died in 1966.

Key Publications

'*Traité de Criminalistique*' (Treatise of Criminalistics, 1931–1936).

This seven-volume series, Locard's *Magnum Opus*, is considered his most significant work. It outlines his methods and theories in forensic science and criminology.

'*Dust and Its Analysis*' (Police Journal, 1928). This paper is an English translation.

'*The Analysis of Dust Traces*' (American Journal of Police Science, 1930),

'*La police et les methods scientifiques*' (Police and Scientific Methods, 1934). This book explores the application of scientific methods in police work.

Motivation for Writing

Locard, like Gross, wished to promote the use of science and the scientific method in criminal investigations. He also agreed that less reliance should be placed on human testimony. The publication was a manual for investigators, which would also promote his laboratory and encourage the use of science in policing.

Contexts

Scientific/Technical

Perhaps the most important scientific/technical context was the incremental developments in microscopy and photography that occurred during Locard's professional life. Carl Zeiss and other instrument makers developed microscopes with improved resolution and image clarity. These improvements provided the tools to better examine and measure the minutiae of fingerprints and documents, including handwriting.

One example of such developments occurred in 1925. Calvin Goddard (1891–1955), while at the Forensic Ballistics Bureau in New York, United States, developed the comparison microscope for the examination and comparison of firearms ammunition. The instrument permitted side-by-side comparison and the superimposition of images. The comparison microscope also found application in document examination.

Locard's life and particularly his professional life spanned a period of major development in forensic science, which he himself either initiated or advanced, particularly in France. The era was marked by developments in the identification of criminals, initially using anthropometry (measuring and recording certain dimensions of the body of criminals) and fingerprint classification systems such as the Henry system.

Locard's establishment of the laboratory in Lyon was followed in 1923 by the establishment of the first laboratory in the United States by August Vollmer in Los Angeles, which is discussed in Chapter 3 on the Ontogeny paper. The FBI laboratory was established almost a decade later in 1932 and the London Police laboratory in 1935.

As mentioned earlier, Locard spent some time with the Paris Police learning the anthropometric identification system from Alphonse Bertillon.

Outside forensic science, the world witnessed Einstein's Theory of Relativity published in 1915 and Fleming's discovery of penicillin in 1928, accompanied by developments in physics and molecular biology, which are recorded in other chapters of this book.

Alphonse Bertillon (1853–1914) and Anthropometry

Given Bertillon's role in the development of forensic science, it is worth devoting a few sentences to Bertillon and the rise and fall of anthropometry.

Bertillon joined the Paris Police in 1879 and was first employed in a junior position. Between then and 1881, he developed his now famous anthropometric system of identification, 'Bertillonage' or 'Le Portrait Parlé' (the word portrait), based on certain measurements of the human body. In 1891, he published his method in the Annales de démographie internationale.

In 1883, Bertillon's system was used to identify a repeat offender and thereby gained acceptance by the Paris Police and began to be adopted and adapted by other police forces. The Chicago Police Department adopted Bertillonage in 1888; the New York City Police Department followed suit in 1896.

Bertillon's method was promoted at the 1889 International Congress of Criminal Anthropology in Paris. The Congress recommended its application to all police forces worldwide. In the same year, Bertillon presented his system of identification at the Universal Exhibition in Paris, and the international jury awarded him a gold medal.

In 1893, the 'Judicial Identity Service' was created at the Paris Police Prefecture. It was headed by Bertillon and had 35 employees. The Service combined anthropometry, photography, and judicial records (a collection of custodial sentences handed down in France). In that year, Bertillon was appointed to the rank of Knight of the National Order of the Legion of Honor.

However, 1893 was to mark the zenith of Bertillon's career and influence. By applying the principles of Bertillonage to handwriting examination, Bertillon helped falsely convict Alfred Dreyfus in one of the most famous cases in history, and certainly in France. Bertillon had no experience in handwriting examination. In 1904, a group of mathematicians issued a report exposing Bertillon's lack of expertise, and Dreyfus was acquitted in 1906.

The ease with which fingerprints could be taken, examined, and stored eventually led to the abandonment of Bertillonage, which required specialist training and

(Continued)

(Continued)

equipment; it was resource-heavy. By the turn of the century, fingerprints had pretty much totally displaced anthropometry as a means of identification.

A more complete set of the reasons for the decline in anthropometry and the rise of fingerprints is given in Chapter 1 of the book.

Criminocorpus Museum published on 11 July 2016 and consulted on 12 March 2025. Permanent link: https://criminocorpus.org/fr/ref/25/17518/

Historical

The major historical events during Locard's professional life were, of course, the two world wars. World War I (1914–1918) was largely fought on French soil, with France, Britain, and America allied against Germany. World War II (1939–1945) saw France invaded by Nazi forces, with part of southern France becoming a puppet state under the Vichy regime. Lyon, at that time, was a major city in Vichy, France.

The growth of National Socialism in Germany brought about the end of the International Academy of Criminalistics. The German-speaking members leaned more towards social Darwinism in their view of crime and supported the racial purity ideas of the Nazis that led to the Holocaust. The French-speaking members, Bischoff and Locard, wished to distance themselves by relying on a more scientific and less sociological approach to the investigation and study of crime. However, these differences were amplified by the impact of the rise of Nazi Germany, its antisemitic policies and the cult of the 'Fuhrer'. It is no coincidence that the breakup of the Academy coincided with the 'Anschluss', the annexation of Austria by Nazi Germany in 1938.

During World War II Lyon fell under the Vichy regime, which collaborated with the Nazis. Given the breakup of the Academy on what were essentially ideological grounds, one can only wonder at Locard's attitude to the collaborationist government as Lyon's Jews were rounded up and deported, as they were in the rest of France. It is important to note that Locard was a student of Lacassagne, who rejected social Darwinism and was of the view that criminals were the product of the environment and not biology. He must have been greatly disturbed, given this criminological perspective. Perhaps Locard was a member of or otherwise assisted the French Resistance; some sources claim he was a member (Frappa 2024). Until recently, the history of the Vichy regime and the activities of members of society living under that regime was a 'closed book' in France. So, there is little available evidence to shed light on Locard's role during that period and any developments he may have made in the practice of forensic science.

Social/Society

As has been highlighted and discussed, the 1920s witnessed a significant presence within society of social Darwinism, particularly in the form of Eugenics (selective breeding). It appears evident that Locard and the 'French' school of forensic science viewed crime investigation more as a scientific endeavour, while the 'German' school adopted a social Darwinist approach, embracing a sociological perspective for crime investigation and study. Conversely, the 'French' school rejected this approach, which aligned itself with the racial purity ideologies espoused by Nazi Germany. As recorded earlier, this ideological divergence played a pivotal role in the dissolution of the International Academy of Criminalistics prior to World War II.

Structure of the Publication

'*Criminal Investigation*' has 303 pages and seven chapters, and a conclusion section. The structure is detailed as follows. The titles of chapters are roughly translated into English, as are most of the section titles, unless the meaning is clear. The purpose of the translation is to enable non-French-speaking readers to gain a better understanding of the scope of Locard's publication.

As mentioned earlier, a digitally scanned version of the book may be found at https://criminocorpus.org/fr/bibliotheque/doc/2555/

Chapter I – L'ENQUÊTE CRIMINELLE (The Criminal Investigation). P5–27

A. La découverte du crime (The discovery of the crime). p6
B. Poursuite du criminal (Criminal prosecution). p9
C. Théorie de la preuve dans le procès penal (Theory of evidence in criminal trials). p10
D. Modes de prevue (Methods of evidence). p12
E. Les méthodes scientifique et la prevue technique (Scientific methods and technical evidence). p18

As the title indicates, this chapter sets out the nuts and bolts of the scientific investigation of crimes.

Chapter II – LE TÉMOIGNAGE (The Testimony). P27–101

§1. Analyse du témoignage (Analysis of testimony). p30
  A. Sensations
  B. Perception
  C. Fixation
  D. Expression
§2. Phénomènes collectifs (Collective phenomena). p55
§3. Le faux témoignage (False testimony – motives). p58
§4. Le faux témoignage pathologique (Pathological false testimony). p68
§5. Le témoignage des enfants (The testimony of children). p76
§6. L'interrogateur (The interrogator – necessary qualities). p80
§7. Technique de l'interrogatoire (Interrogation technique). p83
  A. Technique de l'interrogatoire des témoins (Witness interrogation technique)
  B. Technique de l'interrogatoire du prévenu (Technique for interrogation of the defendant)

CONCLUSIONS. p101

This chapter, echoing Gross, highlights the weaknesses of witness testimony. Those weaknesses, including poor observational skills, poor memories, relying on second-hand accounts and deliberate false testimony, are recognised and discussed. Despite those weaknesses, the fact remains that such evidence may contain elements that are truthful and accurate. Therefore, the purpose of interrogation is to elicit the truth from witness testimony, to distinguish the signal from the noise. To achieve that aim, recourse is made to psychology to identify interrogation strategies that might reveal the truth.

Like Gross, Locard argues that because of the weakness of witness testimony, more reliance should be placed on physical evidence and the use of the scientific method in the investigation of crime.

The introduction of psychology makes this chapter the most criminological section of Locard's publication.

Chapter III – LES EMREINTES DIDGTALES (Fingerprints). P102–138

Recherche des empreintes sur le lieu du crime (Search for fingerprints at the crime scene). p106

Nature et valeur de la prevue dactyloscopique (Nature and value of fingerprint evidence). p124

This chapter is a treatise on fingerprint examination with statistical analysis and several case examples in support of the methods described.

Chapter IV – TRACES ET TACHES (Traces and Stains). P139–170

From the perspective of this history, this is the most important chapter as it contains the text that later becomes Locard's exchange principle, expressed as 'every contact leaves a trace'.

Given its subject matter, this chapter is also a foundational treatise of traceology discussed in Chapter 10, the Sydney Declaration.

The structure is as follows.

This chapter discusses at length how trace evidence might be transferred during the commission of a crime and how science can be used in the investigation of crime, with practical examples.

On page 139 is a description of the exchange principle as introduced earlier, which can be roughly translated as follows.

> *The truth is that no one can act with the intensity of criminal action without leaving multiple marks of its passage ... sometimes the criminal left on the scene the marks of his passage, sometimes, by a reverse action, he took away on his body or on his clothes the clues of his stay* [or his action].

Chapter V – L' EXPERTISE DES DOCUMENTS ÉCRITS (Document Examination Including Handwriting). P171–204

This chapter gives a detailed description of Locard's graphometric techniques for measuring and comparing certain features of handwriting, e.g. slopes and angles.

Chapter VI – DÉCHIFFREMENT DES ÉCRITURES SECRÉTES (Deciphering Secret Codes). P205–235

Chapter VII – METHODOLOGIE DE LA PREUVE INDICIALE (Methodology of Indirect or Circumstantial Evidence[1]). P236–294

Impact at the Time

'Criminal Investigation' echoed Gross's position that the investigation of crime was a scientific endeavour guided by the scientific method.

There is no doubt of the significant impact of 'Criminal Investigation' among French-speaking peoples, particularly in traceology, fingerprints and document examination, including graphometry. However, as pointed out elsewhere, its non-translation into English and other languages weakened its impact outside the francophone world, apart from the exchange principle.

Impact Today

Every student of forensic science is aware of 'Locard's Exchange Principle' that 'every contact leaves a trace' and that it is a fundamental principle applied in forensic science.

However, as mentioned earlier, it cannot be tested, and one exception would undermine the principle.

The power/status of the principle has weakened somewhat over time. As forensic science has developed, so has the understanding of transfer and persistence. The 'silent witness' may be absent or misleading. For example, gunshot residue deposited on the hands of a shooter is rapidly lost and today, given the sensitivity of DNA analysis techniques, finding someone's DNA at a scene is not proof of activity or even presence; the trace can be misleading. It is ultimately a court of law or other tribunal of fact that decides on the interpretation of scientific findings and observations, which is certainly the case in common law jurisdictions.

The fact that little of Locard's work was translated into English at the time probably accounts for its limited impact outside the francophone world.

Contribution to Current Practice

'Criminal Investigation' is a treatise on various disciplines in forensic science, particularly fingerprint and document/handwriting examination and the examination of dust and stains. The publication is now mostly of historical interest and has had little impact on current practice.

However, it does introduce poroscopy in fingerprint examination and the principle of standardising procedures. In addition, the publication must be considered a foundational document in traceology, which will be discussed further in Chapter 10 on the Sydney Declaration.

Concluding Remarks

L'Enquête Criminelle et les Méthodes Scientifiques (Criminal Investigation and Scientific Methods) is the source of the exchange principle quoted in most forensic science textbooks as 'every contact leaves a trace'.

Key Takeaways

'Criminal Investigation'

- Introduced an exchange principle usually expressed as 'every contact leaves a trace', although Locard never wrote that phrase.
  - The principle can never be tested, and one exception would undermine it.
  - The principle has weakened over time as the understanding of transfer and persistence has improved.
- Introduced poroscopy, recording the pattern of sweat pores, which has been incorporated into fingerprint examination.
- Helped sow the seeds of traceology.
- Standardised procedures.
- Promoted the scientific investigation of crime.

Note

1 This is evidence that cannot directly prove a fact in issue.

Bibliography

Frappa, Amos. 2024. *Edmond Locard, le fondateur de la police scientifique*. AFFIT Editions.

Locard, Edmond. 1928. "Dust and Its Analysis: An Aid to Criminal Investigation." *The Police Journal* 1: 177–192.

Lonsea. n.d. *International Academy of Criminology*. Accessed March 14, 2025. http://www.lonsea.de/pub/org/419.

3

The Ontogeny of Criminalistics – Questions and an Agenda

THE ONTOGENY OF CRIMINALISTICS

PAUL L. KIRK

Paul L. Kirk, Professor of Criminalistics, University of California, Berkeley, California, is well known to the readers of this journal and to all active in the field of criminalistics. Professor Kirk has published a number of articles in this and other technical journals, and is the author of *Crime Investigation* (Interscience Publishers, 1953). His present paper has been prepared from material presented before the California Association of Criminalists of which he is an active member.—EDITOR.

Image 3.1 Publication.

Name of the Publication

The Ontogeny of Criminalistics was written by Paul Leland Kirk (9 May 1902 to 5 June 1970) in 1963 when he was Professor of Criminalistics (and Biochemistry) at the University of California, Berkeley, CA, United States, and was published in the US Journal of Criminal Law and Criminology and Police Science in 1963.

The reference is as follows. Kirk, Paul L. 1963. "The Ontogeny of Criminalistics." *Journal of Criminal Law, Criminology and Police Science* 54: 235–38.

According to Semantic Scholar, the paper has been cited 139 times and is classified as highly influential. ResearchGate records 147 citations.

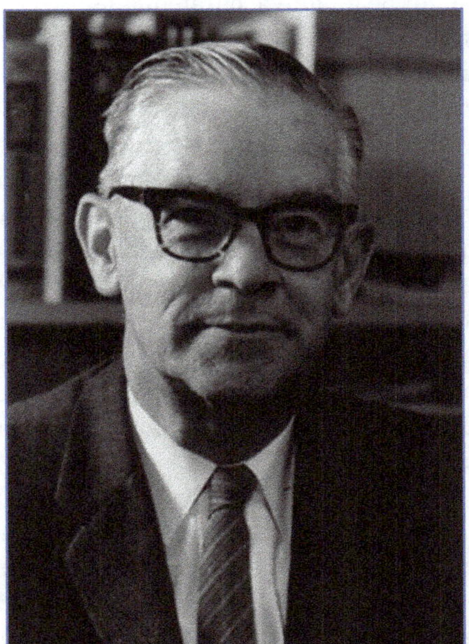

Image 3.2 Paul Leland Kirk. Mgm Paul L Kirk/Wikimedia Commons/Fair use.

A History of Forensic Science in 10 Publications: How They Established Current Practice, First Edition.
Sean Doyle.

Introduction

The relationship between the term 'criminalistics' as used by Kirk in the paper and 'forensic science' was discussed in the section on Terms, Definitions and Explanations, and is again in Chapter 10 on the Sydney Declaration. Some argue, such as the California Association of Criminalists (California Association of Criminalists 2024), that there is a difference, criminalistics perhaps being a sub-discipline of forensic science. The distinction is certainly unclear. Nevertheless, in his paper, Kirk accepts that for many the terms are synonymous and, in this chapter, they are treated thus.

Kirk himself defines criminalistics as follows.

> *... the application of the techniques and principles of the basic sciences, particularly chemistry and physics, to the examination and interpretation of physical evidence ...*
>
> *(Kirk 1955)*

This definition closely corresponds to the definition given in 'Interpreting Evidence' Chapter 6, that forensic science is the 'science of interpretation', but differs from that given in Chapter 10, the 'science of the trace'.

Professor Kirk borrows the term 'ontogeny' from the science of biology. Ontogeny is the developmental history of an individual organism or a functional entity such as an ecosystem in its lifetime, from conception onwards. Ontogeny is distinct from phylogeny, which refers to the evolutionary history of a species. Indeed, although the unity that Kirk anticipated has not yet come to be, understanding forensic science as an ecosystem might be a more accurate model. According to some, forensic science is a collection of scientific disciplines, sometimes interacting with each other and with the legal/judicial environment in which they operate (Fraser 2020a), and to others, it is the science of the trace. These issues will be discussed at length in Chapter 10.

Essentially, in the ontogeny paper, Kirk seeks to define what forensic science is, questions what its origins and components or fundamental principles might be, what its purpose is and sets out a developmental agenda. It also considers whether forensic science qualifies as a profession. As will be clear from this book, those issues remain debated and contested. However, in this paper, Professor Kirk argues that forensic science is the science of individualisation; that is, attributing the source of a trace to a unique origin, a means of determining whether two items of evidence have a common source. One example given is whether a bullet has been fired by a particular firearm to the exclusion of all others. Another is whether a fingerprint[1] lifted at a crime scene is that of a suspect and no one else.

In the paper, Kirk seeks to shed some light on the basic laws, theories and principles of forensic science and encourage others to do the same. He claims that forensic science is a science, and its practice is a profession and offers some evidence in support. However, he concludes that forensic science lacks the necessary development to find general acceptance as either.

Biography of the Publication

The paper cites no earlier works, indeed no works at all. It expresses Kirk's desire to establish forensic science as a scientific discipline and a profession. It is both a call to action and a developmental agenda.

Professional Biography of the Author

Paul Leland Kirk (1902–1970), formerly Professor of Criminalistics (and Biochemistry) at the University of California, Berkeley (UCB), was well-known to his contemporaries active in the field of forensic science. Professor Kirk published numerous articles in many technical journals and was the author of 'Crime Investigation: Physical Evidence and the Police Laboratory' (Kirk 1953)[2] among other works.

Paul Leland Kirk was born in Colorado Springs, Colorado, United States, in 1902. He was first and foremost a scientist, but, as recorded by some, he was also a man of practical application as opposed to pure theory (Chisum and Turvey 2011). He studied first at Ohio State University, where he received a bachelor's degree in chemistry. He obtained a master's degree in chemistry from the University of Pittsburgh and a doctoral degree in biochemistry from UCB.

Volmer and Kirk Establishing Criminalistics at UC Berkeley

In 1916, the then Berkeley police chief, August Volmer (1876–1955), established a criminology course at UCB to train his police officers in the use of science in the investigation of crime.

In 1937, Kirk, a professor of biochemistry since 1929, assumed leadership of the Criminology[3] program at UCB. The program gained momentum and grew in its reputation under his charge (Chisum and Turvey 2006).

In 1950, Volmer, after much lobbying, established the School of Criminology at UCB, and Kirk was appointed to chair the criminalistics department. According to Peter De Forest and colleagues.

> *The program grew to be well-known, and Kirk developed a substantial reputation in forensic science, devoting his time to instruction, research, and casework.*
>
> *(De Forest et al. 1983)*

Therefore, Kirk, in collaboration with Volmer, established the first academic program in criminalistics in the United States. In addition to advocating for the discipline of criminalistics and advising several schools in the development of their departments, Kirk was a frequent consultant for both prosecution and defence, giving expert evidence on, for example, fire investigation, glass, fibres and bloodstain pattern analysis (BPA).

Several sources relate that he would tell students that he was initially drawn to forensic science when a biochemistry student approached him with a question about a deceased dog and whether it could be determined whether the dog had been poisoned. Investigating this matter sparked Kirk's interest. Soon after, he was instructed to examine the clothing of a complainant alleging rape. The investigators wanted to know whether anything on the clothing could be found at the microscopic level to link the alleged perpetrator to the complainant and support the allegation of rape. Kirk's finding of fibres from the suspect's shirt and the subsequent conviction sealed Kirk's interest and secured his reputation for reliable results based on careful examination.

Kirk's War Years 1942–1945

Perhaps Kirk's greatest claim to fame, certainly outside the realm of forensic science, was his involvement in the Manhattan Project, the development of the first atomic bombs. The physicist J. Robert Oppenheimer (1904–1967) and the US Army officer Major General Leslie R. Groves (1896–1970) led the project. Kirk initially worked at the so-called 'Rad Lab' with Ernest Lawrence (1901–1958) at Los Alamos, New Mexico. He then used his skills as an analytical chemist in the analysis of minute quantities of material in the production of the fissile element plutonium at Hanford Engineering Works, Richland, Washington State. The Manhattan Project aimed to produce two fissile materials, uranium-235 and plutonium-239. Hanford was the plutonium production facility.

Ultramicroanalysis

At Hanford, Kirk and a team of chemists employed this analysis of minute quantities of material called ultramicroanalysis. This involved using a microscope to observe and monitor the procedures. These analytical techniques were used to study microgram[4] quantities of material, which, during the early production of plutonium, was about all the scientists had available. Ultramicroanalysis was used to determine the chemical properties of plutonium so that it might be isolated from uranium.

It is beyond the scope of this book but the full story of the development of atomic weapons is fascinating; from Lise Meitner (1878–1968) and her 'splitting' of the atom to the realisation that an atomic bomb was feasible by Otto Frisch OBE FRS (1904–1979) and Sir Rudolf Peierls (1907–1995)[5] at the time refugee Jews at the University of Birmingham, England, and the involvement of Albert Einstein (1879–1955), Niels Bohr (1885–1962), Enrico Fermi (1901–1954), all 'rock star' physicists. The success of the project also depended on the entire industrial might of the United States. Together with Kirk and others of the brightest and best scientists and engineers, all played some part in the Manhattan Project. A very readable and comprehensive account is given by Rhodes (2012).

UC Berkeley Criminology/Criminalistics

On his return to UCB after the war, he established a course in technical criminology and was appointed Professor of Biochemistry and Criminology and then Professor of Criminalistics from 1954 onwards. Returning with him were the analytical techniques developed at

Hanford, which he would apply to forensic investigations. The methods were published in 'Quantitative Ultramicroanalysis' (Kirk 1950) and applied to the scientific investigation of crime, truly trace analysis.

Ultramicroanalysis is a complex title for a set of analytical chemical techniques for analysing and detecting very small amounts of a chemical or substance of evidential value, i.e. micrograms. It is of interest to note that analytical chemistry today can detect amounts as low as nanograms (one thousand millionths of a gram) and in some cases even femtograms (one million millionths of a gram)! One wonders what superlatives Kirk might have employed to express that level of quantitation.

The Birth of Criminalistics

In one of his books, Kirk credits Volmer as giving birth to 'modern criminalistics' (Kirk and Bradford 1965). Various accounts record Volmer being given a copy of Hans Gross' book on Criminal Psychology (Gross 1918), which cites the journal edited by Gross, 'Archives of Criminal Anthropology and Criminalistics' (Kell 2017). However, in the title of this journal, Gross is using the term criminalistics as an approximation, if not a synonym, of criminology. So, while Volmer was exposed to Gross's criminology, it remains unclear how Kirk arrived at adopting the term 'criminalistics' to mean the examination of physical evidence applying the natural sciences. However, Kirk does argue strongly for the use of 'criminalistics' in a paper written in 1947 (Kirk 1947). The first use of the term in English is given to be in 1910 in the US Journal of the American Institute of Criminal Law and Criminology, but this only includes a review of the 1906 English translation of Gross's Handbook with the subtitle 'System der Kriminalistik' (E.L. 1910). The origin of the term 'criminalistics' is mentioned in the section on Terms, Definitions and Explanations and discussed in some detail in Chapter 10 on the Sydney Declaration.

Kirk's First Book

In 1953, Kirk published the first edition of his book 'Crime Investigation: Physical Evidence and the Police Laboratory' (Kirk 1953), a treatise on criminal investigation, crime reconstruction, and forensic examination, which is very much a handbook for police investigators along the lines of Gross's Handbook. Like Gross, Kirk relies very much on the 'silent witness' of physical evidence and recognises the unreliability of eyewitness and human testimony.

The following quote is attributed to Kirk.

> *This is evidence that does not forget. It is not confused by the excitement of the moment. It is not absent because human witnesses are. It is factual evidence. Physical evidence cannot be wrong; it cannot perjure itself; it cannot be wholly absent. Only its interpretation can err.*
>
> *–Dr Paul Kirk, p4 (Kirk 1953)*

It echoes the ideas of both Gross and Locard. Indeed, it is an expanded form of Locard's exchange principle, which is usually paraphrased as; 'every contact leaves a trace', which was discussed in Chapter 2. In this paper, Kirk laments the lack of '*architects*', which prompts the question: why is the paper silent on these two major figures in the development of forensic science?

The paper promotes the role of the scientific generalist with an understanding of the fundamental principles of forensic science who can help realise the full potential of forensic science. These remain issues today and are further discussed later in this chapter and again in Chapter 10 on the Sydney Declaration.

In 'Crime Investigation', Kirk emphasises the distinction between identification and individualisation, which is one of the main messages of the Ontogeny paper.

> ... *the real purpose of the criminalist* [or forensic scientist]*: to determine the identity of source. That is, two items of evidence, one known and the other unknown, must be identified as having a common origin.* (page 16)

Famous Case

Kirk, applying science and the fundamentals of forensic science as he understood them to be, then turned his mind to several different evidence types, including fibres and BPA.[6] It was in the investigation of a murder utilising BPA that Kirk was involved in the famous case of the murder of Marilyn Reese Sheppard in 1954 and the conviction of her husband, Dr Sam Sheppard. Kirk was instructed by the defence as part of Dr Sheppard's appeal against conviction. Kirk investigated the crime scene and conducted experiments to establish the cause of different patterns of blood staining using the laws of physics. Kirk's examination, experiments and report supported Dr Sheppard's innocence (Cleveland State University 2024). Nevertheless, the initial appeal in 1955 failed. However, intense media pressure resulted in the US District Court overturning the conviction in 1964, and in 1966, the US Supreme Court upheld that decision. Kirk's BPA report, a crime scene report *par excellence* (emphasis added), was considered decisive (Kirk 1955; Cleveland State University 2024).

Kirk Awards

Interestingly, in that case, he crossed swords with a medical practitioner, Dr Samuel Gerber, instructed by the prosecution, who apparently suffered from some of the flaws highlighted by Gross and later Kirk, particularly a lack of an open mind. In addition, having been instrumental in Sheppard's appeal and crossing Gerber, Kirk was denied membership of the American Academy of Forensic Sciences (AAFS). Gerber was then a senior and influential member of the AAFS. Given the treatment of Kirk by the AAFS, it is ironic to note that one of the highest honours now awarded by the AAFS is the Paul L Kirk Award for Criminalistics[7]. Confusingly, another US forensic science society also gives a Paul Kirk Award. The California Association of Criminalists (CAC), in conjunction with the Chartered Society of Forensic Sciences, offers the award biennially (California Association of Criminalists 2024).

Other Publications

In addition to 'Criminal Investigation', Kirk also authored a standard textbook on fire investigation, 'Kirk's Fire Investigation', later editions of which remain in print today, edited and revised by others (Icove and Haynes 2017).

Kirk also authored some other textbooks, 'Density Refractive Index – the Application to Criminal Identification' in 1951, published by Charles C Thomas Company and 'The Crime Laboratory: Organization and Operation' (1965), co-written with Lowell W. Bradford, Director, Laboratory of Criminalistics, Santa Clara County, California.

Paul L. Kirk became a giant in the field of forensic science. His academic research, teaching, casework, literature and sheer pioneering energy stand testament to the brilliance and impact of this early 'criminalist'.

Kirk died at the age of 68 in 1970, sadly, before his dream/ambition to use blood as the most powerful evidence type in the process of 'individualisation'. That moment came when Sir Alec Jeffreys, in the late 1980s, discovered highly variable parts of the DNA molecule and realised that such variability might be used to identify individuals. That is the subject of Chapter 4.

Contexts

History

Kirk certainly lived in interesting and turbulent times. He grew up during the First World War. The Great Depression (1929–1939) began with the US stock market crash of 1929. Other significant events included the influx of Midwest farmers into California to escape the Dust Bowl (1930–1936), Roosevelt's 'New Deal' in 1933 and the Japanese attack on Pearl Harbour on the 7th of December 1941. The attack against Pearl Harbour brought the United States into World War II, which had begun in September 1939. After the defeat of Nazi Germany in May 1945, World War II ended with the nuclear destruction of Hiroshima and Nagasaki in August 1945. The Nagasaki bomb 'Fat Man' utilised plutonium, which, as recorded earlier, Kirk helped to produce.

This post-war period was characterised by living under the threat of nuclear extinction. The Soviet Union developed its own nuclear weapons and drew the Iron Curtain in 1946 to begin the Cold War, which came to a head with the Cuban Missile Crisis in October 1962.

Two other major conflicts marked Kirk's life: the US military intervention in Korea and Vietnam.

It is of interest to speculate that if Kaiser Wilhelm II had not marched into neutral Belgium on the 14th of August 1914 on his way to wage war against France, World War I may have been avoided. With no World War I, no Adolf Hitler, no rise of the Nazis and no World War II. Given the magnitude of the resources needed to develop and manufacture nuclear weapons, and with no requirement to do so, they might never have been produced. What a different world we might now live in!

Science

War and conflict have historically accelerated scientific development, primarily in the advancement of weapons. Even so, many of those developments had peacetime applications, such as the jet engine and improved methods of industrial production.

Advances in nuclear physics led to the building of nuclear power stations, and less obvious but equally impactful was the consequent production of radioactive isotopes.

Isotopes are different forms of the same chemical element. For example, hydrogen has two stable isotopes: hydrogen itself with one particle in its nucleus and a slightly heavier form, often called deuterium, which has two particles in its nucleus.

Radioactive isotopes are unstable and, as they fall apart, emit radiation which can be detected and measured. Hydrogen has a radioactive isotope often called tritium; as expected, it has three particles in its nucleus. Having different forms of the same chemical element that can be detected and measured means that chemical reactions can be studied, e.g. phosphorus-32 for enzyme reactions, together with metabolic and biochemical pathways; examples include Iodine-131 for thyroid function, drugs containing carbon-14 and tritium (hydrogen-3) for studying their fate in the body. This has led to a better understanding of chemical and biological processes and resulted in advances in diagnostic testing in medicine and a better understanding of how the human body metabolises nutrients. In addition, radioactive isotopes such as cobalt-60 have had a major impact on the treatment of cancer.

As discussed in Chapter 4 on DNA 'fingerprinting', the radioactive isotope phosphorus-32 was used in early DNA 'fingerprinting'. The isotope helped visualise the DNA patterns used to identify individuals.

The development of nuclear reactors also made possible a technique known as neutron activation analysis (NAA), a powerful analytical tool. Neutrons are subatomic particles generated by a nuclear reactor. NAA can detect up to 70 elements simultaneously at amounts in the nanogram[8] range and below. It involves irradiating a sample of an unknown material and monitoring the radioactive decay induced to identify the major and trace components. NAA has found some application in the analysis of Gunshot Residues and environmental forensics.

As mentioned earlier, Kirk himself applied the ultramicroanalysis developed on the Manhattan Project to the investigation of crime. Several other analytic tools and techniques advanced significantly in meeting the needs of the Project, including mass spectrometry and infra-red spectroscopy, again powerful analytical tools used to identify and quantify substances. War accelerated the development of these and other analytical tools, which are now put to routine use in forensic science laboratories around the world to identify and quantify illicit substances, for example.

The totality of scientific advances resulting from World War II is too large to catalogue but includes the mass production of the antibiotic penicillin, the use of radar for weather forecasting and its technology for microwave ovens, advances in computing from breaking the enigma code, and advances in surgery such as skin grafting, reconstructive surgery and blood transfusions.

During the post–World War II period, the Space Race started. It was essentially a competition between German scientists and engineers in the United States and those in the USSR.

Society

Social Darwinism Gone

The racial hygiene policies of Nazi Germany, the mistaken notion of the survival of the fittest and eugenics, all popular before World War II, were dealt an almost fatal blow by the holocaust. Social Darwinism, discussed in Chapter 1, became stigmatised. However, eugenics, trying to breed out human weakness to promote human 'betterment', maintained some respectability until the 1950s (Wilson 2024). The rejection of various forms of social Darwinism profoundly affected criminology. There was no longer a criminal type to be identified, racist assumptions regarding certain ethnic groups being more likely to commit crime were undermined; criminality was not a product of biology. Regarding forensic science, the rejection of social Darwinism further underlined the scientific approach of Gross, the reliance on unbiased and rigorous science to solve crime.

Ethics

The Manhattan Project also introduced ethics into the scientific arena. The question of using atomic bombs, the original weapons of mass destruction, against the civilian population of Japan troubled many involved in the Project. Unfortunately, ethical considerations have yet to firmly take root in forensic science, as the numerous examples of forensic fraud and malpractice demonstrate. These include so-called dry labbing – not analysing samples and fabricating results, giving misleading evidence. Malpractice is often driven by misunderstood objectives, which again is probably related to forensic science being understood by some as police science, at the service of law enforcement and not justice.

There also remains a lax approach to or an absence of regulation. There are many rules and regulations that remain unpoliced, unenforced and lack deterring sanctions.

Structure and Relevant Contents

Introduction

In broad terms, the Ontogeny paper seeks to address the terminological ambiguity that plagued forensic science in 1963 and continues to do so.

In the paper, Kirk seeks to define what forensic science is, and questions what its origins and components/fundamental principles might be, and what its purpose is. He sets out a developmental agenda. He also considers whether the practice of forensic science qualifies as a profession.

Although the term criminalistics is used in the paper, Kirk considers it synonymous with forensic science. He does not seek to distinguish between the two, another example of the fluidity in forensic science terminology. Therefore, while accepting there might be a nuanced distinction, criminalistics being a subdiscipline of forensic science, the term forensic science is used throughout this chapter unless clarity demands otherwise.

Extraordinarily, the paper cites no works supporting the arguments and claims made.

Structure

The paper begins with a historical sketch of the early development of selected disciplines, including fingerprints for the identification of persons, linking spent ammunition to a firearm, and handwriting to an author. It names and praises those who pioneered these disciplines. However, surprisingly, there is no mention of Hans Gross or Edmond Locard.

Kirk claims that employing fingerprints as a means of identification was the '*starting point*' for forensic science. It might be argued that identifying the criminal by any means was the starting point. This is expanded on later.

On the issue of the 'criminalistics' v 'forensic science' debate, in the paper Kirk states that both are fundamentally '*a law-science profession*' and recognises that for many the terms are synonymous. This further justifies the use of 'forensic science' in this chapter.

The paper goes on to chart the progress of laboratory methods in the early twentieth century in support of the investigation of crime. The acceptance by criminal justice stakeholders, courts, litigators, law enforcement, etc., of the validity of the results generated by laboratory methods.

The paper then introduces one of the main subjects, elucidating the fundamental principles of forensic science.

In the paper, Kirk characterises recent progress as follows.

> *... technical rather than fundamental, practical rather than theoretical, transient rather than permanent.*

Progress thus far comprised technical procedures, effective as they have been, with little regard for the fundamentals of forensic science. Kirk draws attention to this deficiency and the resultant need to elucidate the laws, theories and principles of forensic science. The stated aim is to find the '*simple and brief*' laws underpinning forensic science.

However, what Kirk is doing is laying the foundations for his assertion that forensic science is the science of individualisation.

The example of the examination of a bullet and linking it to a particular firearm is used to illustrate the point that, while the procedure is understood, the fundamental principles of firearms identification are not. This is reinforced by a reference to handwriting examination.

The paper next looks to the natural sciences for an example of the fundamentals: Newton's laws of motion, the laws of thermodynamics and Einstein's relationship between energy and mass. In the paper, Kirk argues that even though they describe complex phenomena, these laws are simply and briefly stated. It is worth emphasising that Kirk was seeking simple and brief laws, i.e. not complex and long-winded. This aim will find resonance in Chapter 10 on the Sydney Declaration.

Kirk holds up the examples of Sir Isaac Newton (1642–1727) and Albert Einstein (1879–1955) as '*architects*' of the natural sciences, having elucidated the fundamentals. In his paper, Kirk draws attention to what he considers to be the lack of such architects of forensic science, although at this point in history, both Gross and Locard might be considered as such. The omission of these pioneers seems odd, and it may be that their absence can be explained by the fact that neither advances the contention that forensic science is the science of individualisation. Returning to the Ontogeny paper, Kirk proposes that the absence of architects may be due to the non-acceptance of forensic science as a science in its own right. He then outlines what he thinks is the nature of forensic science, in terms of its fundamental principles and offers advice on what direction future development might take as part of the ontogeny.

His first task is to distinguish between the terms 'identity' and 'identification' and, in doing so, define forensic science as the science of individualisation, e.g. attributing a fingerprint recovered from the scene of a crime to a particular individual to the exclusion of all others.

In the paper, Kirk claims that 'identity' is defined as uniqueness, only one of a kind, which supports the process of individualisation. Kirk contrasts this with 'identification', which, because of common usage, is defined as placing an item of evidence in a class of similar objects, e.g. identification of a mark as a fingerprint or an object as a bullet. The paper points out the lack of forensic utility of such a broad classification. The only purpose of 'identification', or broad classification, is a prelude, a step that precedes 'individualisation'. This leads to the bold statement that forensic science is the '*science of individualisation*', the science of individuality.

There follows a discourse on what Kirk believes is the incorrect use of 'identification' when 'individualisation' is the correct term. This attempts to address one of the many ambiguities in forensic science terms, a recurring topic in this book.

Kirk then records the contrast between the poor forensic utility of identifying blood groups at the time, which places blood recovered from a crime scene in a class of a particular human blood group and other evidence types where the evidence is 'individualised', assigning spent ammunition to a particular firearm. The complaint is made that by not understanding the difference between 'identity' and 'individualisation', certain disciplines in forensic science might not develop as they otherwise might. Identification, as defined by Kirk in the paper, is of little probative value and, as stated earlier, should be seen as a step towards individualisation. Kirk concludes that all disciplines should aim for individualisation. Kirk concludes that this is the developmental direction forensic science should take.

Consequently, understanding the difference between 'identification' and 'individualisation' is essential for the development of forensic science. In addition, without a clear idea of what forensic science is, development will be hindered.

Profession?

Having defined forensic science as the science of individualisation in the Ontogeny paper, Kirk now turns his attention to the question of whether forensic science is a profession.

The paper lists three candidate categories for consideration: a profession, a science or an occupation. Kirk points out the ambiguity of the word 'profession', which has more than one meaning; the opposite of an amateur and 'the professions', such as medicine and the law, are given as examples.

In the paper, Kirk formally defines a profession by three criteria: an extensive period of education and training, a code of behaviour and possessing a means of demonstrating competence. The paper criticises the slow rate of the development of university-level courses of study in forensic science, which hinders its development. This developmental aim has been met. There are forensic science courses of one type or another available at a multitude of universities around the world.

The paper refers to the code of ethics of the California Association of Criminalists (CAC 2015), which Kirk, a CAC member, promotes as an exhaustive model. In his experience, even those practitioners not bound by a code are objective, fair and just, an assessment that will be challenged in Chapter 8 on 'Observer Effects'. Kirk concludes that this criterion is met.[9]

Regarding demonstrating competence, in the paper, Kirk highlights the fact that having completed a relevant and suitable university course, at whatever level (bachelor, master or doctoral), does not demonstrate competence in professional practice. Some form of licensing or certification is suggested. Of particular relevance is the point that qualification by a court as an expert witness is no guarantee of competence. A fact that has grown in recognition and importance as the number of miscarriages of justice to which unreliable scientific evidence has contributed increases.

Surprisingly, given its novelty and the limitations he sets out, Kirk concludes that forensic science could be considered a profession even in 1963!

A Science?

In the paper, Kirk characterises a science as a body of knowledge based on fundamental principles that allow prediction and interpretation. Science is supported by research, which adds to the body of knowledge. 'Individualisation' and 'Individuality' are again listed as the fundamental principles of forensic science, which Kirk describes as simple in concept but not clearly expressed. These fundamentals separate forensic science from other sciences. Later authors argue that it is the use to which science is put that makes it forensic science and that distinguishes it from other sciences, or argue that there is no such thing as forensic science (Fraser 2020b).

Kirk laments the uncoordinated and unsystematised '*great body of knowledge*' produced by a moderate research effort, which he considers technical rather than theoretical. To that body of knowledge, casework should be added.

The conclusion is reached that forensic science meets the criteria of a science, but at the time of writing, it lacks the development necessary to be generally recognised and accepted as such.

The subject of research is considered, and the paper sets out a research agenda identifying the areas requiring development. The need to define objectives and broaden the scope beyond technical advances to encompass theoretical advances is mentioned, a requirement echoed in the Sydney Declaration Chapter 10. The most important research objective is 'interpretive', which requires a sound probabilistic approach to the evaluation of evidence supported by relevant statistical studies[10].

One of the outcomes sought was to reduce the scope for honest disagreement between forensic scientists acting as expert witnesses, thereby weakening the reputation of forensic science as an aid to the criminal justice system. This is an aim never likely to be achieved, particularly in common law jurisdictions in which an adversarial approach to uncovering the truth is employed. This concern may have been prompted by crossing swords with Gerber in the Sheppard case, referred to earlier.

The paper concludes with a rallying cry. It highlights the importance of forensic science and its responsibilities with some lofty analogies. It asks the question where is forensic science headed? A goal needs to be defined for forensic science so that it commands respect as a science and generates pride in its achievements.

Developmental Agenda Summary

In summary, the Ontogeny paper sets out the developmental agenda as follows:

- Accept that forensic science is the science of individualisation, recognise the distinction between identification, placing an object in a restricted class, and identity, meaning uniqueness, only one of a kind.
- Agree on a common terminology.
- Adopt a code of conduct or ethics.
- Create university-level courses in forensic science.
- Define research objectives and agree on a systematised research program.
- Devise and put in place a means of independently demonstrating competence using some form of post-graduate certification or assessment.
- Codify/systematise/coordinate the body of knowledge generated from disparate research and practice.
- Devise and introduce a probabilistic approach to the interpretation of scientific evidence.

Impact at the Time

Among other things, Kirk's Ontogeny paper was perhaps one of the first serious attempts to define what forensic science was. Many readers will wonder what the issue is, as it should be clear what it is, on the basis that 'I know it when I see it'. However, practitioners and academics continuously and sometimes hotly debate whether there is such a thing and, if there is, what it is. To many, this might seem to be a discussion akin to debating the number of angels that can dance on a pinhead. However, as the Sydney Declaration, Chapter 10, argues, echoing the Ontogeny paper, if we do not know what forensic science is, then how can it be taught, and how can an appropriate research program be constructed? Nevertheless, whatever the debate, forensic science continues to serve justice and relevant research is carried out.

The paper certainly established the use of the term criminalistics to describe the recovery, examination and interpretation of physical evidence applying the natural sciences. The origin of the term is discussed in Chapter 10. However, there can be little doubt that the subtitle of Gross's' Handbook 'als System Der Kriminalistik' played some part.

In the early days after its publication in 1963, Kirk's Ontogeny paper received little attention and only started gaining interest as 'traceology'[11] began to (re)gain ground around 2010, as this citations-per-year graph from Semantic Scholar reveals. Sadly, most citations occurred after he died in 1970 (Semantic Scholar 2024). Figure 3.1 depicts the citations per year according to Semantic Scholar.

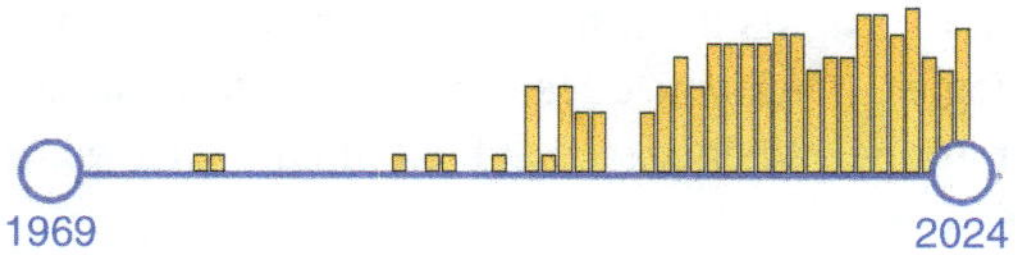

Figure 3.1 Citations per year – the maximum being 10.

Impact Now

Development Agenda and Need for Basic Theory

The 'Ontogeny of Criminalistics' is now considered a landmark paper in forensic science. As discussed earlier, the paper claimed that forensic science was a science – the science of individualisation, and a profession, but lacked recognition as such because of insufficient development, particularly the absence of basic theory.

One of the main impacts of Kirk's paper was the setting of a sound developmental agenda. Many of the items on the agenda have been addressed. In addition, Kirk's identification of the need for fundamental principles continues to provide a reference point for discussion, as demonstrated by the Sydney Declaration, the subject of Chapter 10.

Create University-Level Courses in Forensic Science

The number of universities offering forensic science-related courses at both undergraduate and postgraduate levels now numbers in the hundreds (Hotcoursesabroad 2024).

Many organisations that provide forensic science prefer to recruit graduates in the natural or life sciences and provide internal 'apprenticeships'. Many begin as technicians and then move to research before a progressive involvement in casework (Broome and Todd 2012). It is interesting to note that Gross and Locard were self-taught in terms of science.

Coordinated Research Effort/Agenda

Forensic science research remains disparate and uncoordinated, reflecting the silos of practice and the variation in scientific content from DNA analysis at one end of the spectrum, through forensic chemistry and the feature comparison disciplines, such as fingerprints, at the other. Large bodies of knowledge remain in silos unshared, and risk being forgotten.

Research undertaken 'in-house' by forensic science laboratories, which must conduct bespoke research to meet court deadlines, is not always shared, resulting in instances where academic research lags by sometimes a decade. This is an example of how a lack of information exchange slows development.

Probabilistic Interpretation

The call for probabilistic interpretation has been met, initially in the field of DNA analysis, where evidence could not be interpreted in any other way. In addition, a probabilistic approach is beginning to be adopted, or at least considered, for some feature comparison disciplines. However, there is still resistance to such an approach, as discussed in Chapter 6 'Interpreting Evidence'.

Common Terminology

Some initiatives are addressing the issue of terminological ambiguity, which blights forensic science and was one of the issues that Kirk sought to deal with when defining 'identity' as uniqueness and 'identification' as a broad classification. He also contributed to the ambiguity by not distinguishing between criminalistics and forensic science.

The Organisation of Scientific Area Committees (OSAC) now has its lexicon (OSAC 2024), and ISO's Technical Committee 272 on forensic science is producing a standard ISO121043-1 'Forensic science – Terms and definitions'.

A Profession?

Certifying Competence

The Ontogeny paper records the requirement for demonstrating competence as a forensic scientist in addition to university-based education and training.

That requirement has been addressed in several ways. In the United Kingdom, the government initially established a register of competent practitioners, the Council for the Registration of Forensic Practitioners (CRFP). However, that scheme proved unsustainable (Doyle 2019).

In the USA, several 'boards' assessed and certified practitioners as competent in specified disciplines. However, the independence of those 'boards' was questionable.

In the absence of independent bodies assessing and certifying individual competence, the most widespread approach has been to rely on conformance to the international standard ISO/IEC 17025, the subject of Chapter 7. Conformance to this standard requires accredited organisations to have measures in place to ensure the competence of their staff and to certify that status. This hands responsibility for competence to the organisation. In which case, competence is not being independently assessed.

There has been recent progress in the United States with certification bodies becoming accredited to the international standard ISO/IEC 17024 'Conformity assessment – General requirements for bodies operating certification of persons' (Forensic Specialties Accreditation Board 2024).

The increasing complexity of scientific evidence, for example, probabilistic genotyping[12] and genealogy, will generate new challenges for establishing competence.

Code of Conduct/Practice Directions

Most forensic science providers require their staff to abide by a documented code of conduct, however named[13]. In addition, most forensic scientists are members of professional bodies which also document a code and require members to conform. How that is policed and what sanctions are in place for breaches is sometimes not entirely clear and remains a weakness. In many jurisdictions, there are legal practice directions for expert witnesses and their evidence, conformance is a requirement for the admission of evidence.

A Science?

The debates around whether forensic science is a science and what precisely it is continue with some claiming it is beyond definition (Fraser 2020b) and some that it is the science of the 'trace' (Margot 2017), a concept which will be discussed in Chapter 10 on the Sydney Declaration. Nevertheless, it is clearly the use of science to investigate crime and help resolve legal disputes. In this respect, Kirk's '*law-science profession*' was about right. Chapter 10 of this book will include a closer look at the issue of fundamental principles that are '*simple, brief and to the point*'. Certainly, at this point in the story, the fundamentals of forensic science as sought by Kirk are far from clear.

The Science of Individualisation

In his Ontogeny paper, Kirk asserts that identifying persons using fingerprints was the '*starting point*' for forensic science. However, it is more accurate to state that the need for identification 'full stop' was the starting point. It may be recalled from Chapters 1 and 2 that Bertillon's Anthropometry, which for a time was widely adopted, preceded fingerprints. Nevertheless, this acceptance that fingerprint examination was a starting point may explain Kirk's choice of individualisation as the aim of forensic science. Fingerprint examiners at that time, and ever since, have claimed individualisation – identity to the exclusion of all others. This claim, now considered to lack cogency, may have provided the basis for Kirk's fundamental principle of individualisation. As mentioned often in his book, there is no scientific or logical bias for this claim. It seems to have been considered a self-evident truth, accepted without challenge.

And so it was that Kirk's assertion that forensic science was the science of individualisation went unchallenged for over two decades. It was not until the advent of DNA evidence, the subject of Chapter 4, which engaged statisticians in forensic science, that the principle of individualisation began to be questioned.

Interestingly, just as DNA analysis sounded the death knell for individualisation, it simultaneously advanced the cause of probabilistic interpretation, one developmental aim recorded by Kirk in his paper.

Why did this logical fallacy originally take root, and when did it finally fall?

Take Root

As Kirk asserts, forensic science had its origins in law enforcement, which was certainly the case in common law jurisdictions such as those of the United States. What is understood today as forensic science was sometimes called 'police science' and forensic science laboratories 'police laboratories'.

In feature comparison disciplines, such as fingerprint examination, there is no need for any scientific knowledge or training to compare one fingerprint to another, and so the discipline could develop in the absence of an underpinning body of scientific knowledge based on scholarship and research. There was an absence of experimental support for the assertion of individualisation made by fingerprint examiners.

It seems to have been an immutable law that no two prints are identical. Fingerprints were thought to be unique to each individual and an infallible means of identification. These views remained unchallenged until the advent of DNA analysis, e.g. in 1982 (Odell 1982).

The Scottish Fingerprint Inquiry (Campbell 2011) is quite revealing about the non-scientific and fallacious logic of fingerprint examination, certainly in Scotland at the time (2009–2011). The inquiry records how examiners, during the progress of their examination, soon reach an '*inner conviction*' or a '*personal point of certainty*' regarding individualisation or a common unique source. Reverse or circular reasoning – comparing the reference print to the questioned print, and side-by-side comparison are also part of the process, each increasing the risk of cognitive bias as discussed in Chapter 8.

The logical reality is that as a proportion of the world's population, both current and past, very few fingerprints have been examined and so it may be that the fingerprints of two people may be sufficiently similar that a fingerprint examiner might conclude they have a common source, which would undermine, certainly in the case of fingerprints, the claim to individualisation. In addition, even if it were the case that the fingerprints of no two people can 'match', the false positives in the case of Brandon Mayfield and Shirley McKie (Cole 2016) demonstrate that unqualified conclusions regarding the source, that questioned and reference fingerprints are from the same person, are not justified. Fingerprints are not the infallible means of identification once claimed.

The Utility of Individualisation/Before the Challenge/the Heyday of Individualisation

As evidenced by Gross' Handbook, demonstrated by the career of Kirk and the establishment of the school of criminology at UCB for the training of police officers and as argued earlier, the Ontogeny of forensic science began in a law enforcement environment. Its purpose was to identify criminals by acquiring biometric data from criminals/prisoners, such as physical characteristics (Bertillon in 1883) or fingerprints (Francis Galton in 1892) for subsequent identification. So, this notion of 'identification' became central to the scientific investigation of crime, which, in common law jurisdictions such as those of the United States, was initially conducted by police, for the most part. Police officers are not prone to equivocation; among their fundamental beliefs is that a suspect charged with a crime is guilty. Police examiners, as many early forensic scientists were (and in many jurisdictions still are), tended to give their evidence firmly, and so the principle of individualisation probably suited the police mentality. The fingerprint on the knife was that of the accused, the bullet was fired from that gun, etc.

It was this early relationship with law enforcement that gave shape to early forensic science, as Kirk acknowledges and argued above. To be fair, it could not have happened in any other way, and for many decades, highly qualified and trained, through courses such as those at UCB, and experienced experts gave evidence of individualisation without challenge.

Juries found no issue with the claim by the fingerprint expert that the questioned and reference prints 'matched', and the questioned print could not be that of anyone other than the accused. The evidence was unequivocal, the jury was clear, and the justice system was satisfied. In addition, the expert did not have to enter the messy and untidy realms of statistics, probability and experiment.

Kirk's successors at UCB went on teaching and accepting that forensic science was the science of individualisation. Many examples have been given in support of the principle of individualisation, offering calculations that demonstrated, for example, the astronomically small probability of two persons having the same fingerprints.

The concept, having been born at UCB, was strongly supported and defended by Kirk's successors even in the light of the advances in DNA analysis and interpretation.

> *The concept of individualization is clearly central to the consideration of physical evidence .... Our belief that uniqueness is both attainable and existent is central to our work as forensic scientists.*
>
> *(Inman and Rudin 2001)*

Fall

The concept of individualisation came under pressure with the advent of DNA evidence in the late 1980s. The history, development and impact of this evidence type is the subject of Chapter 4. It was during this period that the world of science began to significantly interact with the interpretation of physical evidence. One of the last redoubts of individualisation was and remains fingerprint examination.

DNA was an evidence type unlike many of its predecessors. It was scientific in origin, required statistics for interpretation and conclusions were expressed probabilistically rather than categorically. A firearms examiner might conclude that the weapon in question was the murder weapon to the exclusion of every other firearm in the world, a categorical opinion of individualisation. In contrast, a DNA scientist, when reporting that, for example, the bloodstain at the scene was highly likely to be that of the suspect, would consider the likelihood that it was of someone other than the suspect. The probabilistic approach always accepts that a different source might exist and seeks to quantify that likelihood and take it into account when expressing an opinion. To this day, many fingerprint experts and firearm examiners make no such allowance (Edmond 2020).

As discussed earlier, up until the advent of DNA evidence, fingerprint evidence, and similar feature comparison evidence of individualisation had been accepted by courts almost without question, and the notion of individualisation was accepted by most forensic scientists. As detailed in Chapter 4, DNA evidence was immediately recognised for its power and therefore was initially subject to rigorous challenge, which included a demand that it demonstrate, as it were, its scientific credentials. This entailed providing experimental evidence that DNA evidence could be relied upon by courts in making decisions. One of the requirements for demonstrating reliability is 'validation', which means providing objective evidence of fitness for purpose. Validation will be discussed in more detail in Chapters 7 and 9. In terms of individualisation, the scrutiny to which this new DNA evidence was initially subjected was rigorous, and the obvious question arose: why have fingerprints and the other feature comparison evidence types not been subject to similar scrutiny?

> *The increased use of DNA analysis, which has undergone extensive validation, has thrown into relief the less firmly credentialed status of other forensic science identification techniques (fingerprints, fiber analysis, hair analysis, ballistics, bite marks, and tool marks). These have not undergone the type of extensive testing and verification that is the hallmark of science elsewhere.*
>
> *(Kennedy and Merrill 2003)*

Another aspect of the DNA attack against individualisation was its use by the Innocence Project (2023) to exonerate those whose wrongful conviction was in part based on these feature comparison evidence types.

The Aftermath

Kirk's role in the history of individualisation is explored in some detail by Simon Cole, recorded in his paper published in Law, Probability and Risk (Cole 2014). The paper asserts that Kirk's distinction between individualisation and identification was ambiguous and that ambiguity has not helped fingerprint examiners trying to find an alternative to individualisation, '*the print is that of the suspect to the exclusion of all others*'. Cole argues that, having accepted the weaknesses in the concept of individualisation, fingerprint examiners are attempting to find a rationale to support retaining the conclusion, to explain it in some other way, starting with the aim of retaining the term and trying to find support; to quote Cole.

> *It is difficult to avoid concluding that the common cause of the* [sic] *all of the semantic and conceptual difficulties outlined above is the backward process of starting with a historically embedded reporting term ('individualization') and making serial efforts to devise a defensible justification for that term.*

Fingerprint examiners are essentially trying to have their cake and eat it. They wish to continue to use the term and concept of 'individualisation' but accept the fact that it cannot mean '*the print is that of the suspect to the exclusion of all others*'. This seems to be pure sophistry in trying to maintain conflicting positions.

Cole's paper is a decade old, but the term 'individualisation' is still in use (NIST OSAC 2023). So, certainly, in the feature comparison disciplines, Kirk's legacy lives on. In some disciplines, forensic science remains the science of individualisation as claimed by Kirk in his Ontogeny paper.

The reactionary attitude of fingerprint examiners will be touched on again in Chapter 8 on Observer Effects and more fully explored in Chapter 9 on the 2009 NAS report.

The Generalist

Kirk must be credited with raising the possibility of a scientific generalist, similar to the roles of Gross and Locard, but operating in a common law jurisdiction. It was a role played by Kirk in his involvement in the investigation of crime, giving expert evidence on BPA and fibres, for example.

Kirk's seminal text 'Crime Investigation: Physical evidence and the police laboratory' (Kirk 1953) also calls for the education of forensic generalists, which chimes with the Sydney Declaration, the subject of Chapter 10.

The question today is, would a biochemist with expertise in analytical science be accepted as an expert in BPA and/or fibres? The answer by the authors of the Sydney Declaration would be: if the generalist was so trained and educated, then – yes! The follow-up question would be, but how has competence been demonstrated?

Another possible weakness in the role of the generalist is exposure to potentially biasing information during the investigative phase of the forensic science process. Cognitive bias is discussed in Chapter 8. The investigative phase includes the recognition and recovery of evidence and the generation of explanations. Cognitive bias, Gross's '*pre-conceived theories*', risks sending the investigation in the wrong direction.

When the forensic science generalist works hand in glove with the police, the risk is that the forensic scientists will see their role as supporting the police and prosecuting authorities in their tasks of identifying a prime suspect, gathering evidence against that suspect and securing a conviction. This issue is also discussed in Chapter 10 on the Sydney Declaration.

Current good practice is to shield the examining scientist from any information that is not directly relevant to the examination. For example, a fingerprint examiner should not be informed that the firearm being examined is registered to the suspect or that the suspect's DNA has been found on it.

One model that could accommodate a generalist and a shielded examining scientist is one based on Case Assessment and Interpretation (CAI), which is discussed at length in Chapter 8.

The Search for Fundamental Principles

Kirk's Ontogeny paper recorded the need for fundamental, theoretical and permanent principles to form the basis of forensic science. The lack of basic theory was a '*serious deficiency*'. This is a deficiency that some claim remains to this day, and judging by the Sydney Declaration, the statement of this requirement is probably Kirk's most significant contribution to the ongoing debate as to what forensic science is. Good philosophers do not provide answers but ask the right questions. In the Ontogeny paper, Kirk certainly asks some good questions.

Contribution to Current Practice

Several items on Kirk's developmental agenda are now part of current practice, some through the adoption of and conformance to quality standards. Two of the most important standards are ISO/IEC 17025 for laboratory activities, mentioned earlier and is the subject of Chapter 7, and ISO/IEC 17020, which applies to crime scene activities. Conformance requires staff to be competent. Their education and training must be specified, as well as the necessary competencies for doing the job, which would include abiding by a code of conduct. As reported earlier, for an independent assessment of competence, some certification bodies have gained accreditation to ISO/IEC 17024 for evaluating and certifying the competence of the individual.

Another item on Kirk's agenda is adopting a probabilistic approach to interpretation. This has now been refined to the likelihood ratio approach, which is the subject of Chapter 6 on interpretation.

Other items on the agenda relate to research and would only impact current practice on fruition. However, it is fair to state that any advances through research would be mostly discipline-specific and lead to incremental improvements in factors such as speed/turnaround time, sensitivity – getting more information from less material, or cost reduction.

The Sydney Declaration responds to Kirk's call for the elucidation of fundamental principles. If the model presented by the authors of that publication is ever adopted, then that would have a profound effect on practice. However, as will be discussed, implementing that model may be an uphill struggle.

Concluding Remarks

In his Ontogeny paper, Kirk recognised some of the fundamental issues in forensic science, principally the questions of what it is and what its purpose is.

He argued that forensic science is the science of individualisation, attributing an item of evidence, such as a fingerprint, to a unique source to the exclusion of all other sources.

Kirk's concept of individualisation is either dead or at least on its last legs, fatally wounded by the advent of DNA analysis (Chapter 4), the 2009 NAS Report (Chapter 9) and subsequent scholarship (Saks and Koehler 2008; Cole 2014; Champod 2015; Evett 2015). However, by starting the debate, Kirk's Ontogeny paper has led inexorably to a better understanding of the strengths and weaknesses of forensic science and scientific evidence and consequently the reliability of that evidence.

Despite overwhelming and compelling scholarship to the contrary, it is unfortunate that even in papers published more recently, the fallacious myth of individualisation still finds resonance. Some authors still accept without question the concept of individualisation (Chen et al. 2022; Gomes et al. 2023). This is perhaps more a symptom of one of the main weaknesses of forensic science identified by Kirk, its disparate nature. This results in interdisciplinary blindness and ignorance and a lack of awareness; to put it colloquially, the left hand does not know what the right hand is doing.

Having suggested the origins of forensic science lay in fingerprint examination, Kirk went on to set an agenda for the development of forensic science, with hindsight a remarkable example of forward-thinking. Among the requirements are the need for validation, regulation and the probabilistic interpretation of evidence. Unfortunately, the development of forensic science has been driven, in part, by the need to respond to continuing miscarriages of justice.

The issue of terminological ambiguity is raised in the paper. However, until recently, there has been little progress on that front. What has been revealed is the need for a precise, common vocabulary easily understood by non-scientific criminal justice system stakeholders, particularly lawyers, judges and jury members. A standard vocabulary is still some way off.

Despite Kirk's musings in his paper, no 'Einstein' or 'Newton' of forensic science has emerged as an 'architect'. This may support the view that forensic science is not a single science but a syncretic activity.

Nevertheless, there have been some important contributors. In addition to all the authors of the publications selected for this book, there are major figures in certain disciplines; in interpretation, Ian Evett CBE (Principal Forensic Services, England), John Buckleton

(ESR, New Zealand), Colin Aitkin (Professor at Edinburgh University, Scotland) and Franco Taroni (Professor at the University of Lausanne, Switzerland). In addition to Sir Alec Jeffreys CH FRS (Emeritus Professor, Leicester University) in DNA, should be added Peter Gill (Professor at Oslo University Hospital, Norway) and John Butler (NIST, United States), with Suzanne Bell (Emeritus Professor at West Virginia University, United States) in analytical science. This is very far from an exhaustive list, and apologies to the many unnamed contributors to the development of forensic science.

Before leaving the subject of architects, a strong case could be made that Hans Gross, the designated father of so many offspring, is the 'Einstein' of forensic science and the principles and practices he introduced are the fundamentals of forensic science. These include applying the scientific method to the investigation of crime, documenting scene procedures, which are still in use today, and keeping an open mind, unsullied by preconceived theories.

With the rejection of forensic science as the science of individualisation so eloquently argued by Kirk in his paper, his aim to find the '*simple, brief and to the point*' fundamental laws of forensic science is yet to be realised. This topic will be taken up again in Chapter 10 on the Sydney Declaration.

Key Takeaways

The Ontogeny paper.

- Is now considered a landmark publication in forensic science.
- Uses the term 'criminalistics' to mean the application of the natural sciences to the recognition and examination of physical evidence.
- Defines forensic science as the science of individualisation, which is no longer accepted.
- Calls for the fundamental principles of forensic science to be elucidated.
- Argues that forensic science is both a science and a profession.
- Initiates the debate as to what forensic science is, while that is in doubt, Kirk argues that development will be hindered.
- Identifies the requirement for a common vocabulary understood by all stakeholders.
- Sets out a developmental agenda which has largely been completed.
- Is a continuing reference point for debates regarding the fundamental principles of forensic science (Buzzini 2024), which may be the most enduring legacy of the Ontogeny paper.

Notes

1 Strictly, the marks in question are the friction ridges on the inside of the tip of a finger, thumb or toe.

2 This book is a must-read for forensic science students.

3 Criminology is simply defined as the study of all matters related to crime. Criminology and its relationship with criminalistics and forensic science are discussed in the section on Terms Definitions and Explanations, that relationship is also discussed in Chapter 10 on the Sydney Declaration. Criminalistics didn't emerge until the 1940s.
4 A microgram is one millionth of a gram or one thousand-millionth of a kilogram.
5 The so-called Frisch-Peierls memorandum which essentially sparked the Manhattan Project.
6 Also called blood spatter, the distribution of a victim's blood following a violent attack.
7 Given that Kirk's exclusion from membership of the AAFS was based on work for the defence, it would be of interest to note how many Kirk awards have been given for a body of case works mostly devoted to exposing wrongful convictions.
8 A nanogram is one billionth (10^{-9}) of a gram.
9 Many jurisdictions have codes of conduct and practice directions, which bind forensic scientists.
10 Significant progress has been made in this area with the introduction of the likelihood ratio approach to interpretation.
11 The science of the trace, the trace being a remnant of an earlier activity.
12 Using statistical and biological models to generate virtual DNA profiles of individual contributors from mixed and degraded DNA.
13 Sometimes termed a code of conduct or practice.

Bibliography

Affidavit of Paul Leeland Kirk. 1955. 64571 (1954–1955 Post-Trial Motions and Ohio Eighth District Court of Appeal. 10, 26 April).

Broome, Sharon and Clifford Todd. 2012. "The Management of Casework within the United Kingdom Forensic Explosives Laboratory." In *Forensic Investigation of Explosions. Second Edition*, edited by Alexander Beveridge, 159–195. Boca Raton, FL: CRC Press.

Buzzini, Patrick. 2024. "Kirk's 'Ontogeny of Criminalistics' revisited under the lens of the Sydney Declaration." *Forensic Science International* 359: 112023.

CAC. 2015. "Code of Ethics." *California Association of Criminalists*. 2015 September. Accessed September 26, 2024. https://www.cacnews.org/membership/California-Association-of-Criminalists-Code-of-Ethics-09-23-2015.pdf.

California Association of Criminalists. 2024. *Criminalistics Information*. Accessed September 20, 2024. https://www.cacnews.org/membership/criminalistics.shtml.

—. 2024. *Paul Kirk and President's Award*. Accessed September 21, 2024. https://www.cacnews.org/awards/paulkirk.shtml#:~:text=The%20award%20is%20granted%20in,recipient%20of%20the%20Presidents%20Award.

Campbell, Anthony. 2011. *The Fingerprint Inquiry Report*. Edinburgh: APS Group Scotland.

Champod, Christophe. 2015. "Fingerprint Identification: Advances Since the 2009 National Research Council Report." *Philosophical Transactions of the Royal Society B* 370: 1–10.

Chen, Hongyu, Rongliang Ma, and Meigin Zhang. 2022. "Recent Progress in Visualization and Analysis of Fingerprint Level 3 Features." *Open Chemistry* 11 (e202200091): 1–19.

Chisum, Jerry W., and Brent E. Turvey. 2006. "A History of Crime Reconstruction." In *Crime Reconstruction*, edited by Jerry W. Chisum and Brent E. Turvey, 28–33. London: Elsevier Science.

Chisum, W. Jerry, and Brent E. Turvey. 2011. "A History of Crime Reconstruction." In *Crime Reconstruction, Second Edition*, edited by W. Jerry Chisum and Brent E. Turvey. Waltham, MA: Elsevier.

Cleveland State University. 2024. "1954–1955 Post-Trial Motions and Ohio Eighth District Court of Appeal." Accessed October 9, 2023. https://engagedscholarship.csuohio.edu/sheppard_eight_district-1950s/10.

Cleveland State University. 2024. *Engaged Scholarship @ Cleveland State University*. Accessed October 4, 2024. https://engagedscholarship.csuohio.edu/kirk_photos/.

Cole, Simon A. 2014. "Individualization is Dead, Long Live Individualization! Reforms of Reporting Practices for Fingerprint Analysis in the United States." *Law, Probability and Risk* 13: 117–50.

Cole, Simon A. 2016. "Scandal, Fraud, and the Reform of Forensic Science: The Case of Fingerprint Analysis." *West Virginia Law Review* 119 (2): 523–48.

De Forest, P., H. Lee, and R. Gaensslen. 1983. *Forensic Science: An Introduction to Criminalistics*. New York: McGraw Hill.

Doyle, Sean. 2019. "A United Kingdom Register." In *Quality Management in Forensic Science*, edited by Sean Doyle, 164–67. London: Academic Press.

E.L. 1910. "Reviewed Work(s): Criminal Investigation: A Practical Handbook for Magistrates, Police Officers and Lawyers by Hans Gross, John Adam and J. Collyer Adam." *Journal of the American Institute of Criminal Law and Criminology* 1: 156–57.

Edmond, Gary. 2020. "Fingerprint Evidence in New Zealand's Courts: The Oversight of Overstatement." *New Zealand Universities Law Review* 29: 1–24.

Evett, Ian. 2015. "The Logical Foundations of Forensic Science: Towards Reliable Knowledge." *Philosophical Transactions of the Royal Society B* 370: 1–10.

Forensic Specialties Accreditation Board. 2024. *Conformity Assessment*. Accessed July 18, 2024. https://thefsab.org/cabs/.

Fraser, Jim. 2020a. *Forensic Science: A Very Short Introduction. Second Edition*. Oxford: Oxford University Press.

Fraser, Jim. 2020b. "Preface and Acknowledgements to Second Edition." In *Forensic Science: A Very Short Introduction*, edited by Jim Fraser, xviii. Oxford: Oxford University Press.

Gomes, Francisco M., Claudio Martin Pereira de Pereira, Kristiane de Cassia Mariotti, Thieres Magaiver Pereira, Nayara Araujo dos Santos, and Wanderson Romao. 2023. "Study of Latent Fingerprints – A Review." *Forensic Chemistry* 35: 100525.

Gross, Hans. 1918. *Criminal Psychology – A Manual for Judges, Practitioners and Students*. First English. Translated by Horace M. Kallen. Boston: Little, Brown, and Company.

Hotcoursesabroad. 2024. *401 Universities Offering Forensic Science*. Accessed September 26, 2024. https://www.hotcoursesabroad.com/study/training-degrees/international/forensic-science-courses/cgory/b18-3/sin/ct/page/5/programs.html.

Icove, David J., and Gerald A. Haynes. 2017. *Kirk's Fire Investigation, Eighth Edition*. Pearson.

Inman, Kieth, and Nora Rudin. 2001. *Principles and Practice of Criminalistics: The Profession of Forensic Science (Protocols in Forensic Science)*. Boca Raton: CRC Press.

International Association for Identification. 2011. *The Report of the International Association for Identification, Standardization II Committee.* National Criminal Justice Reference Service (NCJRS).

Kell, Gretchen. 2017. "August Vollmer Biography Explores Famous Police Chief's UC Berkeley Ties." *Berkeley News*, 19 April.

Kennedy, Donald, and Richard A. Merrill. 2003. "Assessing Forensic Science." *Issues in Science and Technology* 20 (1): 33.

Kirk, Paul L. 1947. "Standardization of Criminological Nomenclature." *Journal of Criminal Law and Criminology* 38 (2): 165–67.

Kirk, Paul L. 1950. *Quantitative Ultramicroanalysis.* New York: John Wiley & Sons.

Kirk, Paul L., and Lowell W. Bradford. 1965. *The Crime Laboratory: Organization and Management.* Thomas.

Kirk, Paul Leland. 1953. *Crime Investigation: Physical Evidence and the Police Laboratory.* New York: Interscience.

—. 1950. *Quantitative Ultramicroanalysis.* New York: John Wiley and Sons.

Margot, Pierre. 2017. "Traceology, the Bedrock of Forensic Science and Its Associated Semantics." In *The Routledge International Handbook of Forensic Intelligence and Criminology*, edited by Quentin Rossy, David Décary-Hétu, Olivier Delémont and Massimiliano Mulone. London: Routledge.

NIST OSAC. 2023. "OSAC Lexicon." *The Organization of Scientific Area Committees for Forensic Science.* 12 June. Accessed May 8, 2024. https://www.nist.gov/glossary/osac-lexicon.

Odell, Robin. 1982. "Fingerprints." In *Science Against Crime*, edited by Russell Stockdale, 114. London: Marshal Cavendish.

OSAC. 2024. "OSAC Lexicon." *NIST OSAC.* Accessed July 17, 2024. https://www.nist.gov/glossary/osac-lexicon.

Rhodes, Richard. 2012. *The Making of the Atomic Bomb.* Simon & Schuster.

Saks, Michael J., and Jonathan J. Koehler. 2008. "The Individualization Fallacy in Forensic Science Evidence." *Vanderbilt Law Review* 61: 199–219.

Semantic Scholar. 2024. *The Ontogeny of Criminalistics.* Accessed September 26, 2024. https://www.semanticscholar.org/paper/The-Ontogeny-of-Criminalistics-Kirk/c80575ce3a0c67ac288cfd220a477a2be9e7ce5b#citing-papers.

The Innocence Project. 2023. *The Innocence Project.* Accessed October 19, 2023. https://innocenceproject.org/.

Wilson, Philip K. 2024. *Eugenics.* 26 August. Accessed September 21, 2024. https://www.britannica.com/science/eugenics-genetics.

4

DNA 'Fingerprinting' – Putting the Science in Forensic Science

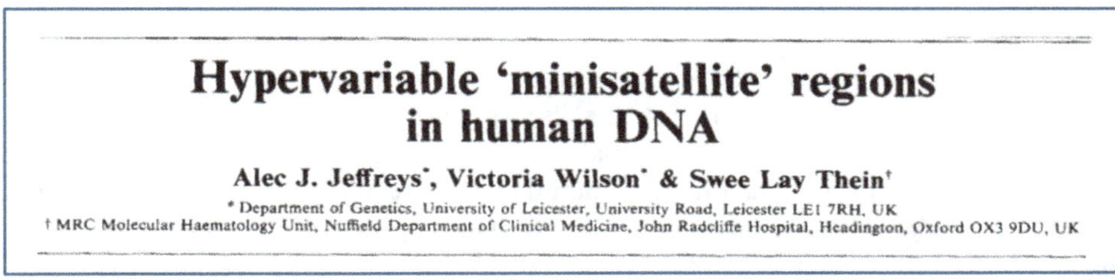

Hypervariable 'minisatellite' regions in human DNA

Alec J. Jeffreys*, Victoria Wilson* & Swee Lay Thein†

* Department of Genetics, University of Leicester, University Road, Leicester LE1 7RH, UK
† MRC Molecular Haematology Unit, Nuffield Department of Clinical Medicine, John Radcliffe Hospital, Headington, Oxford OX3 9DU, UK

Image 4.1 The header of the publication.

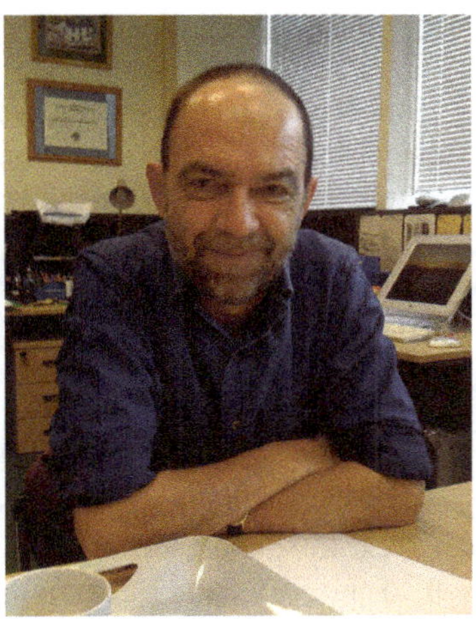

Image 4.2 Sir Alec Jeffreys. Jane Gitschier/Wikimedia Commons/CC BY 2.5.

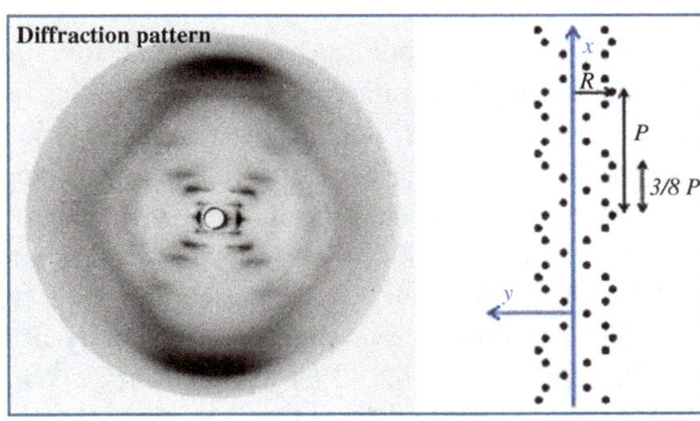

Image 4.3 Photo 51. Raymond Gosling/Wikimedia Commons/Public Domain.

A History of Forensic Science in 10 Publications: How They Established Current Practice, First Edition.
Sean Doyle.

Name of the Publication

The publication is titled *Hypervariable 'minisatellite' regions in human DNA*. It was jointly authored by Alec Jeffreys and his colleague Victoria Wilson, then at the University of Leicester's Department of Genetics, together with Swee Lay Thein at the Medical Research Council's Molecular Haematology Unit, John Radcliffe Hospital, Oxford.

The paper was published in the prestigious journal Nature in March 1985 (Jeffreys et al. 1985) and is just seven pages in length.

According to Semantic Scholar, the paper has been cited 3598 times, including 164 highly influential citations. According to ResearchGate, it has 3802 citations.

Introduction

In simple terms, the publication reports the discovery of repeated sequences of DNA code, which vary in number between individuals and how such variation might be exploited to identify individuals and shed light on familial relationships. This novel and scientific means of identifying individuals profoundly affected forensic science, as recorded in this chapter. Indeed, the effect of DNA analysis on the development of forensic science is a major theme running through this book.

The Science

Before introducing the publication, some understanding of the underlying science is necessary. The paper is highly technical, and a detailed understanding is only accessible to a molecular geneticist. Nevertheless, with an introduction to some of the scientific terms and concepts, the general reader will gain a better understanding and appreciate the significance of this publication. There should still be sufficient technical detail to satisfy the more scientific reader.

The structure of the DNA (deoxyribonucleic acid) was first elucidated by James D. Watson (1928–) and Francis Crick OM FRS (1916–2004) at Cambridge University in 1953 'standing on the shoulders' of many others including the crystallographers Rosalind Franklin (1920–1958) and Maurice Wilkins CBE FRS (1916–2004) both at King's College London (Pray 2008). Watson, Crick and Wilkins were awarded the Nobel Prize for Physiology or Medicine in 1962 for elucidating DNA's structure, controversially without mention of Franklin's contribution. Sadly, Franklin had died in 1958. Rosalind's now-famous Photo 51, demonstrating the helical nature of the DNA molecule, is shown in Image 4.3.

The structure of the molecule is a double helix and is most simply thought of as a twisted ladder, as depicted in Figure 4.1. The frame of the ladder is formed by sugar and phosphate (PO_4) molecules. The rungs of the ladder hold the so-called genetic code, the four chemical bases adenine (A), guanine (G), cytosine (C) and thymine (T).

To understand the processes that follow, it is not necessary to remember the names of the bases, just the abbreviating letters: A, C, G and T. The bases that form the rungs of the ladder are held together by weak chemical bonds called hydrogen bonds. The weakness

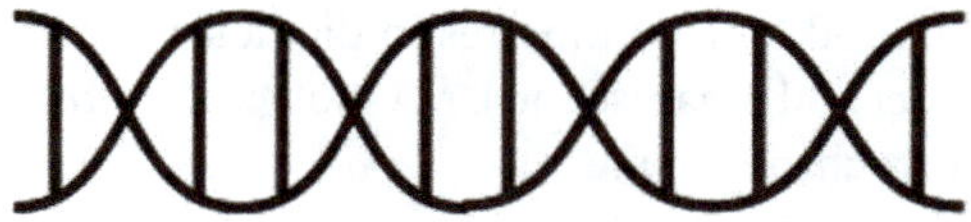

Figure 4.1 The twisted ladder or double helix.

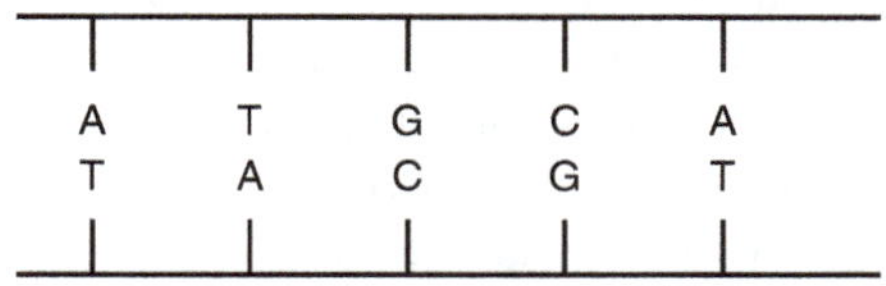

Figure 4.2 The rungs of the ladder and the complementary base pairing.

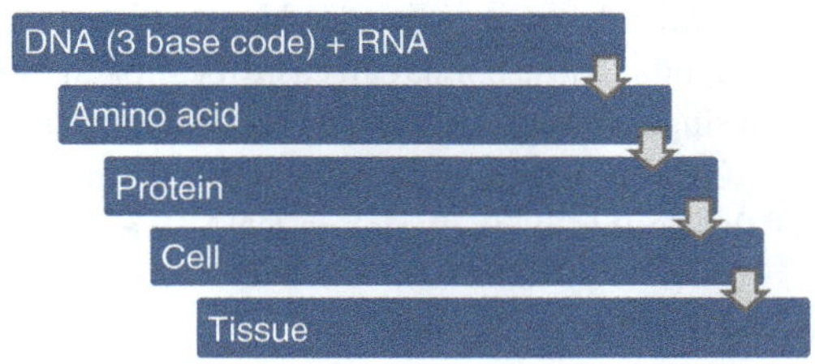

Figure 4.3 Steps in making tissue.

of these bonds enables one strand of the double helix to be easily separated from the other. In DNA analysis, this is achieved simply by heating. Because of the shape and size of the bases, only C and G fit together, as do A and T. This is known as the complementary base pairing of the DNA molecule. This complementarity, A with T and G with C, is the property of the DNA molecule that facilitates analysis. These properties are depicted in Figure 4.2.

Most cells in the human body have DNA in two locations, the nucleus of the cell and the mitochondria. The mitochondria are the parts of the cell that generate the energy the cell needs to function. While the DNA in the mitochondria has forensic utility[1], this chapter will focus on the DNA in the nucleus. The DNA in the nucleus is inherited from both mum and dad, the biological parents.

Most living things, including human beings, are generally composed of proteins of different types. Proteins make up tissues such as hair, nails, muscle, etc., and, in turn, organs such as skin and lungs. Proteins are made up of smaller molecules known as amino acids.

Returning to the bases, A, T and C, G; a sequence of these bases will code for a particular amino acid. The code will be transferred by RNA (ribonucleic acid) to another part of the cell called a ribosome, where proteins are assembled out of the amino acids. Thus, DNA is a molecular blueprint for a living thing. The DNA code is effectively an instruction to build proteins. These steps are represented in Figure 4.3.

Terminology

The DNA molecule inside the nucleus is very long, about 2 metres. It is wrapped around proteins to form chromosomes to enable it to be packed into a cell nucleus, which is around 0.01 millimetres in diameter (about 100 000 times smaller). Chromosomes compact and organise the DNA molecule within the cell nucleus. Figure 4.4 is a representation of a chromosome.

It is important now to think of chromosomes as packets or units containing DNA. In the nucleus of a human cell, there are 46 chromosomes in 23 pairs, one of which determines sex, as shown in Figure 4.5. One of each pair is either from Mum or Dad.

Another term to introduce is locus (plural loci)[2]. A locus is a specific location on a chromosome where there is a particular sequence of bases on the DNA molecule.

In the analysis of DNA, other terms encountered are probe and locus probe. A probe comprises a short sequence of bases from a single strand of the DNA molecule, which targets a complementary sequence at a specific location or locus on another DNA molecule. So, if the target is, say, A-A-C-T-T, then the probe will be T-T-G-A-A. It should be recalled that the rungs (A-T and G-C) of the twisted ladder that is the DNA molecule are held together by weak hydrogen bonds. Those bonds can easily be broken by heating, and the DNA molecule then 'unzips' into single strands, which enables the probe to find the target sequence.

To repeat, the genetic code is the sequence of the bases, A, T, C and G on each strand of the double helix, which is DNA. We get half our DNA from mum and half from dad.

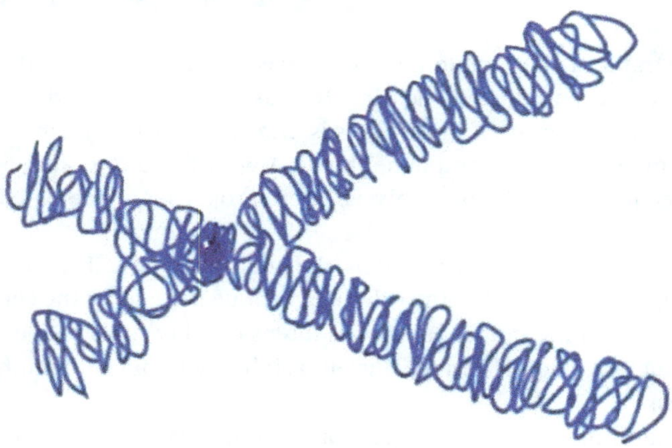

Figure 4.4 A chromosome, a packet of DNA.

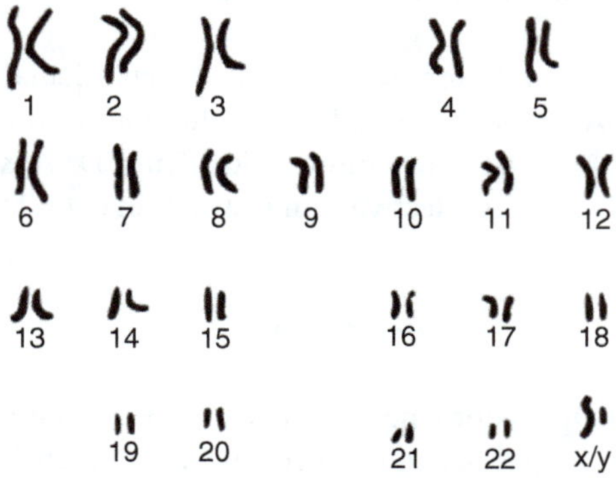

Figure 4.5 23 pairs of chromosomes, the x/y determining sex. Mikael Häggström/Wikimedia Commons/Public Domain.

Chromosomes are how DNA is packaged and organised within the cell's nucleus. A locus is a specific location on the chromosome with a particular sequence of bases.

Another term in this limited vocabulary is allele. An allele (or allelomorph) is a variant of the sequence of bases at a particular location, or locus, on a DNA molecule. In DNA analysis, it is only the variation in the number of repeated sequences at the selected locus that is of interest. Normally, there will be two alleles at each locus of interest, one from the mother and another from the father.

The final term to be familiar with is genome. The human genome is a complete set of genetic information in human cells, encoded as DNA within the 23 chromosome pairs in cell nuclei and in a small DNA molecule found within individual mitochondria. These are usually treated separately as the nuclear genome and the mitochondrial genome.

As humans, we share over 99% of our DNA, with most of us having two eyes, feet, hands, and so on. However, Jeffreys began to focus on those parts of the DNA molecule that differ from person to person – the unique genetic code of an individual.

The Publication

Turning now to the publication itself, the text of the abstract is as follows.

> *The human genome contains many dispersed tandem-repetitive 'minisatellite' regions detected via a shared 10–15-base pair 'core' sequence similar to the generalized recombination signal (χ)* [chi] *of Escherichia coli. Many minisatellites are highly polymorphic due to allelic variation in repeat copy number in the minisatellite. A probe based on a tandem-repeat of the core sequence can detect many highly variable loci simultaneously and can provide an individual-specific DNA 'fingerprint' of general use in human genetic analysis.*

The final sentence being the most important, a means has been found of identifying persons with a very high degree of certainty.

As mentioned earlier, the paper was published in 1985 in the journal Nature, one of the world's most widely read and prestigious academic journals, which only publishes work of very high impact and quality. The paper is extremely technical and only fully intelligible to experts in the field of molecular genetics. It built on the research by Alec Jeffreys into the protein myoglobin and its gene, i.e. the sequence of bases in the DNA molecule that codes for that protein. Myoglobin plays a role in the transport of oxygen in the muscles of mammals.

The paper reports the discovery of repeat units of base sequences, which vary in number from individual to individual. The fact that they can take different forms between individuals means they are polymorphic. These repetitive sequences are called in the paper 'minisatellite' regions and the repeats 'tandem-repeats'. The marked degree of variation between individuals is termed 'hypervariable'. The paper reports that the previously isolated/discovered minisatellite probe from myoglobin was found to be capable of detecting other minisatellites, some of which were highly variable – the paper concludes that this is a '*powerful probe*' for highly variable regions of the DNA molecule. As discussed earlier, a probe comprises a sequence of bases that would detect a complementary target sequence or core unit. Core sequences are usually 10–15 bases in length. Other probes were developed, and the paper goes on to demonstrate the power of DNA 'fingerprinting' as a means of paternity/maternity testing and individual identification.

In summary, Jeffreys and his co-workers discovered the variability in these repeated sequences of bases by accident and then put together probes to detect those sequences. He then found that the number of repeat units could vary significantly between unrelated individuals but not between related individuals. These repeat sequences and their variation in number between unrelated individuals are the basis for DNA 'fingerprinting' and indeed later DNA analysis.

Alec Jeffreys' ground-breaking discovery initiated the forensic exploitation of the DNA molecule, which continues to this day.

Jeffreys' motivation was a combination of academic ambition, a desire to learn more about how the DNA molecule might store information and generate new knowledge. He was specifically looking for genetic markers that might find application in medicine. As Jeffreys himself says, the discovery of DNA fingerprinting was the result of '*messing about in the lab*'.

Later that year, Alec Jeffreys, together with Peter Gill and Dave Werrett at the Central Research Establishment of the Forensic Science Service (FSS) in Reading, England, published a joint paper in Nature (Gill et al. 1985). The FSS was then part of the UK Home Office, the Government department responsible for the police. The paper, titled 'Forensic application of DNA "fingerprints"', highlighted Jeffreys' method of identification, particularly in cases of alleged sexual assault, and demonstrated the stability of the DNA molecule over long periods. The abstract concludes with the following claim.

> *It is envisaged that DNA fingerprinting will revolutionize forensic biology, particularly with regard to the identification of rape suspects.*

In his research, Jeffreys postulated and then found a sequence of bases that repeated variously between unrelated individuals. He originally called this repeating sequence, such as -ACTGCAACTT-ACTGCAACTT-ACTGCAACTT-ACTGCAACTT-, a 'stutter'[3], given the name 'minisatellite' in the paper and elsewhere named 'variable nucleotide tandem repeats', abbreviated as VNTR. These repeated sequences vary in number, such that one individual might have ten repeats, or $[ACTGCAACTT]_{10}$, and another, say, forty $[ACTGCAACTT]_{40}$. Therefore, the number of repeats might be used to distinguish one person from another[4].

Now, to better understand the phenomenon of stutter, Jeffreys needed to cut DNA up into segments for closer study. This proved to be a challenge overcome by using restriction enzymes, molecular scissors. Restriction enzymes are proteins that recognise specific sequences of bases along the DNA molecule and cut the molecule at the beginning and end of the repeated sequences, essentially targeting and separating those sequences. This resulted in varying lengths of DNA fragments specific to an individual. The fact that the DNA was cut into fragments of different lengths according to the number of repeat units by restriction enzymes gave the name to Jeffreys' method of Restriction Fragment Length Polymorphism, abbreviated as RFLP[5].

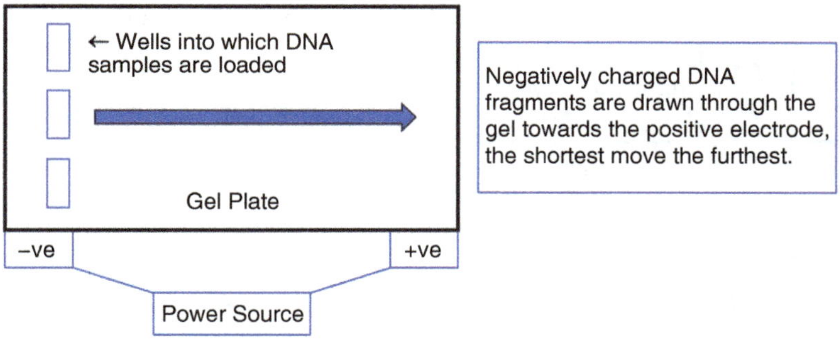

Figure 4.6 Gel electrophoresis apparatus from above.

The DNA fragments were then separated according to size using a technique known as gel electrophoresis. DNA samples are loaded into wells or indentations at one end of a gel plate, and an electric current is applied. The DNA fragments are negatively charged and so move through the gel towards the positive electrode, with shorter fragments moving faster and further than longer ones, as depicted in Figure 4.6.

The separated DNA fragments were then transferred from the gel to a material membrane using a technique known as Southern Blotting, involving direct contact. A radioactive probe was then introduced to bind to the repeat sequences. As mentioned earlier, a probe is a short segment of DNA that can be used to help find and bind to specific sequences of bases in a DNA molecule.

The membrane was then exposed to an X-ray film in a process known as autoradiography. The radioactive probes created dark bands on the film corresponding to the position of the separated repeat units. The pattern of the bands, resembling a barcode, is unique to everyone. This was a person's DNA 'fingerprint'. The RFLP workflow is set out in Figure 4.7, and the autoradiography results showing the visualised bands are depicted in Figure 4.8.

In September 1984, Jeffreys took a DNA sample from one of his lab technicians and placed it alongside DNA from her mother and father as well as the DNA from a tobacco plant, a cow and a seal.

What he found was that the probe had bound to all the stutter sequences that had a similar sequence. This resulted in a pattern of dark bands that was unique to the individual. The technician also shared parts of her pattern with her mother and father, showing that they were related.

It was by using this probe that Jeffreys finally had his eureka moment at 9:05 a.m. on 10 September 1984.

In contrast, the tobacco, cow and seal all had completely different patterns, demonstrating the applicability of DNA 'fingerprinting' in wildlife and environmental forensics.

Jeffreys, therefore, had developed a technology of identification by comparing the number of repeat units in sections of an individual's DNA with the number of repeats in a DNA sample.

Forensic science, with its primary aim of identification, particularly of criminals, quickly recognised the potential of DNA 'fingerprinting' in the investigation of crime and rapidly exploited it.

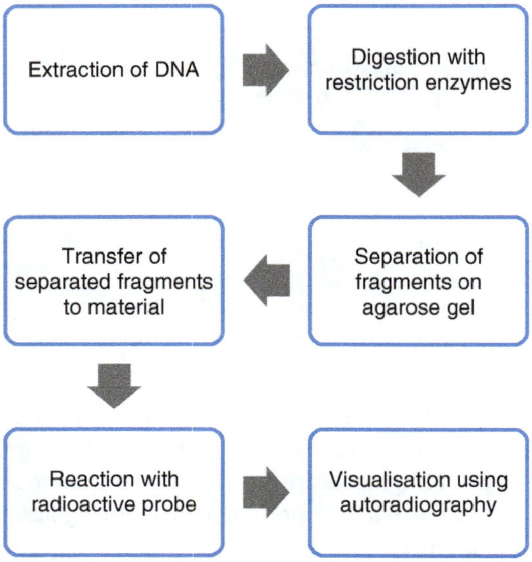

Figure 4.7 The RFLP workflow.

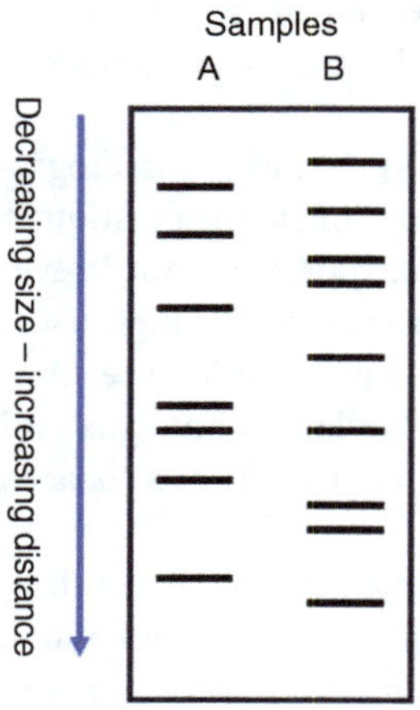

Figure 4.8 Representation of an autoradiograph showing a typical barcode DNA 'fingerprint'.

Biography of the Publication

The genesis of the paper is a product of the serendipitous scientific journey of Jeffreys. Sir Alec Jeffreys (as he now is) was born into an inventive and curious family. He became disillusioned with biochemistry at Merton College, Oxford, and changed his focus to genetics for his doctoral studies. Another stage in Jeffreys' journey was his relationship with Dick (Richard) Flavell FRS (1945–)[6] at the University of Amsterdam, prompting another change in direction, or focus, from yeast to haemoglobin and its gene. Returning to England, Jeffreys was attracted by the academic freedom offered by Leicester University and having arrived with not much by way of resources, Jeffreys thought there was little point in following or addressing popular and therefore highly competitive lines of research in molecular genetics. He therefore decided to study variations, or polymorphisms, in the DNA molecule, having developed some tools to do so. The final steps were the discovery of highly variable stutters, or repetitive DNA sequences, and then how the number of repeats varied between individuals and immediately realising that DNA could be used for identifying individuals. This was a very surprising and unanticipated result given that human beings share over 99% of their DNA. As mentioned earlier, the original 'eureka' moment on the 10th of September 1984 was followed by refining the technology to produce better quality results, essentially a clearer autoradiogram, the bar code visualisation, and conducting other experiments to demonstrate the power of the technology to the extent that the technology was sufficiently developed for publication in Nature in March 1985.

Professional Biography of the Author

Sir Alec John Jeffreys, CH, FRS, MAE, has been described as an ordinary man who did an extraordinary thing. However, like many true giants, Jeffreys is a man of great humility and generosity and, as a Brit, a lover of understatement, e.g. describing his 'Eureka' moment as the product of '*messing around in the lab.*'

Unlike the previous authors who engaged with justice systems, Hans Gross, an examining magistrate, and Paul Kirk, a criminalist or forensic scientist, Jeffreys was a pure academic in fields unrelated to forensic science. He was at first a biochemist, then a molecular geneticist, planning and following a career in academia. He had no plan or motivation to develop technologies of forensic utility and certainly not DNA 'fingerprinting'. They were born from the pure search for new knowledge and, ironically, the constraint of limited resources. Although Jeffreys's discovery rapidly found forensic utility, that was a surprise to him. Often, the greatest of scientific discoveries wait years to find practical use, for example, laser light and microwave radiation, but not in the case of DNA 'fingerprinting'.

Sir Alec was born in Oxford, England, on the 9th of January 1950 into a family of inventors, acquiring the characteristics (through Mendelian inheritance?) of curiosity and inventiveness. Receiving a microscope and a chemistry set at a young age sparked his interest in biochemistry.

With the encouragement of a schoolteacher, he applied and won a scholarship to Merton College, a constituent college of the University of Oxford, England, where he followed a four-year biochemistry course and graduated in 1971–1972 with a first-class honours degree.

However, while studying biochemistry, he became interested in genetics and decided that would be his focus. In 1975, he completed his doctoral degree in genetics at Merton, his thesis titled 'Studies on the mitochondria of cultured mammalian cells' (1975). He was then awarded a European Molecular Biology Organization (EMBO) research fellowship (1975–1977) to work with Piet Borst CBE (1934–)[7] at the University of Amsterdam in the Netherlands to study yeast.

At Amsterdam, he met Dick (Ricard) Flavell, who was studying mammalian genes, specifically for the protein haemoglobin, which supplies oxygen to the muscles of vertebrates (animals with backbones)[8]. With Professor Flavell, Jeffreys developed a method for detecting the gene in humans. In simple terms, he had developed technologies that could unlock information stored by the DNA molecule.

Once that post-doctoral term ended, and with a desire to obtain an academic position back in the United Kingdom, Jeffreys applied to several UK universities. He was invited for an interview for the position of lecturer (temporary) at the University of Leicester, England, by the founder of the genetics department, Professor Robert (Bob) Hugh Pritchard (1930–2015). Realising the academic freedom he would be given at Leicester, he accepted the position. He addressed the question of whether inherited variation can be detected directly at the DNA level or, more simply, how information is stored within the DNA molecule. That began his study of variation in human DNA and eventually led him to stumble upon the stutters or minisatellites that would be the basis for DNA 'fingerprinting'.

The numerous awards and honours given to Professor Jeffreys included election to the Royal Society in 1986 (FRS), election to the Academia Europaea in 1989 (MAE), and a knighthood for services to science and technology in 1994 with the title 'Sir'. Sir Alec was made a Member of the Order of the Companions of Honour in 2017 (CH). He was also made a freeman of the City of Leicester in 1992–1993. Freeman is a position of medieval origin, then conferring certain rights, privileges and responsibilities, but it is now mostly honorific.

As an interesting aside, the Conservative government at the time had put up a famous footballer, Gary Lineker[9], a son of the City of Leicester, as a candidate for Freeman. Professor Bob Pritchard, a political activist in another party of a different political persuasion and very much involved in the government of the City, put up Jeffreys as a candidate (Liberal Democrat Voice 2015).

Sir Alec Jeffreys retired in September 2012 and continues his association with the University of Leicester as an Emeritus Professor.

Contexts

Scientific

Science is not like art, where only Van Gogh could have painted 'The Starry Night' or Beethoven composed 'Ode to Joy'. On the contrary, if Einstein had not derived the relationship between matter and energy as $E = mc^2$, some other physicists would have. Similarly, if Darwin had not developed a theory of evolution, someone else would. So, if Jeffreys had not invented DNA 'fingerprinting', it would have fallen to someone else. Nevertheless, those who first uncover new knowledge are deservedly lauded for their discoveries, particularly one as highly consequential as DNA 'fingerprinting'.

The early part of the twentieth century was perhaps the era of physics in which huge advances were made in science, admittedly on the back of the Second World War. Ironically, World War II was preceded by many German Jewish scientists fleeing the Third Reich and, among other things, contributing to the production of atomic bombs for the Allies.

The latter half of the century might be thought of as the era of biotechnology, including molecular biology and genetics. It could be argued that this era began in 1953 with the elucidation of the double-stranded, helical, complementary and antiparallel model for the DNA molecule by James D Watson and Francis Crick, building on the work of Maurice Wilkins, Rosalind Franklin and others.

As mentioned earlier, the contribution of Franklin initially went pretty-much unrecognised, a lack of recognition she shared with the physicist Lise Meitner (1878–1968), mentioned in Chapter 3 of the Handbook, who discovered nuclear fission, the splitting of the atom. These are two of the many 'forgotten women in science'.

Developments in the understanding of the DNA molecule in molecular biology made possible the study of molecular genetics, i.e. studying inheritance at the molecular level. The knowledge generated facilitated genetic engineering and an understanding of the genetic code of three bases coding for an amino acid, the building blocks of proteins, tissues and organs. Perhaps the most consequential advance was the sequencing of the entire human genome, completed in 2003, revealing genetic factors that affect human life, diseases and genetically related disorders.

Other notable advances were improving the efficiency of antibiotic and vaccine production. Examples of such advances include making antibiotic production more efficient through microbial fermentation and producing new vaccines for diseases through genetic engineering.

These advances at the time Jeffreys was finding his way gave him a sufficient understanding of the DNA molecule and the tools necessary for exploring how it might store information.

However, the particular contexts for Jeffreys' invention of DNA 'fingerprinting' were the tools he had developed to unlock information stored in the DNA molecule and the academic freedom he enjoyed at Leicester to pursue that exploration.

Historical

For this and the remaining publications, events are not yet 'over the historical horizon'; they have yet to move from memory to history. The author and readers will have directly experienced contemporaneous events, and it is difficult to bring a neutral or detached perspective to any assessment of potential historical impact. Major scientific questions have been broadly answered; we have a theory of evolution, a knowledge of quantum mechanics, cosmological models, theories of relativity, and an understanding of the information stored in the DNA molecule, the genetic code. What remains is an increasingly granular or 'in the weeds' research effort to uncover knowledge that is mostly beyond the comprehension of non-specialists. This knowledge will only reach the public domain if it finds practical application in everyday life.

Social

As with history, societal impacts on the development of 'DNA fingerprinting' were minimal. The granular detail of the research leading to the discovery of minisatellites/tandem repeats in trying to unlock the 'secrets' of the DNA molecule kept these matters away from society in general. In the case of DNA 'fingerprinting', the existence of tandem repeat units was discovered by accident. It is not society that in any way encouraged, facilitated or prompted the development of DNA 'fingerprinting', except perhaps in providing academic freedom in the search for new knowledge. In this, there is a very important lesson: academic freedom, in the sense of setting no boundaries to academic research, is essential for generating new and useful knowledge. Society did not affect DNA research, but the opposite; DNA analysis continues to have a profound and major effect on society, which is explored later in this Chapter and in the remainder of the book.

Structure of the Publication

The structure of the paper is as follows.

- Introduction
- Probe for variable human DNA
- Isolation of minisatellites
- Highly polymorphic minisatellites
- A χ [chi] sequence in minisatellites?
- Probe for hypervariable regions
- Pedigree analysis
- A new mutant allele
- Conclusions

As recorded earlier, the abstract is as follows.

> *The human genome contains many dispersed tandem-repetitive 'minisatellite' regions detected via a shared 10–15-base pair 'core' sequence similar to the generalized recombination signal* (χ) [Chi] *of Escherichia coli [a bacterium]. Many minisatellites are highly polymorphic due to allelic variation in repeat copy number in the minisatellite. A probe based on a tandem-repeat of the core sequence can detect many highly variable loci simultaneously and can provide an individual-specific DNA 'fingerprint' of general use in human genetic analysis.*

As already emphasised, the publication is highly technical and only fully accessible to a molecular biologist, i.e. experts in the field. Nevertheless, what follows should aid a general understanding of the various studies reported in the publication.

Introduction

There is an introduction setting the scene, as it were. The publication begins by asserting that most of the DNA molecule in humans does not vary much between individuals. Other authors claim that 99.9% of human DNA is in common. It then points to the need for and benefit of probes for highly variable regions of the DNA molecule. It reports the chance discovery of these highly variable regions. It then explains that the variable regions consist of tandem repeats, and the variation is in the number of repeat units. It calls these tandem repeats 'minisatellites'. It is worth emphasising that tandem repeat, minisatellite, and stutter are essentially synonymous. The variation in the number of repeat units can then be detected using the RFLP method explained earlier.

The introduction then refers to earlier work with the protein myoglobin and its gene, and that repeat sequence is capable of detecting minisatellites and could be used as the basis of a probe.

Probe for variable human DNA

This section reports the construction of a tandem-repetitive probe derived from a tandem-repetitive section of the human myoglobin gene. A probe relies on the complementary nature of the DNA molecule explained earlier, whereby A always binds to T and C to G, forming the 'rungs' of the 'twisted ladder'. Using this probe to detect sequences in DNA from a daughter, her mother and father demonstrated length variation of minisatellite regions.

Isolation of minisatellites

This short section describes the isolation of minisatellites, demonstrating that they contained an integral number of repeat units.

Highly polymorphic minisatellites

The DNA of 14 unrelated British 'Caucasians' was used to study more broadly the variability, or polymorphism, of minisatellites. Four of the eight minisatellites showed variation, and three a high degree of variation with between five and eight tandem repeat units per location. It was also found that the greater the number of repeat units, the longer the length of the segment of DNA, the more easily the probe could 'find' the required segment of DNA.

There follows the report of a study on the likely causes of the variability in the number of repeat units. The biology of mutations is particularly important in the study of cancer.

A χ [chi] sequence in minisatellites?

This section reports a study to determine which region(s) of the probe were detecting each minisatellite. The study suggests a model predicting that isolated core sequences may also be hotspots for initiating human chromosome recombination. These contain a core sequence resembling the chi sequence of the bacterium *Escherichia coli*, which is a binding site for recombination proteins. This study is essentially an attempt to explain biologically the variation in the number of repeat units.

Probe for hypervariable regions

This covers the selection of a probe capable of producing a DNA 'fingerprint'. The paper reports that the repeat length of each minisatellite region is usually half, the same or double the length of the probe from the human myoglobin gene. The consequence of this finding is that a probe consisting only of a tandem-repeated core sequence '*should be able to detect not only the human DNA fragments but additional minisatellites*'. This enabled the selection of a suitable repeated core probe. The complexity of the profile produced provides an individual-specific DNA 'fingerprint'.

Pedigree analysis

To establish that these variants are stably inherited, being passed from one generation to the next without confounding mutation, DNA was analysed from an extensive Asian–Indian pedigree of Gujarati origin, including 54 individuals from four generations.

Results showed that variation between individuals is so great that all individuals, even in a single sibship of a first cousin marriage, could be distinguished. In addition, that inheritance is Mendelian, i.e. traits are passed from one generation to the next. Each child has half of Mum's DNA and half of Dad's, providing a set of stably inherited genetic markers.

A new mutant allele

The discovery of a new mutation in a separate study is reported. This is a new allele (a variant DNA sequence) not from Mum or Dad. This enables a mutation rate to be predicted. The theory is that these variations in the number of repeat units are the product of changes in the DNA molecule from one generation to the next. This allows the biological processes that drive the instability to be studied. However, such mutations can cause difficulties in familial casework.

Conclusions

The publication concludes that a probe targeting a core sequence can be used for the simultaneous analysis/detection of multiple highly variable regions, or loci, of the DNA molecule. The paper predicts that the use of these DNA 'fingerprints' provides a powerful method for paternity and maternity testing and forensic applications, in addition to applications for the study of diseases.

Impact at the Time

The forensic exploitation of DNA 'fingerprinting' met with some early success and challenges. It did not take long for the forensic utility of this new means of identification to find practical application. Shortly after the first reports of DNA 'fingerprinting' appeared in the popular press, it was pressed into service.

A lawyer representing a party to a UK immigration dispute read about the discovery that DNA could be used to identify human beings and determine paternity/maternity. She approached Jeffreys for help. At the heart of the dispute was a contested mother–son relationship.

It should be recalled that half your DNA comes from Mum and half from Dad. However, in this case, the identity of the boy's father was unknown. To overcome this problem, advantage was taken of the fact that the DNA of biological siblings, i.e. those having the same mother and father, will collectively represent a wider scope of the parents' DNA. This allowed the DNA 'fingerprint' of the father to be reconstructed from the mother and the boy's siblings. The DNA results established that the boy in question was a member of that family. He was allowed to remain in the United Kingdom.

Perhaps the most famous early case was in the search for the perpetrator of the rape and murder of two teenage girls in Enderby, Leicestershire, England. Lynda Man was found dead on the 21st of November 1983, and Dawn Ashworth on the 31st of July 1986. There are numerous popular accounts of the investigation. However, regarding DNA, a suspect, Richard Buckland, had confessed to the second murder but denied murdering Lynda Man. The police turned to Jeffreys in the hope of tying Buckland to both murders. However, the DNA 'fingerprinting' results conclusively demonstrated that Buckland did not rape or murder either girl. A result that greatly surprised the police. Therefore, the first use of DNA analysis in a criminal case led to the exoneration of the then prime suspect.

It is worth just pausing to consider the outcome of the case had DNA analysis not been available. With the police strongly suspecting that Buckland was the double murderer and having a confession to one of the murders, a miscarriage of justice may well have resulted.

As the popular accounts go on to record, a mass screening of men in the area was conducted with no 'matches' to the crime scene samples found. It was only a chance overhearing of remarks made by someone claiming to have provided blood samples in the place of Colin Pitchfork that led to his arrest and DNA analysis identifying him as the rapist and murderer.

According to Jeffreys, within a year, the demand for DNA 'fingerprinting' had exceeded his capacity to provide the service, and it was commercialised by the private company Cellmark, which was established in 1987 (Cellmark 2024).

DNA 'fingerprinting' was hailed as a means of delivering the certainty required by the law. A certainty not delivered by a person expressing a subjective opinion, as with fingerprints, but by objective science. However, the power of DNA 'fingerprinting' raised ethical concerns and questions about its claims.

These early 'successes' and the probative power of DNA evidence led to resistance, scrutiny and challenge, most notably in the United States. In reality, DNA analysis was 'rushed into service' with quality requirements lagging.

In 1989, Eric Lander, then a molecular biologist who served as an expert witness in early DNA analysis cases, wrote.

> *At present, forensic science is virtually unregulated – with the paradoxical result that clinical laboratories must meet higher standards to diagnose strep throat than forensic labs must meet to put a defendant on death row.*
>
> *(Lander 1989)*

Some US jurisdictions at the time applied what is known as the *Frye* or general acceptance test. If a scientific technique is generally accepted within the relevant scientific community as valid and produces reliable evidence, then evidence based on the technique is admitted. Initially, US judges decided that this novel evidence type was generally accepted and therefore admissible. That was until the case of *People of New York v. Castro* in 1989.

In that case, the court recognised the difficulty of applying the *Frye* test to complex evidence and advanced a three-part refinement of the *Frye* test. It was decided that a court should address the following questions in ruling on the admissibility of DNA 'fingerprinting'.

Prong 1. Is there a theory which is generally accepted in the scientific community, which supports the conclusion that DNA forensic testing can produce reliable results?

Prong 2. Are there techniques or experiments that currently exist that are capable of producing reliable results in DNA identification and which are generally accepted in the scientific community?

Prong 3. Did the testing laboratory perform the accepted scientific techniques in analysing the forensic samples in this particular case?

These questions might be translated into generic requirements for sound science, valid methods and documented compliance with relevant quality standards.

In the case of *Castro*, the testing laboratory's procedures were called into question, and expert testimony revealed that it had failed to use generally accepted and reliable techniques that could prove that the blood in question was that of the victim. DNA 'fingerprinting' had failed Prong 3. DNA fingerprinting had satisfied Prongs 1 and 2 but not 3, so the evidence was not admitted.

For a deeper dive into the early challenges faced by DNA 'fingerprinting', the reader is directed to the account in Quality Management in Forensic Science (Doyle 2019).

An example of a later historical challenge to DNA evidence in the State of Colorado in the case of *People of Colorado v. Michael Eugene Shreck* in 2001, in which it was successfully argued pretrial that recent advances in DNA analysis[10] were not yet sufficiently reliable to warrant admission of the results as expert evidence. Thus, the trial court issued an order barring that evidence. However, the Colorado State Supreme Court overruled the lower court, and the evidence was admitted. Nevertheless, this demonstrates how advances in technology can raise questions of admissibility. This is an example of the constant tension between law enforcement wanting to use the latest tools in the 'fight against crime' and the courts' aim of delivering justice.

What these legal and technological issues demanded were standardised operating procedures (methods) and quality management, particularly quality control and assurance.

In addition to early challenges to the reliability and consequent admissibility of DNA-based expert evidence, there were also the practical issues of resources, time, effort, and cost, together with issues with the analysis method itself. Jeffreys' RFLP method to identify and measure variations in the length of repeat sequences is shown in the workflow Figure 4.8 and may be summarised as follows. Extracting the DNA from cells. Cutting DNA into fragments using restriction enzymes. Separating the resulting fragments of tandem repeats of various sizes using gel electrophoresis. Transferring the separated fragments in the gel to an appropriate medium. Visualising the separated fragments by adding the DNA probe, which includes a radioactive isotope and exposure of the radioactive DNA fragments to an X-ray film (all called autoradiography). This results in the familiar 'barcode' usually having more than 30 lines.

In the early 1980s, Jeffreys' DNA 'fingerprinting' was revolutionary. It introduced the concept of identification via DNA, which relied on his discovery of the highly variable mini-

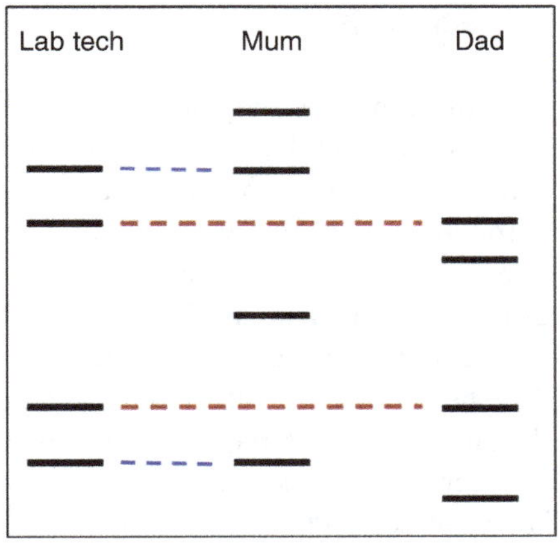

Figure 4.9 Representation of Jeffreys' results – probe detects repeat units, and correspondence of bands with Mum and Dad.

satellite regions of the human genome. The RFLP method might be considered the first generation of DNA analysis. However, that method suffered from several weaknesses. The method was time and effort-heavy. It required a relatively large amount of DNA. The DNA needed to be fresh, not degraded. It involved the use of radioactive materials. The entire sample was consumed. Interpreting the barcodes could be a challenge. And, as the RFLP method was commercialised, the lack of standard methods meant results could not be compared. Considering those weaknesses in turn.

The RFLP method described above was time-consuming and labour-intensive. It took between days and weeks to produce a result.

The RFLP method needed a relatively large amount of DNA for success. In criminal cases, this required sufficient DNA to be recovered from the crime scene, usually from visible quantities of body fluids such as blood or semen. This is because a fairly large amount of the DNA probe must bind to the target DNA sequence to make visualisation via autoradiography possible. It was often the case that insufficient DNA was collected.

The source of the DNA needed to be fresh. The repeat sequences targeted by RFLP were quite long (Figure 4.9). As mentioned earlier, these were termed variable number tandem repeats, abbreviated as VNTR. These repeats ranged in length from about 10 to 100 base pairs. Now, DNA can be degraded by environmental conditions such as sunlight, heat and humidity. DNA recovered from crime scenes was often degraded by those conditions into shorter lengths, making it difficult to distinguish between fragments resulting from degradation or those from restriction enzyme cuts. Therefore, the sample might be of insufficient quality for successful analysis.

DNA 'fingerprinting' results were visualised by exposure of the radioactive species to an X-ray film. Working with radioactive materials raised health and safety concerns.

The interpretation of the bands on the autoradiograph could be tricky. The bands could be indistinct or have unclear boundaries, risking differences of interpretive opinion.

As DNA 'fingerprinting' expanded and began to be conducted by an increasing number of providers, the lack of standardisation meant that DNA results from Lab 1 could not be compared with those from Lab 2.

Impact Today

Of course, the discovery of minisatellites and identification using an individual's DNA by Jeffreys was not the end of the journey. If Jeffreys' RFLP method is thought of as the first generation, the technology has now advanced to at least the third generation.

To follow that journey, a few more terms need to be introduced: 'sensitivity', 'discrimination power' and 'turnaround time'. These factors are not only important in DNA 'fingerprinting' but in all areas of analytical science.

'Sensitivity', in the context of DNA 'fingerprinting', is how much DNA is needed to produce useful evidence. It should come as no surprise that, as the technology has advanced, the amount of DNA required has massively reduced.

'Discriminating power'; again, in this context, it is related to the likelihood that two unrelated people will have matching DNA profiles or fingerprints. In DNA analysis, a random match is extremely unlikely, and so it is highly discriminating.

One strength of the RFLP method was its discriminatory power; there was an astronomically low chance of a random match[11]. This is because RFLP targeted numerous loci simultaneously, and the precise number could be selected.

'Turnaround time' is essentially analysis time, how long it might take to obtain a useful result. Again, this has massively reduced.

By far the biggest advance in technology was the discovery in 1983 of the polymerase chain reaction (PCR) by the American biochemist Kary Mullis (1944–2019). Mullis received the Nobel Prize in Chemistry in 1993 for his discovery.

In 1986, Mullis published a paper on PCR (Mullis et al. 1986). The process involves unzipping the DNA molecule by breaking the weak hydrogen bonds between the bases, exploiting the complementarity of the molecule to create new strands and then zipping the new strands together, which creates a copy of the original DNA. The process requires thermal cycling, heating to unzip the DNA and cooling to zip together the new DNA. The heat-tolerant enzyme T*aq* polymerase[12] and short, single-stranded DNA molecules that flank the region to be copied are the necessary ingredients. The copying process is known as amplification. With each cycle, the amount of DNA doubles, such that after 4 cycles there are 16 copies and after 32 cycles over a billion copies! There is a trade-off, though, as the number of cycles approaches 32, so-called transcription errors start creeping in. These errors are the result of environmental contamination and the amplification of non-target DNA, generating false signals or noise.

The inclusion of PCR in the workflow of DNA analysis resolved most of the weaknesses of the RFLP method. Very little DNA was now required for successful analysis; nanogram[13] quantities of DNA could be analysed. That has lately been reduced to picogram[14] quantities. PCR amplified shorter repeat sequences of DNA, which meant that degraded DNA could yield useful results. These shorter repeated sequences, often around five base pairs long, are called short tandem repeats or STRs. PCR-based STR analysis was also much faster at producing results, usually within a day and currently within hours.

The initial utilisation of PCR for so-called second-generation DNA analysis targeted only a few loci, and so there was an initial reduction in discrimination power compared to RFLP. However, as the number of simultaneously targeted loci increased, that improved such

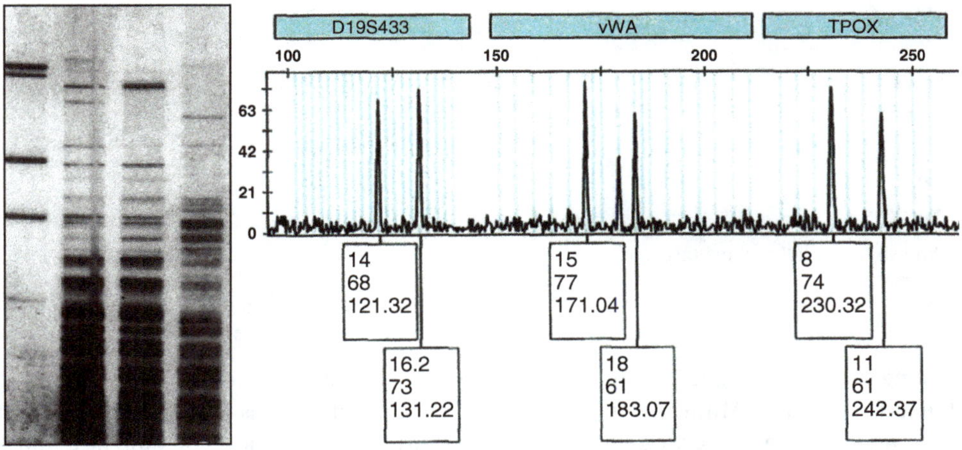

Figure 4.10 Comparing the results of DNA 'fingerprinting' using the RFLP/VNTR method and modern STR profiling.

that with 10 or more loci targeted, PCR-based STR analysis approached the discriminating power of the RFLP method. The current simultaneous targeting of 13 or more loci is sufficiently discriminating.

The incorporation of fluorescent dyes, which effectively replaced the radioactive probes, and the use of capillary electrophoresis[15] have transformed the analysis and interpretation of the repeat sequences, now STRs. The analysis is mostly automated, and interpretation is increasingly so, especially as AI is adopted.

Figure 4.10 depicts the stark contrast between early DNA 'fingerprinting' as developed by Jeffreys and modern DNA analysis. The signals are the dark bands on the autoradiograph on the left and the peaks in the graphical output, called an electropherogram or EPG, on the right. As explained earlier, a dark band represents a repeat sequence; those at the top have not travelled far in the gel and are of the larger number of tandem repeats. Those towards the bottom have travelled the furthest and have fewer repeat units. The band's intensity, i.e. how dark it is, represents the quantity of a particular number of repeat units.

In addition to the signals being far clearer, the output of modern DNA analyses, now all software-driven, is far more informative. The name of each locus is given, e.g. D19S433. The 'D' represents a unique, non-coding sequence of DNA, in this case, sequence 433, and the number 19 identifies the chromosome on which the locus is found. The loci identified as vWA (von Willebrand factor) and TPOX (human thyroid peroxidase) are both genes in that they code for proteins. In modern DNA analysis, the number of loci targeted is usually between 13 and 15; only three are shown here. One of the loci not shown, Amelogenin on the x/y chromosome, identifies the sex of the individual.

The horizontal or *X* axis is molecular weight. The vertical or *Y* axis is the intensity of the signal in relative fluorescent units (RFU); like the autoradiograph, it is a function of the quantity of a particular number of repeat units. The faint blue vertical lines represent the possible number of variations, or alleles, at a particular locus. The numbers in the box represent, in order: the variant, or allele number; the RFU and the molecular weight.

Table 4.1 Part of a genotype.

Locus	Genotype	
D19S433	14	16.2
vWA	15	
TPOX	8	11
And so on, for all the loci targeted.		

Taking the locus D19S433 as an example, as expected, there are two variants or alleles at the locus, one from Mum and one from Dad. They are identified as allele numbers 14 and 16.2, meaning that there are 14 and 16.2 of the short tandem repeats. It should be emphasised that modern DNA analysis is almost fully automated, including the interpretation of results. There are three peaks at the locus vWA. The software has decided that the second of the three peaks is a false positive or drop-in and has ignored it.

The final output will be the genotype or genetic makeup of the individual whose DNA has been analysed. This is in the form of a table of all the loci targeted and the two alleles at each of those loci, as represented in Table 4.1, based on the information in Figure 4.10 above.

The genotype of the suspect will be compared to the questioned genotype, originating, say, from the crime scene. If those genotypes are in agreement, then the data will be statistically analysed and a likelihood ratio (LR) assigned. The LR is a measure of the strength of the DNA evidence in supporting the contention that the DNA found at the crime scene was that of the suspect. The LR is discussed in detail in Chapters 5 and 6, and the section on Terms, Definitions, and Explanations.

In conclusion, it is fair to state that without PCR amplification, DNA analysis may have remained a niche method of limited forensic utility.

Current Technological Progress

Significant technological advances are occurring as this book is written, e.g. Next Generation Sequencing (NGS), which can sequence the bases in repeats and will increase the forensic utility of sequencing mitochondrial DNA. Another advance is forensic genealogy – a combination of familial searching and genealogy.

Already in place and developing is the profiling of STRs on the male-only Y chromosome (Y-STR), establishing male/paternal relationships and the sequencing[16] of the large quantity of DNA in the numerous mitochondria of the cell for establishing female/maternal relationships.

Y-STR profiling has proven forensic utility in cases of alleged sexual assault by a male, as post-coital intimate samples may be awash with female DNA, making the detection of male DNA difficult. As Y-STR only profiles male DNA, this challenge is overcome. However, Y-STR profiling has far less discrimination power than full DNA profiling, which might generate likelihood ratios with magnitudes of 10^{13}, in comparison to Y-STR of about 10^{2}.

National DNA Databases

The effect on society has been significant. European, North American and Australasian countries have national DNA databases, as do China and Japan, with many others in operation or being planned. The first was created in the United Kingdom in 1995. The establishment of these databases has prompted ethical concerns and requires conformance with quality standards for methods used to produce DNA profiles loaded onto databases. In the United States, the standard was first set in 1994 by the DNA Advisory Board (DAB) and later by the Specialist Working Group of DNA Analysis Methods (SWGDAM). Adherence to quality standards is required by US Federal Law as a condition of a laboratory's participation in the national DNA database. In Europe, the requirement is conformance to the international standard ISO/IEC 17025 (the subject of Chapter 7) as set out in the Prüm Convention[17]. Conformance to the same standard ensures that DNA evidence produced in one jurisdiction can be used as evidence in another and aids cross-border cooperation in the investigation of international crime.

Regulations vary by jurisdiction regarding whose DNA profile may be loaded onto a database. Some restrict the population of the database to profiles of those convicted of crime, and some to those arrested or charged. Some impose limits on how long DNA profiles might be stored. Most jurisdictions permanently store DNA profiles obtained from crime scenes.

On a broader note, now that the entire human genome can be sequenced as a matter of routine, several ethical questions are arising. One of the main ones is, should the genome of newborns be sequenced? This would have the benefit of identifying disease-causing mutations and facilitating early diagnosis and treatments. While it might be possible to restrict this information to medical practitioners, it is easy to see how it could be exploited by the state for other purposes.

Wrongful Convictions

Perhaps the greatest impact of DNA profiling today is helping to identify those wrongly convicted. Looking back to the first use of DNA in a criminal case as clearing a suspect, it emphasises the point that forensic scientific evidence is at its strongest when excluding an individual or a particular line of inquiry.

The ongoing impact of the Innocence Project is to expose the earlier weakness of expert scientific evidence and testimony (The Innocence Project 2023).

Increased Sensitivity, an Issue

The DNA results/profiles from less and less DNA has had its drawbacks. It may not be possible to specify the cellular origin of the profile; was it from blood, semen, etc.? While DNA remains very strong evidence of identity, it is now weaker evidence of presence, and activity and therefore less helpful in crime reconstruction. An individual's DNA may have been innocently transferred to a crime scene. In a case of alleged sexual assault, where the complainant and alleged perpetrator are the only witnesses, the finding of one party's DNA on the other may not support an allegation of sexual assault, particularly if the parties were recently socially engaged in non-sexual activity.

Starting with a very small amount of DNA, say from a few cells, requires a greater number of PCR amplification cycles to produce enough DNA for analysis and, in turn, produce a useful profile. However, as mentioned earlier, as the number of amplification cycles increases, the chances of errors occurring also increase. These errors are essentially false-positive and false-negative signals. False negative signals are technically called drop-out, and false positives are called drop-in. Drop-in was encountered earlier and is depicted in Figure 4.10. These false signals make interpretation more challenging.

In addition, increased sensitivity means that mixed DNA profiles are more common. This issue has largely been resolved by what is known as probabilistic genotyping software (PGS)[18]. The software is based on complex mathematics and statistics. The first step is for an analyst to decide how many individuals are contributing to the mixed DNA profile. In simple terms, this is decided by looking at the number of signals at any one location, which is a function of the number of alleles. Remember that there should be two per individual, one from Mum and one from Dad. So, if there are, say, six, then the number of contributors is likely to be three. Once that decision is made, the software then generates virtual profiles based on the signals detected and then applies an interpretational process to determine which profiles best explain the mixed profiles. Essentially, the software separates the virtual profiles of individual contributors. These profiles are then compared to those of suspects, and a likelihood ratio is assigned as a measure of how certain it is that a separated questioned profile is that of a suspect. This software can also make allowance for drop-in and drop-out. Again, given the sensitivity of the technology, the finding of such a low level of someone's DNA at a scene may not support allegations of presence or activity, let alone proof of such.

Finally, because of the sensitivity of modern methods, one of the main issues is contaminating DNA. Modern DNA analysis involves the processing of many samples simultaneously and sequentially. DNA from one investigation has been known to contaminate samples from a separate investigation, falsely implicating the innocent. In addition, a lack of effective contamination avoidance procedures can result in general contamination by extraneous DNA. DNA laboratories are now effectively clean rooms with stringent contamination avoidance measures in place, including the wearing of full barrier clothing; hats, masks, suits, boots and gloves, which are changed often. As a contamination avoidance measure, full barrier clothing is now regularly worn by those at the crime scene.

Contribution to Current Practice

DNA has become the standard evidence-type template against which all other disciplines are compared. It has become the 'gold standard' of forensic scientific practice, calling into question the principles and practices of all other disciplines or evidence types. It could be argued that DNA analysis has put the 'science' into forensic science. The effects of DNA analysis on forensic science will become even clearer in the chapter on the International Standard ISO/IEC 17025 on the US National Academies of Sciences 2009 Report, Chapters 7 and 9, respectively.

Where DNA has led, others have followed, and now conformance to ISO/IEC 17025 by forensic science laboratories for most of their activities has become the norm.

Although fingerprint examiners had and, in some quarters, still do claim the power of individualisation, DNA evidence had the statistical power to meet that standard as the chance of a random match based on profiling 13 or more STRs is infinitesimally small. However, DNA analysis is science, and no scientist would ever claim certainty. Therefore, great efforts were made to accurately measure the discriminatory power of DNA evidence and find a way of conveying the level of certainty to a tribunal of fact, such as a court of law. In the case of a 'match' between a profile recovered from a crime scene and that of the suspect, forensic scientists merely report along these lines.

> *... the DNA evidence provides extremely strong support for the proposition that the questioned DNA is that of the suspect.*

In addition, DNA has led the way in interpretation, adopting a logical and probabilistic approach, which is fully explored in Chapter 6 on interpretation.

So, in addition to raising standards in forensic science generally, it also promoted probabilistic interpretation, called for in the Ontogeny paper (Chapter 3), and the introduction of the logical and balanced approach to interpretation based on the assignment of a likelihood ratio, as discussed in Chapter 6 on interpretation. Logical and balanced interpretation and probabilistic reporting are now considered to be standard practice.

DNA analysts giving expert evidence are acutely aware of the risk of transposing the conditional (or should be!) and, in addition to conforming to the principle of balance and logic in practice, also conform to the principles of transparency and robustness. These issues are discussed in Chapters 5 and 6.

DNA, CCTV (closed-circuit TV – essentially video surveillance) and seized digital devices are perhaps the most impactful sources of evidence used in the investigation of crime today. Therefore, there has been a huge investment in the technological advancement of DNA analysis to the extent that it is now a technology of *'first resort'*, to quote Sir Alec Jeffreys. However, as is clear from earlier sections, the science underpinning that technology is quite remarkable in its complexity.

Concluding Remarks

Sir Alec Jeffery's highly technical publication detailing his eureka moment while experimenting in the lab began a revolution in forensic science and arguably has put the science in forensic science. DNA analysis has impacted all other evidence types and has led to the standardisation of forensic practice. The discovery of hypervariable 'minisatellite' regions in human DNA has provided a powerful tool in the investigation of crime and the delivery of justice, which has been for the benefit of society at large.

Key Takeaways

Alec Jeffreys and his team at Leicester University discovered tandem repeats of DNA sequences that varied in number from individual to individual, leading to a revolution in forensic science. That discovery has transformed forensic science and criminal investigations.

The discovery was completely scientific in origin and nature, coming from pure 'blue-sky' research.

It was a new and fundamentally different means of establishing identity, a role previously and exclusively held by fingerprints.

The forensic exploitation of the DNA molecule began with 'fingerprinting' and continues to this day, with the entire human genome now available for interrogation.

DNA 'fingerprinting' required a new set of standards regarding operating procedures/methods, proof of validity, quality control, and quality assurance; in addition, results had to be reported probabilistically. Fingerprints and some other feature comparison disciplines still do not meet these standards. The standards apply to all other forensic science disciplines.

DNA 'fingerprinting' laid the foundation for the establishment and maintenance of national DNA databases. The exchange of DNA data facilitated cross-border cooperation in the investigation of international crime.

DNA analysis has proved a powerful tool in the uncovering and prevention of miscarriages of justice, particularly in exonerating those wrongly convicted.

DNA analysis can establish familial relationships and, together with genealogy, provides a new forensic/investigative tool.

Technological advances bringing increased sensitivity, being able to process less and less DNA, have been a mixed blessing. Not knowing the cellular source of DNA has weakened it as evidence of presence and activity, increased the likelihood of mixed profiles, mostly resolved with probabilistic genotyping software, and increased the risk and impact of contamination, requiring stringent contamination-avoidance measures.

DNA 'fingerprinting' might be considered first-generation DNA analysis based on RFLP and longer minisatellites/VNTRs, radioactive probes and visualisation with autoradiographs. Generation 1 was labour-intensive and time-consuming, i.e. expensive in time and money. Current technology is perhaps third generation and based on STRs or microsatellites, amplification with PCR, separation with capillary electrophoresis, and visualisation with fluorescent-coloured dyes, with the processing and interpretation conducted mainly by machines in hours, i.e. quickly and cheaply. Therefore, DNA analysis together with fingerprints and CCTV has now become the discipline of first, and often only, choice in the investigation of crime and identifying the criminal.

The contribution of DNA analysis to society has been overwhelmingly positive, which is evidenced by the many honours and awards given to Sir Alec Jeffreys, CH FRS MAE.

Notes

1 The DNA in the mitochondria is inherited from mum only and so helps reveal maternal links.

2 The singular 'Locus' is usually pronounced with a hard C and the plural 'Loci' with a soft C.

3 The term 'stutter' has taken on an entirely different meaning in modern DNA analysis; it now means a false positive signal produced by the polymerase chain reaction (PCR) discussed later in this chapter.

4 It should be noted that in minisatellites, the number of bases in the repeat sequences are usually between 5 and 30+ and the number of repeat sequences is between 5 and 50.
5 It should also be noted that RFLP is a generic term applying to any method used to study variations in the restriction fragments of DNA, whatever the cause of variation.
6 Currently, Sterling Professor of Immunobiology at Yale School of Medicine.
7 Emeritus professor of clinical biochemistry and molecular biology at the University of Amsterdam.
8 Richard Flavell and Alec Jeffreys were among the first to discover split genes, also known as introns, which are non-coding sequences within genes. Their work almost won them a Nobel Prize! (Dong et al. 2005).
9 Gary Lineker is a cofounder of Goal Hanger Podcasts, which has in its 'stable' 'The Rest Is History'.
10 An increase in the number of loci targeted.
11 Some authors claim there is a less than 10^{18} chance of two unrelated individuals having a matching DNA 'fingerprint' using RFLP.
12 T*aq* = Thermus aquaticus.
13 One billionth of a gram or 10^{-9} g.
14 A trillionth of a gram or 10^{-12} g.
15 A method of separation far more effective than gel electrophoresis and able to separate the minute quantities of DNA involved.
16 The sequence of bases of mtDNA is analysed rather than STRs.
17 A treaty between several European Union member states stepping up cross-border cooperation in the fight against crime, particularly terrorism.
18 There are complex unresolved issues around PGS, e.g. different packages can produce different results (Thompson 2023).

Bibliography

Cellmark. 2024. *Info About Us*. Accessed October 23, 2024. https://www.cellmark.co.uk/info/about-us/#:~:text=Established%20in%201987%2C%20Cellmark%20is,quality%2C%20reliability%20and%20service%20excellence.

Dong, Chen, Shomyseh Sanjabi, and Elizabeth Eynon. 2005. "Gene Regulation and Function: It's Rocking Science – Meeting Report." *Immunity* 23: 557–60.

Doyle, Sean P. 2019. "4.4 The Forensic Exploitation of DNA and Its Development as an Evidence Type." In *Quality Management in Forensic Science*, edited by Sean P. Doyle, 196–207. London: Academic Press.

Gill, Peter, Alec J. Jeffreys, and David J. Werrett. 1985. "Forensic Application of DNA 'Fingerprints'." *Nature* 318: 577–79.

Jeffreys, Alec J., Victoria Wilson, and Swee Lay Thein. 1985. "Hypervariable 'Minisatellite' Regions in Human DNA." *Nature* 314: 67–73.

Lander, Eric S. 1989. "DNA Fingerprinting on Trial." *Nature* 339: 501–05.

Liberal Democrat Voice. 2015. *Obituary: Bob Pritchard*. 14 April. Accessed June 11, 2024. https://www.libdemvoice.org/obituary-bob-pritchard-45478.html.

Mullis, Kary, Fred Faloona, Stephen Scharf, Randall Saiki, Glenn Horn, and Henry Erlich. 1986. "Specific enzymatic amplification of DNA in vitro: the polymerase chain reaction." *Cold Spring Harbor Symposia on Quantitative Biology* 51: 263–73.

Pray, Leslie A. 2008. "Discovery of DNA Structure and Function: Watson and Crick." *Nature Education* 1: 100.

The Innocence Project. 2023. *Our Work. Restoring Freedom*. Accessed August 22, 2023. https://innocenceproject.org/restoring-freedom/.

Thompson, William C. 2023. "Uncertainty in Probabilistic Genotyping of Low Template DNA: A Case Study Comparing STRmix™ and TrueAllel™." *Journal of Forensic Science* 68 (3): 1049–63.

5

Statistical Evidence and Fallacies

Interpretation of Statistical Evidence in Criminal Trials

The Prosecutor's Fallacy and the Defense Attorney's Fallacy*

William C. Thompson† and Edward L. Schumann†

Image 5.1 Publication header.

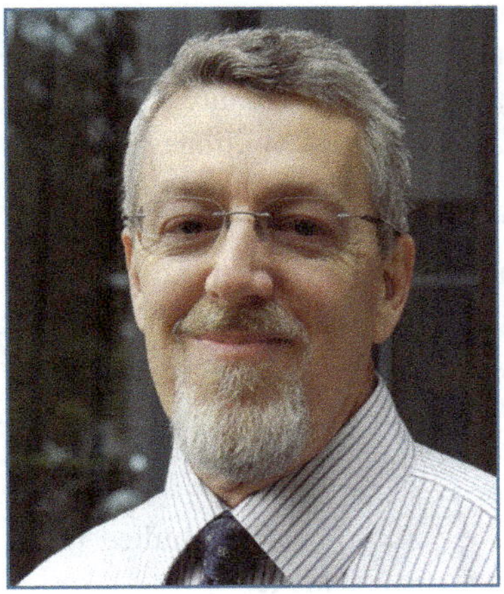

Image 5.2 William C. Thompson. With permission of William C. Thompson.

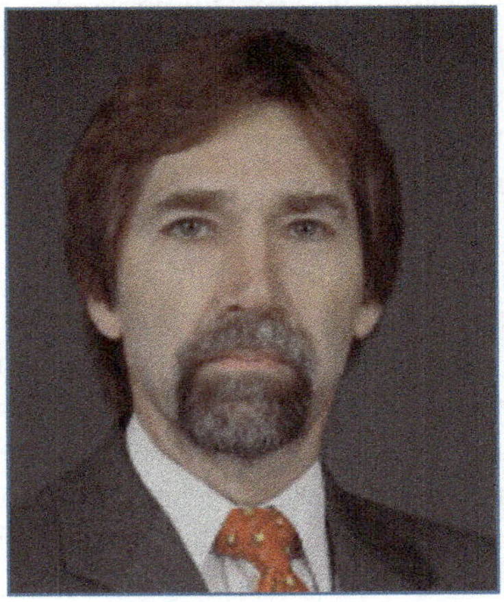

Image 5.3 Edward L. Schumann. With permission of Edward L. Schumann.

A History of Forensic Science in 10 Publications: How They Established Current Practice, First Edition.
Sean Doyle.

Name of the Publication

The publication is titled *Interpretation of Statistical Evidence in Criminal Trials: The Prosecutor's Fallacy and the Defense Attorney's Fallacy.*

William C. Thompson and Edward L. Schumann (of the University of California, Irvine).

Law and Human Behaviour, Vol. 11. No. 3. 1987, p22.

According to Semantic Scholar, the publication has been cited 109 times, including 12 which were highly influential. According to ResearchGate, it has been cited 419 times.

Introduction

The publication is credited with inventing the terms Prosecutor's and Defence Attorney's fallacies and introducing them into the lexicon of forensic science. The paper's main purpose was to determine the degree to which those involved in criminal proceedings might be prone to such fallacies and, consequently, to gauge how much weight the fact-finder or jury[1] might attach to statistical evidence and whether that weight is warranted. The fallacies, or logical errors identified, as the names imply, unfairly favour the prosecution or defence case.

In simple terms, the defence attorney's fallacy decreases the perception of guilt by the fact-finder by falsely giving less weight to probative evidence. Conversely, the prosecutor's fallacy falsely increases the perception of guilt by the fact-finder by giving more weight to probative evidence.

In discussing these fallacies and their potential impact on criminal justice, it is important to bear in mind that there are four groups to consider: the litigating lawyers, forensic scientists acting as expert witnesses, lay fact-finders/juries and judges.

Regarding forensic science, the subject of this paper represents a major milestone in the development of presenting scientific evidence probabilistically, the probability of a 'match', rather than categorically, 'match/no match/inconclusive'. Probabilistic reporting was a necessary development identified by Kirk in his ontogeny paper, the subject of Chapter 3. The next stage of this development will be discussed in Chapter 6 'Interpreting Evidence'.

When reading the publication, it is important to note that it is focused on the entire judicial/trial process, which includes stages that a forensic scientist plays no part in, specifically the weighing of evidence by the fact-finder or jury. Throughout a trial, the fact-finder will be presented with all the evidence considered relevant, much of which a forensic scientist giving expert evidence will be unaware of. Thus, the scope of the publication is broader than just the role forensic scientists play in the judicial/trial process.

However, as the title implies, very much central to the judicial process studied in the publication is the presentation and communication of statistical evidence.

Presenting statistically sound evidence to a court of law or any tribunal of fact presents significant challenges in communication. The publication addresses these challenges and how they might be overcome. Unfortunately, despite best efforts, communication remains a challenge. The paper was published in 1987; to indicate the scale of the challenge, below is a quote from 2011!

> *Indeed, we believe that for most people – and this includes from our own experience highly intelligent barristers, judges and surgeons, any attempt to use Bayes theorem* [explained later in this chapter and again in Chapter 6] *to explain a fallacy is completely hopeless.*
> *(Fenton and Neil 2011)*

The reality, as exposed by the psychologists Daniel Kahneman (1934–2024) and Amos Tversky (1937–1996) in their Nobel Prize-winning work 'Judgment under uncertainty: Heuristics and biases', (Tversky and Kahneman 1974)[2] is that human beings have problems assessing information presented numerically and/or probabilistically. As Gross observed in the Handbook, the subject of Chapter 1, and as developed in Chapter 8, 'Observer Effects', humans are susceptible to any number of confounding biases and therefore prone to errors in reasoning.

Essentially, the brains of humans are wired to rely on rules of thumb, mental shortcuts, which have served the species well as it has evolved, and so the potential for confusing the fact-finder and indeed the lawyers and judges is significant.

That being said, this chapter will rise to the challenge. As it is as much aimed at the non-specialist as the specialist reader, an attempt will be made to tease out the essential concepts and present them in an easy-to-understand manner.

The main concern is that the logical fallacies, or errors in thinking, highlighted in this publication could go unnoticed and potentially lead to miscarriages of justice. Indeed, as the cases cited demonstrate (R v Clark 2003; Batty 2005), this has already happened.

Terms, Definitions and Explanations

Before exploring the publication in more detail, it is important to have some grasp of what the various terms used in the publication mean.

The subject of the publication is logical fallacies, invalid or faulty reasoning, which might contribute to a miscarriage of justice.

The two fallacies that the authors introduce are errors in thinking that could be made by litigating lawyers, expert witnesses and even judges. In addition, these errors increase the risk of misinterpretation by the fact-finder. As the title states, the logical errors are called the prosecutor's and defence attorney's fallacies. Introducing, raising awareness, and the potential impact of these fallacies on criminal justice are the reasons this publication appears in this book. Others would go on to further develop and add knowledge in the interpretation of scientific evidence; Robertson and Vignaux, the authors of the publication discussed in Chapter 6, are two such figures.

Justice Systems

The publication was authored by American academics and is therefore framed by the judicial systems of the United States. In the United States, there are federal and state laws, and each state is, to some degree, a separate jurisdiction.

First, the United States, in common with all jurisdictions that are based on medieval English law – essentially former colonies of what was the British Empire – employs a common law system of criminal justice. As explained in the section on Terms, Definitions and Explanations, common law is based on precedent, i.e. case law rather than being documented or codified. It is evolutionary and adopts an adversarial approach to weighing evidence, uncovering the truth and delivering justice. In this system, lawyers act for the prosecution. Their role is to present the facts to prove the crime with which a defendant is charged. The prosecutor represents the state, whereas the defence lawyer, or attorney, acts primarily as the protector of the defendant's rights and interests. Perhaps the most important right is the presumption of innocence, which applies in most jurisdictions. It is important to note in passing that these role differences produce divergent ethical responsibilities.

In the adversarial system, the burden of proof usually lies with the prosecution. The defence is not required to prove anything, and the defendant is not required to give or present evidence.

So, in the adversarial system/model of criminal justice, there are two sides: the prosecution, advocating for and representing the state, and the defence, advocating for and representing the defendant.

The other major system of criminal justice is civil law, which is codified, i.e. written down, and has its roots in Roman law and, more recently, the Napoleonic Code of 1804. This system applies in continental Europe and the former colonies of non-British European powers. Civil law is inquisitorial in approach. In contrast with the adversarial system, which has many rules that exclude certain types of evidence, an inquisitorial system is inclusive and considers all evidence that might be relevant.

However, even though there are significant differences between the adversarial and inquisitorial approaches to criminal justice and the paper is framed by the adversarial model, the fallacies which are the subject of Thompson and Schumann's publication can equally affect the outcome of criminal trials in both justice systems.

Probability and Likelihood

In addition to terms relating to criminal law, there are terms relating to probability, which is the likelihood of an event occurring. A likelihood of zero means that the event will not occur, and a likelihood of one means it certainly will. Values between 0 and 1 represent degrees of certainty or uncertainty. The degree of certainty can be expressed as a percentage, certainty being a probability of 100%. Likelihood and probability are synonymous, and each term is used as seems appropriate according to convention.

Associative Evidence and 'Match'

The paper mentions 'associative evidence', which is evidence that links a suspect to a crime. Examples of associative evidence include hair pulled from the head of a perpetrator 'matching' the suspect's hair, and fibres found on a victim's body 'matching' those in the suspect's house.

The word 'match' is in parentheses because, as discussed in Chapter 3 on the 'Ontogeny of Criminalistics', there can never be a 'match' in the sense of assigning a unique source; one source to the exclusion of all others. The term 'match' used in this book means some marked degree of resemblance between a questioned item of evidence originating from the crime scene or linked to a crime and the reference item of evidence originating from, or linked to, a suspect. So, the term associative evidence is to be preferred to 'match'. However, given the caveat that 'match' means a degree of resemblance, the term will continue to be used as it aids understanding.

Bayesian Reasoning and Bayes' Theorem

The area of interpreting scientific evidence can be a quagmire of confusing terminology and hard-to-grasp concepts, which result in logical errors made by forensic scientists and others and the consequent presentation of misleading evidence.

To better understand the impacts of this publication and avoid peppering this chapter with confusing terms (some of which are now outdated and have been replaced), it is necessary to introduce Bayesian reasoning, which might simply be considered as updating beliefs based on new information.

The Reverend Thomas Bayes (1701/2–1761) gives his name to this form of reasoning. Bayes was an English minister of religion, statistician and philosopher. He imagined a man emerging into the world (Adam perhaps?) and seeing the sunrise for the first time. Initially, the man does not know whether this is a common or a rare event. As each day passes and the sun rises, he becomes ever more certain that the sun will rise on the following day. Eventually, he predicts, with close to 100% certainty, that the sun will rise the next day. This is the essence of Bayesian reasoning; gathering more and more evidence will bring us closer to the truth. In principle, this is just updating current beliefs based on new information and making a prediction. Another example is predicting the weather. In the absence of any information, the chance of rain tomorrow might be predicted to be 50%. However, as information is gathered about previous weather patterns and current meteorological data, it might result in the prediction that it will rain tomorrow, or not, with greater certainty!

It's hard to comprehend how crucial this fundamental concept is in so many human endeavours, from medicine and investment decisions to predicting sporting outcomes, gambling, weather, and forensic science. The philosophical basis for Bayesian reasoning is simple yet powerful, with its consequences being rich. The mathematical basis is equally simple.

Bayesian reasoning can be simply expressed as follows.

$$\text{original belief} + \text{new information} \rightarrow \text{updated belief}$$

This is also a simple expression of a form of Bayes' theorem, which is a formulaic version of Bayesian reasoning.

Here a new term is introduced, 'conditional probability'. Bayes' theorem is concerned with conditional probability. It can be used to predict whether a theory or hypothesis is true IF some event has occurred. In the 'Adam' example, what is the probability of the sun rising tomorrow IF it has risen every day so far? Another simplistic example would be a prediction of whether or not it would rain tomorrow, IF it rained today.

This might be expressed mathematically as

$$p(\text{rain tomorrow} \mid \text{rain today})$$

In words, which is the probability that it would rain tomorrow **IF** it rained today. The letter 'p' represents probability, and the vertical line '|' represents **IF**; **IF,** signalling the condition or conditional which always lies on the right of the vertical line.

Having introduced the concept of conditional probability, Bayes' theorem can be stated with greater mathematical accuracy in the following form.

$$\text{Prior Probability} \times \text{Likelihood Ratio} = \text{Posterior Probability}$$

$$\text{i.e. current belief} \times \text{new information} = \text{updated belief}$$

This is closely similar to the earlier expression. Using the example of a jury considering whether a particular gun was the murder weapon. The prior probability is the probability of the current belief before any evidence is given, e.g. that the gun is unlikely to be the murder weapon, as most guns are not murder weapons. That prior probability is then multiplied by an updating factor known as the likelihood ratio. The likelihood ratio is provided by the forensic scientist giving evidence, e.g. that it is more likely than not that the bullet that killed the victim came from that gun. This new information then updates the prior probability, and the posterior probability is that the gun is now considered more likely to be the murder weapon[3].

In this case, the associative evidence is a 'match' between the bullet that killed the victim and the gun in question. The practical process of updating current beliefs requires the following three probabilities.

The first probability needed is the probability of a 'match' **IF** the gun is the murder weapon. It is assumed to be quite high, say 90%. Next, the probability of the 'match' **IF** the gun is not the murder weapon needs to be estimated. In this example, it is quite low. It should be noted that it may not be 100 − 90 = 10%. In this example, it is assumed to be 1%. Thirdly, the probability that the gun is the murder weapon must be estimated. Yes, guns are sometimes used as murder weapons, but, in the absence of any other evidence, the chance that it is the murder weapon must be quite low, say 5%. This is the prior probability. By plugging these estimated probabilities into an algebraic formula of Bayes' theorem, we get the following.

Prior probability		
Initial estimate of how likely it is that the gun is the murder weapon	x	5%
EVIDENCE		
Probability of the 'match' **IF** it is the murder weapon	y	90%
Probability of the 'match' **IF** it is not the murder weapon	z	1%
POSTERIOR PROBABILITY		
Revised estimate of how likely it is that gun is the murder weapon	$xy/(xy + z(1 - x))$	83%

So, the prior probability of 5% has been updated, and the posterior probability is 83%. In a second example, let's assume that the supporting evidence weakens.

Prior probability		
Initial estimate of how likely it is that the gun is the murder weapon	x	5%
EVIDENCE		
Probability of the 'match' **IF** it is the murder weapon	y	50%
Probability of the 'match' **IF** it is not the murder weapon	z	5%
POSTERIOR PROBABILITY		
Revised estimate of how likely it is that gun is the murder weapon	$xy/(xy + z(1 - x))$	34%

As the supporting evidence weakens, the posterior probability has dramatically reduced, and on the balance of probabilities, even given a 'match', the gun is unlikely to be the murder weapon.

The **'IF'** is highlighted as it is important to keep in mind that this signals the condition or conditional.

Likelihood Ratio

Another term now needs to be explained, the 'likelihood ratio' (LR). This is perhaps the most important term in this chapter and perhaps in the book. The LR needs to be well understood to more fully understand the concept of the prosecution fallacy, introduced and discussed in the publication, as it relates to statistical evidence presented by forensic scientists.

As might be deduced, the likelihood ratio is the evidence that updates the prior probability and results in the posterior probability.

The LR is a ratio of conditional probabilities. In this example, the likelihood or probability of a 'match' **IF** the gun **IS** the murder weapon, divided by the probability of a 'match' **IF** the gun **IS NOT** the murder weapon; the 'EVIDENCE' in the above examples. This might be more generally stated as the probability of the evidence 'E' (a 'match') **IF** the prosecution case is true 'H_P', (that the gun **IS** the murder weapon) divided by the probability of the evidence **IF** the defence case is true 'H_D' (the gun **IS NOT** the murder weapon). This might be expressed mathematically as follows.

$$\text{LR} = \frac{p(E|H_p)}{P(E|H_d)}$$

Although this equation does not appear in the publication, it is important in understanding the concepts introduced, and it is a very important equation in forensic science. It will be encountered often in this book and discussed again in some detail in Chapter 6 'Interpreting Evidence'. The likelihood ratio is also discussed in the section on Terms, Definitions and Explanations.

In the publication, the verbal equivalent of H_P[4] is that the defendant is guilty and H_D, that the defendant is not guilty. These are usually called hypotheses. As emphasised earlier, guilt, or otherwise, is a matter for the fact-finder or jury and not for the forensic scientist. What is a matter for the forensic scientist is the probability of the evidence, $p(E)$. This is perhaps the most important concept to keep in mind; the role of the forensic scientist is to consider the probability of the evidence and not the probability of the hypotheses. In our example, $p(E)$ is the probability of a 'match' between the bullet that killed the victim and the gun.

So, in words, the likelihood ratio in this example is the probability of a match between bullet and gun **IF** the gun is the murder weapon, divided by the probability of a match **IF** the gun is not the murder weapon. Using the estimated probabilities in the first example.

$$\text{LR} = 90/1 = 90.$$

So, the evidence of a 'match' is 90 times more likely **IF** the gun is the murder weapon. With this information, the fact-finder or jury updates its belief in whether or not the gun is the murder weapon and is now more certain that it is, although all the evidence in the case must be considered in addition to the firearms evidence.

The **IF** continues to be emphasised as understanding the condition, or conditional, is key to understanding the publication's relevance in forensic science.

By focusing on the LR alone and ignoring priors, the presentation of forensic scientific evidence can be simplified.

Bayesian reasoning applies directly to the fallacies under consideration. The prosecutor's fallacy is caused by giving too much weight to the associative evidence of a 'match' and ignoring the prior probability (of guilt or not-guilt[5]). The defence fallacy is caused by ignoring the associative evidence and giving too much weight to the prior.

As will become clear in Chapter 6 on interpreting evidence, prior probabilities are for the fact-finder alone. The forensic scientist assigns a likelihood ratio, and this is used by the fact-finder to update the prior probability of guilt or not-guilt.

Incidence Rate

A key term used in the publication that requires an explanation is 'incidence rate', which is the proportion of a population or group of things that share some of the characteristics of the questioned evidence. The example given is that the person who committed the crime and the accused have the same blood type. The expert evidence might include the proportion of the population that has that blood type. Where few members of the population possess that blood type, the fact-finder, or jury, is invited to attach more weight to the associative evidence than would be the case if that blood type were common in the population.

Base Rate

Related to the incidence rate is the 'base rate'. It is a statistic that describes the percentage of a population that has a specific characteristic. It is not case-specific; it is arrived at independently of any case. Superficially, this statistic is similar to the incidence rate. While the paper gives examples to help explain the difference, it is not entirely clear that the paper conveys a satisfactory understanding. It is important to understand the difference.

In the context of a criminal trial, the base rate is essentially the probability of guilt before any evidence is presented. In the Bayesian model, the base rate is the prior probability.

Base rates of significance in forensic science would be the frequency of a particular DNA profile among the general population or the frequency of occurrence among the general population in feature comparison disciplines such as fingerprints and handwriting. However, these rates should have been factored into the opinion reported by the forensic scientist.

Studies show that stereotypes tend to overshadow actual data, known as the base rate fallacy, which is at the heart of the prosecutor's fallacy. A common example is in deciding whether a shy, retiring type is a salesperson or a librarian. Studies show that people are more likely to decide that the type is more likely to be a librarian, even though there are far more salespeople than librarians. The base rate of there being far more salespeople than librarians is ignored in favour of the stereotype. Not enough weight is given to the prior probability.

The Prosecutor's Fallacy

As mentioned earlier, the prosecutor's fallacy involves determining the guilt of the accused based solely on the associative evidence of a 'match' – the incidence rate – and ignoring or giving little weight to the base rate or prior.

The prosecutor's fallacy occurs when the likelihood of an association between the accused and evidence is incorrectly interpreted as the probability of guilt. Returning to the murder weapon example, the association or 'match' between the bullet and the gun. The prosecutor argues that because the likelihood of a 'match' between the bullet and gun is high, the likelihood of guilt is also high. Or, taking a DNA-based example, the likelihood of a 'match' between the DNA recovered from the crime scene and that of the suspect is high, likelihood of guilt is also high. The fallacy is confusing the probability of the evidence with the probability of guilt.

The fallacy in the context of forensic science is known as the 'transposed conditional'. In the Bayesian model, it is the role of the forensic scientist to present an assigned likelihood ratio. Recalling the equation for the LR.

$$\mathrm{LR} = \frac{p(E|H_p)}{P(E|H_d)}$$

It should be noted and emphasised again that the forensic scientist always and only considers the probability of the evidence and never the probability of the hypotheses.

So, the statement of conditional probability becomes the probability of the evidence (a 'match') **IF** the prosecution hypothesis is true (the bullet matches the gun).

The hypotheses are the conditionals, and by considering the probability of the conditionals, essentially guilt or not-guilt, the logical error of the transposed conditional is made.

The logical error of the transposed conditional becomes clear with the following example. The probability that an animal has four legs **IF** it's a cow (a high probability) cannot be equated with the probability that an animal is a cow **IF** it has four legs (a low probability). The error is made by asserting that because an animal has four legs, then it must be a cow: In mathematical terms $pX|Y \neq pY|X$. This absence of logic is so important that it will be repeated often.

As before, the vertical line means '**IF**' as in the probability of X **IF** Y is true, and as X and Y are transposed, the fallacy is called transposing the conditional.

This error remains one of the most common errors made in the interpretation of scientific evidence (Robertson et al. 2016). It is avoided by only considering the probability of the evidence. Assessing the probability of guilt is for the fact-finder. This requires disciplined thinking.

The Defence Attorney's Fallacy

This fallacy occurs when the associative evidence of a 'match' is assumed to be irrelevant, and too much weight is attached to the base rate or prior.

The defence attorney's fallacy occurs when the likelihood of finding individuals with matching characteristics in a specific population (e.g. the population of a city or region) is reported. This assumes that the accused belongs to a large, arbitrary population and that no other information is available, making everyone equally likely to be the perpetrator. Based on these assumptions, it is concluded that there is a small probability that the suspect is the actual perpetrator. It is a fallacy to infer from this that the associative or 'match' evidence is weak.

Returning to the murder weapon example. If it were the case that most guns in existence were used to murder people, say 90% of all guns, then the 'match' between the gun in question and the bullet becomes irrelevant, or so it would be fallaciously argued by the defence.

O.J. Simpson

The defence attorney's fallacy was famously exploited in the trial of the American footballer and actor O.J. Simpson. In 1995, he was tried and acquitted of the murders of his ex-wife, Nicole Brown Simpson, and her friend Ronald Goldman. Blood found at the scene of the crime 'matched' that of Simpson. That blood group was shared by 1 in 400 people, the base rate or prior. The defence argued that a football stadium could be filled with Los Angeles citizens matching the sample. Therefore, the figure of 1 in 400 was useless, of no probative value.

As explained earlier, this is fallacious for two reasons; first, it takes no account of the rarity of the matching characteristic, which massively reduces the pool of suspects, in this case by 400. Secondly, Simpson is the only one charged with murder, a charge supported by other evidence.

Final Comments

The highlighting of these logical fallacies and their impact on delivering justice has had a profound effect on the interpretation of scientific evidence. However, forensic science practitioners have yet to universally accept the existence of these fallacies, and if their existence is accepted, to properly understand them, and even if they are understood, to adequately explain them to fact-finders.

There is much evidence to suggest that many judges and litigating lawyers are unaware of these fallacies, which puts justice at risk.

Some authors, such as David Kaye, contentiously argue that such fallacies do not necessarily harm justice (Kaye 2010). However, even if that were the case, they remain a fallacy and recognising them is important in principle and practice.

Summary

The paper introduces and discusses several key terms and concepts, including those in the title, the prosecutor's and defence attorney's fallacies. It is important when reading the publication to be aware that the process being discussed is the entire trial, including those phases that are outside the bailiwick of forensic science. Having introduced and discussed key terms and concepts, the paper reports two experiments and earlier studies which demonstrate the challenges faced in presenting statistical evidence and ensuring it is logically or non-fallaciously presented to the fact-finder.

Motivation for Writing

In this publication, the authors note the increasing prevalence of statistical evidence being presented in criminal trials. They also report that US appellate courts have been divided in their reaction to the incidence rate of 'matching' characteristics based on concerns about how fact-finders might respond to such evidence.

The authors question whether statistical evidence is being undervalued or improperly interpreted by fact-finders. Their motivation was to examine how fact-finders might utilise incidence rate statistics and highlight how the fallacies put justice at risk by contributing to miscarriages of justice. By raising awareness among relevant groups such as lawyers, judges and forensic scientists, the publication aims to reduce that risk.

Biography of the Publication

The publication draws attention to efforts by forensic scientists over the last 15 years studying the incidence rate of various characteristics of several evidence types: hair, soil, glass, body fluids, etc. Statistical data from these studies is increasingly presented in criminal trials. The studies or experiments conducted and reported in this publication were aimed at examining the understanding of this statistical evidence by fact-finders and other parts of the justice system.

Professional Biography of the Authors

The paper was published in 1987. According to their public biographies, William C. Thompson was then an Assistant Professor of Social Ecology[6], at the University of California, Irvine (UCI), and Edward L. Schumann was a doctoral student.

William C. Thompson

It should be noted that William C. Thompson is a joint author with D. Michael Risinger, Michael J. Saks and Robert Rosenthal of the paper on cognitive bias, the subject of Chapter 8.

William C. Thompson is now Emeritus Professor of Criminology, Law, and Society; Psychological Science; and Law at UCI.

When Professor of Criminology, Law and Society at UCI, he had joint appointments in Psychology and Social Behavior and the School of Law. He has published extensively on the use and misuse of scientific and statistical evidence in the courtroom and jurors' reactions to such evidence.

His research has been funded by the National Science Foundation, the National Institute of Justice, and the National Institute of Standards and Technology (NIST) through the Center for Statistics and Applications in Forensic Evidence (CSAFE).

Professor Thompson is the former chair of the Human Factors Committee of the Organization of Scientific Advisory Committees (OSAC), a federal standards-setting organization for forensic science that the US Department of Justice and NIST jointly sponsor.

Among many other contributions to the understanding of scientific and statistical evidence, Professor Thompson served on the committee that drafted the Royal Statistical Society Report published in September 2022 titled 'Healthcare serial killer or coincidence?

Statistical issues in the investigation of suspected medical misconduct' (Royal Statistical Society – Statistics and the Law Section 2022). The report sought to provide advice and guidance in evaluating cases involving medical professionals suspected of murder. This work was and remains particularly relevant in the controversial case of Lucy Letby[7]. These cases often turn on statistical evidence, which, as this chapter makes clear, can be difficult for fact-finders to weigh accurately.

Education

Professor Thompson obtained a bachelor's degree in psychology in 1976 from the University of Southern California. He received his Juris Doctor degree in 1982 from the Boalt Hall School of Law, University of California-Berkeley. He received a doctoral degree in psychology in 1984 at Stanford University. His dissertation topic was 'Bayesian and intuitive assessment of forensic science evidence in criminal trials'.

Professional

Professor Thompson began his academic career in 1981 as a Staff Fellow on the President's Commission for the Study of Ethical Problems in Medicine and Biomedical and Behavioral Research, Washington, D.C. He began his legal career at the California law firm Clark Deichler, LLC in 1992. In 1983, he was appointed to the Assistant Professor Program in Social Ecology and the Department of Criminology, Law and Society University of California-Irvine, and in 1989, Associate Professor. He was appointed as Professor in the UC-Irvine Department of Criminology, Law and Society in 1995, with joint appointments in: School of Law in 2010.

Edward L. Schumann

According to published biographies, Edward L. Schumann grew up in Texas and graduated from North Texas State University (now the University of North Texas) in 1980. He obtained a master's degree in social psychology from the University of Nebraska-Lincoln, where his focus was on small group decision-making. He then joined UCI, where he obtained his doctoral degree in 1991 in social ecology, specialising in law and psychology. With the idea of continuing in academia, Doctor Schumann went to California Western School of Law and received his Juris Doctor degree in 1992.

While at law school, Doctor Schumann began a legal career with the firm Callahan, McCune and Willis, working with the psychology defence team and automotive group. After about 10 years, he left and went to work as a Superior Court attorney with Riverside County, where he also sat as a judge *pro tem*. He left the public sector and went back into private practice around 2010 and worked in a boutique firm specialising in medical malpractice and personal injury defence.

Throughout his career, Doctor Schumann has kept in touch with academia as an instructor at UCI and UC-Riverside. He served on the Trial Court Judicial Attorneys Education Committee and taught courses at the California Center for Judicial Education and Research (CJER) Trial Judicial Attorneys' Institute.

Doctor Schumann is currently employed at the California law firm Callahan, Thompson, Sherman and Caudill LLP in the law and motion department.

Contexts

Science, Statistics and Psychology

The paper was published in 1987, just before DNA-based evidence began to become available as a means of identifying individuals and reconstructing criminal events. Like other developments in forensic science discussed in Chapter 4, it was the advent of DNA-based evidence that drove the need for a better understanding of statistical evidence and how to interpret it.

Psychology played a major part in gaining that understanding. The authors of this publication and others sat at the interface between science, the law and psychology. The impact of psychology on the development of forensic science is one of the major themes running through this book. Indeed, it should be recalled that a companion work of Hans Gross was on psychology, which at the time of publication, in the late nineteenth century, probably had as much impact as his Handbook. Chapter 8, on cognitive bias, explores more deeply the contribution psychology has made to the development of forensic science and justice more generally.

Our modern understanding of human behaviour and how human beings think began with the Nobel Prize-winning study by Kahneman and Tversky (Tversky and Kahneman 1974). It should be noted that psychology has impacted almost every sphere of human endeavour, from medicine, e.g. establishing a link between stress and heart disease, to justice and a better understanding of criminal behaviour and the limits of evidence and testimony.

History

Perhaps the most important event in 1987 was a speech by the then-US president Ronald Reagan, who, on a visit to what was West Berlin, called on the president of the Soviet Union, Mikhail Gorbachev, to remove the Berlin Wall. The wall came down just two years later in 1989.

October of that year included Black Monday, the stock market crash.

The Iran–Iraq war entered a new phase of increased hostilities, and the US Navy began to engage after the USS Stark was struck by an Iraqi-launched Exocet missile.

In the European Union, the Single European Act was passed, which aimed at removing trade barriers between member states.

However, there was no particular historical event or zeitgeist that prompted or encouraged a recognition of these fallacies. The publication is the product of a pure academic search for new knowledge. One of the multitude of examples of how research outcomes can have a major beneficial impact on society.

Structure of the Publication and Relevant Contents

General Structure

The publication has a total of 22 pages and is in four main sections: a lengthy introduction, the details of two experiments and a general discussion of the implications of the experimental results and the errors in thinking, and the two fallacies of the title. The publication concludes by suggesting some potential safeguards.

The abstract is as follows.

> *In criminal cases where the evidence shows a match between the defendant and the perpetrator on some characteristic, the jury often receives statistical evidence on the incidence rate of the 'matching' characteristic. Two experiments tested undergraduates ability to use such evidence appropriately when judging the probable guilt of a criminal suspect based on written descriptions of evidence. Experiment I varied whether incidence rate statistics were presented as conditional probabilities or as percentages and found the former promoted inferential errors favoring the prosecution while the latter produced more errors favoring the defense. Experiment 2 exposed subjects to two fallacious arguments on how to interpret the statistical evidence. The majority of subjects failed to detect the error in one or both of the arguments and made judgments consistent with fallacious reasoning.*
>
> *In both experiments a comparison of subjects' judgments to Bayesian norms revealed a general tendency to underutilize the statistical evidence. Theoretical and legal implications of these results are discussed.*

A more detailed structure is given further in the text.

Abstract
INTRODUCTION
EXPERIMENT 1
Method
- Subjects
- Procedure

Results
- Fallacious Judgements
- Initial and Final Judgements
- Comparing Subjects' Final Judgements to Model Bayesian Judgments

Discussion
EXPERIMENT 2
Method
Results and Discussion
- Recognition of Fallacious Arguments
- Fallacious Judgements
- Judgements of Probable Guilt

GENERAL DISCUSSION
Theoretical Implications
- Prosecutor's Fallacy
- Defence Attorney's Fallacy
- Underutilization of Associative Evidence

Legal Implications
REFERENCES

Introduction

The lengthy introduction presents the concept of associative evidence and its relationship with 'match'. The first type of statistical evidence discussed in support of evidence of a 'match' is the 'incidence rate'.

As explained earlier, the 'incidence rate' is the proportion of a population that shares a 'matching' characteristic, such as blood type. The authors state that a forensic scientist may give expert evidence that, say, 10% of the US population has a particular blood type. Other evidence types would be hair, glass, paint, etc. It should be noted in passing that today, these would be termed 'feature comparison' evidence types in which a human being is making the comparison. The subjectivity of the process increases the risk of errors in thinking (Spellman et al. 2022).

The next paragraph charts the reaction of US appellate courts (courts of appeal are often the highest courts in a jurisdiction) to that type of statistical evidence, the incidence rate, and introduces one of the questions addressed in the publication, what might a jury of non-specialist fact-finders make of this statistical evidence; would they attach too much or too little weight to such evidence? An equally important question is to what extent the lawyers litigating the case, and indeed the judge, make of this statistical evidence.

The introduction includes a comparative discussion of the related statistics, the 'base rate' and how it differs from the 'incidence rate'. As mentioned earlier, it is important to note that 'base rate' is synonymous with the Bayesian prior probability, the probability of an event or outcome before receiving new knowledge or information. The example given is of assessing the likelihood that an individual working in a particular building and owning a briefcase is a lawyer. The base rate statistic is the percentage of individuals who work in the building who are lawyers. The percentage of individuals who own briefcases is an incidence rate statistic.

A more appropriate example would be a teenage boy on trial for stealing a car. The relevant population is teenage boys. The base rate would be the proportion of teenage boys guilty of stealing a car, which would be quite low. In this example, a hair was found in the stolen car that 'matched' that of the defendant. The percentage of teenage boys with hair that 'matched' would be the incidence rate and would be high. Placing this scenario and these statistics in a Bayesian framework results in the following. The base rate is the prior probability. In the absence of any other information, a jury would initially predict that the probability of guilt would be quite low. However, once given the evidence of the 'matching' hair, the jury would update the prior and arrive at an increased probability of guilt. The earlier model of Bayesian reasoning should be recalled.

Prior Probability	×	**New Information**	=	Posterior Probability
Current Belief	×		=	Updated Belief

The key point is that in deciding guilt or not-guilt, the jury should take account of both the prior probability and the associative evidence of a 'match'. In a real case, the jury will hear other evidence, including other associative evidence, which might be contradictory. A high prior probability of not-guilt might outweigh a weak piece of associative evidence supporting guilt.

The publication draws an important conclusion, that human beings can attach inappropriate weight to base and incidence rate statistics. Indeed, the proposition that human beings are cognitively ill-equipped to process statistical information is one of the main conclusions of the publication. The propensity of human beings to make poor decisions based on statistical information was highlighted earlier, citing the seminal work of Tversky and Kahneman and made accessible in Kahneman's book 'Thinking Fast and Slow' (Kahneman 2012).

Ignoring or undervaluing the base rate or prior contributes to the prosecution fallacy. Undervaluing the incidence rate, the associative evidence of a 'match', results in the defence fallacy.

A simple example of undervaluing the base rate is stereotyping individuals. The example of the shy, retiring type being a librarian is given earlier.

In the publication, the authors offer more evidence of this undervaluing or attaching too little weight but highlight case law which demonstrates that US criminal courts generally reject base rate statistics.

The introduction goes on to raise another common error in reasoning, the notion that the probability of guilt can be calculated by subtracting the incidence rate from one or, as a percentage, 100%. This is an example of the Prosecutor's Fallacy. The example given is of a 'match' between the blood type of the defendant and the perpetrator. This associative evidence only occurs in 10% of the population. The error in reasoning occurs in believing that there is only a 10% chance that this 'match' would occur if the defendant were innocent, therefore, there is a 90% chance that he/she is guilty. The error is to ignore other evidence in the case, which, when weighed by the fact-finder or jury, may significantly alter the strength of the associative evidence. In addition, any evidence that significantly reduces the pool of people who are or could be suspects is highly probative.

These discussions prepare for the introduction of Bayesian reasoning discussed earlier and again in Chapter 6 on interpretation and the prosecutor's fallacy of the title. To recap, Bayesian reasoning involves updating belief (the probability of guilt/not-guilt) as new information (evidence) becomes available.

The defence attorney's fallacy is then introduced and described. As explained earlier, this fallacy arises from attaching too little weight or even ignoring the associative 'match' because even though the chance of the match is small, in population terms, the number of individuals who share that characteristic is large. The publication gives an example based on a rare blood type. The blood type in question is shared by only 1% of a city's population of 1 million. However, that equates to 10 000 people with that blood type. The defence fallaciously argues that the 1% chance of a 'matching' blood group carries little evidential weight as it is found in a large number of individuals. This argument ignores the fact that the great majority of individuals with this blood type are not on trial, accused of a crime supported by other evidence. This fallacy was used in the trial of O.J. Simpson, referred to earlier.

O.J. Simpson Case Again

The trial of O.J. Simpson provided another real-world example of this fallacious argument. The defence argued that there was only one woman murdered for every 2500 women who were subjected to spousal abuse, and that any history of Simpson being violent toward his wife was irrelevant to the trial. However, the reasoning behind the defence's calculation was flawed. According to author Gerd Gigerenzer, the correct

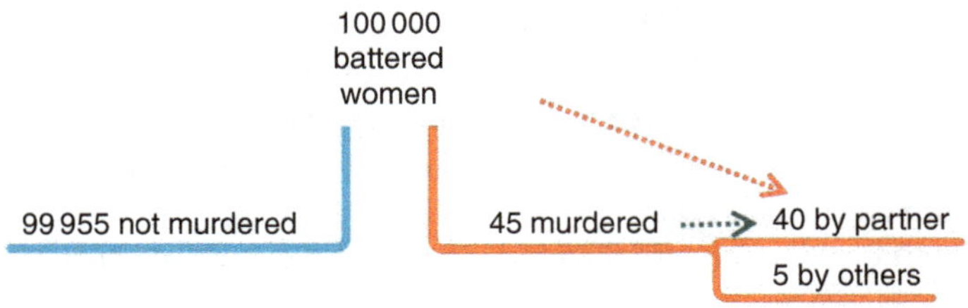

Figure 5.1 Number of women murdered by an abusive partner – after Gigerenzer.

probability requires additional context: Simpson's wife had not only been subjected to domestic violence but rather subjected to domestic violence (by Simpson) and killed (by someone). Gigerenzer writes as follows.

> *[T]he chances that a batterer actually murdered his partner, given that she has been killed, is about 8 in 9 or approximately 90%... While most cases of spousal abuse do not end in murder, most cases of murder where there is a history of spousal abuse were committed by the spouse.*
>
> *(Gigerenzer 2003)*

The correct proportion is 40 of 45 and not 40 of 100 000, as demonstrated in Figure 5.1.

In addition to the O.J. Simpson case, the authors refer to other cases where this fallacious argument may have held sway.

Having identified the fallacies, the introduction goes on to consider how they might arise in the presentation of statistical evidence. However, in doing so, the authors have strayed into an area that is avoided by forensic scientists, presenting evidence in terms of supporting or not supporting guilt. Such considerations are essential for the publication, but examples of experts opining on the chance of the match occurring if the defendant were innocent should not be presented by a forensic scientist giving expert evidence. Having said that, the introduction here gives examples of the potential for both fallacies and their consequences.

To determine whether and to what degree the presentation of statistical evidence might affect the understanding by a jury, the publication records two experiments which lead to the next section of the paper, Experiment 1.

Experiment 1

In this experiment, the subjects were asked to estimate the likelihood of guilt based in part on the incidence rate of a 'match'. The evidence supporting a 'match' was delivered in two ways.

1. The expert presented only the conditional probability that an innocent person would have the 'matching' characteristic.
2. '... the expert stated the percentage of the population who possess the relevant characteristic and the approximate number of people who possess this characteristic in the city where the crime occurred, as a percentage and numbers.'

The details of the experiment are recorded. The subjects were university students playing the role of a fact-finder or jury member[8]. They were provided with instructions and background information and asked to estimate the likelihood of guilt. Relevant information was given in stages. The subjects were first asked to estimate guilt based on the circumstances of the crime, the circumstantial evidence alone.

They were then given expert evidence on hair matching in the ways described above.

1. As a conditional probability) There is only a 2% chance the defendant's hair would be distinguishable from that of the perpetrator, IF he were innocent, the condition.
2. (Percentage and numbers) A study indicated that only 2% of people have hair that would be indistinguishable from that of the defendant and stated that in a city of one million people, there would be approximately 20 000 such individuals.

The subjects then made a final estimate of the probability of the defendant's guilt.

The results demonstrated that about one quarter of the subjects made final estimates of guilt consistent with their having fallen victim to one of the fallacies. Of those, about half fell victim to the prosecutor's fallacy, subtracting the 2% from 100% and estimating the probability of guilt as 98%. The other half fell victim to the defence attorney's fallacy as their final estimate of guilt was the same as the initial estimate, attaching no weight to the associative evidence of a 'match'.

This emphasises the challenge in presenting statistical evidence. Fortunately, some progress has been made since 1987 in communicating this type of evidence to the fact-finder, as discussed in Chapter 6 on interpreting evidence. However, as mentioned earlier and discussed later in this chapter under current practice, there is still work to do to ensure that statistical evidence in forensic science is presented competently, fairly and understood by all parties.

Further analysis demonstrated that the way the statistical evidence was presented made one fallacy or the other more likely. When presented as a conditional probability, the prosecutor's fallacy was more likely (20% compared to 8%). When presented as a percentage and numbers, the defence attorney's fallacy was more likely (17% compared to 4%).

These results and their analysis demonstrated the following.

> *... that the manner in which incidence rate statistics were presented had an important effect on subjects' judgments of probable guilt.*

The authors then analysed the results using Bayesian reasoning. They found that the subjects updating the probability of guilt in the light of the conditional probability of a 'match' was conservative, i.e. their estimate of the probability of guilt (63%) was lower than that calculated using Bayes' theorem (93%). This conservatism is supported by other studies (Edwards 1968).

In the discussion that follows, many of the above points were repeated. However, it did include what is perhaps the simplest expression of the prosecutor's fallacy, the so-called transposition of the conditional and the fallacious equivalence.

> *... falsely assumed the conditional probability of a 'match' given innocence is the complement* [i.e. 1–] *of the conditional probability of guilt given a 'match'.*

Essentially, the probability of the 'match' if innocent is not the same or equal to the probability of a 'match' if guilty, assuming that they are, is the fallacy simply stated. As recorded earlier, this is expressed mathematically as follows.

$$p(X|Y) \neq p(Y|X)$$

This is swapping or transposing the conditional discussed earlier, and to repeat the earlier example, it is the logical equivalent of arguing that the cat is a cow because it has four legs.

Transposing the conditional is a form of the prosecutor's fallacy that occurs in forensic science. Unless the forensic scientist giving expert evidence is competent and understands the evidence presented, it is a very easy mistake to make. To repeat the point, the prosecutor's fallacy can unfairly strengthen the evidence in favour of the prosecution, and so a forensic scientist committing this fallacy is giving misleading evidence and increasing the risk of a miscarriage of justice.

Experiment 2

The scenario presented involved associative evidence of a rare blood group shared by just 1% of the population and an estimated probability of guilt, a prior probability. This was in contrast with the first experiment in which the proxy jury of students was not given a prior but had to estimate it themselves. In this experiment, two arguments were presented to the proxy fact-finders; one in the form of the prosecutor's fallacy, stating the following.

> *Since there is only a 1% chance that someone else committed the crime there is a 99% chance that the suspect is guilty.*

The other argument was in the form of the defence fallacy, arguing that because the population of the city was 200 000, there would be 2000 people with this blood group.

The students were invited to revise the prior probability of guilt in the light of the associative evidence of a 'matching' blood type.

Worryingly, and in support of the view that the concepts in play are hard to understand, the fallacies went unrecognised by most students, and all fell victim.

Most of the responses were consistent with the defence fallacy, apparently disregarding the associative evidence of a 'match' altogether.

Overall, the students gave less weight to the associative evidence than it warranted, as a result, they were biased in favour of the defence. This, to some extent, is comforting in that the proxy jury was more likely to wrongfully acquit than wrongfully convict.

Perhaps O.J. Simpson's defence team had studied this paper as part of their trial preparation! As mentioned earlier, they relied on the defence fallacy to argue their case. Based on blood type, there was a '*stadium full*' of other suspects.

Discussion and Conclusion

Much of the text is a statistical analysis of the results obtained from the two experiments and an interpretation of that analysis. Regarding the experiments conducted, not too much weight can be attached to the results or their interpretation because of the nature of the proxy jury not being representative of a typical jury. In addition, no discussion occurred between the students as would have occurred among real jurors. Furthermore, the outcomes were probabilities rather than the binary decision to convict or acquit. However, in terms of revealing how easy it is to fall victim to these fallacies and the consequent challenges faced by those presenting statistical evidence, the experiments were a success.

The final sentence in the publication is an expression of hope and a call to action as follows.

> *Our hope is that social scientists, building on studies like those reported here, will be able to answer the key underlying behavioral questions so that lawyers and judges may base decisions about mathematical evidence on empirical data rather than unguided intuitions.*

Impact at the Time

At the time of publication in 1987, it found little traction even among lawyers. It wasn't until the advent of DNA analysis (Chapter 4), the adoption by some of the likelihood ratio approach to interpretation (Chapter 6, 1995) and a recognition of the impact of cognitive bias (Chapter 8, 2002) that these fallacies acquired significance in forensic science. The main risk in forensic science is the transposed conditional, which, as mentioned earlier, unfairly strengthens evidence in favour of the prosecution.

Figure 5.2 is a graph from Semantic Scholar which shows that the publication began to get traction in the early 2000s with the first spike in citations in 2009, coincidentally, the year the National Academies report was published, the subject of Chapter 9. DNA profiling took off with SGM (single-gamete multiplex) and six-locus probes in the late 1990s, as charted in Chapter 4.

Impact Today

By all accounts, these fallacies still plague the presentation of statistical evidence (Kilberger 2023). The main contributors to this blight are a lack of competence on the part of scientists presenting such evidence and a lack of awareness on the part of lawyers and judges. Lawyers and judges may rarely encounter scientific evidence in their careers and are therefore ill-equipped to recognise these fallacies and guard against them. Worryingly, if lawyers are competent, then they may advance these fallacies as a means of 'winning' the case, as in the O.J. Simpson trial.

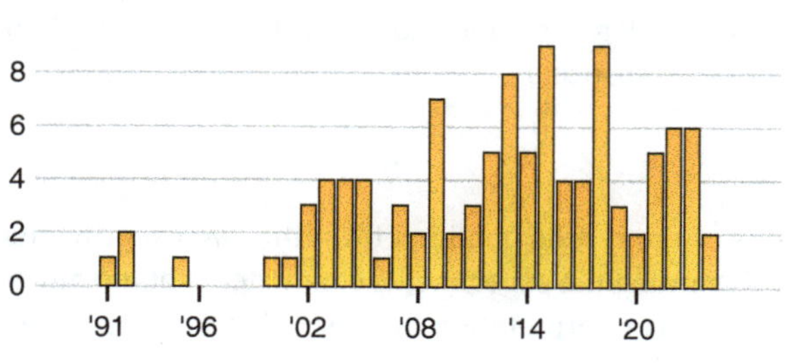

Figure 5.2 Citations.

There is also a lack of complete consensus within the forensic science community as to whether and how probabilistic evidence should be presented. This issue will be discussed further in Chapter 6.

Contribution to Current Practice

The principal contribution of the publication to current practice was to raise awareness among justice system stakeholders of logical errors known as the prosecutor's and defence attorney's fallacies; their nature and how they might be identified, recognised and prevented. The transposed conditional being a particular risk in forensic science.

Despite many treatises explaining the transposed conditional or prosecutor's fallacy and how to avoid it, e.g. Evett (1995), Aitkin et al. (2010) and Hicks et al. (2022), it remains one of the most common errors forensic scientists make when giving expert evidence, e.g. Koehler et al. (2023), Semikhodskii (2022) and courts in understanding the fallacy (Robertson et al. 2011).

It should not be too difficult to recognise that a cow having four legs does not mean that every animal that has four legs is a cow!!!

Responsibility for the lack of competence and awareness rests with universities, forensic science providers, litigators and judges. An awareness and a proper understanding of these logical errors will help to reduce the risk of a miscarriage of justice. There is much guidance available. In the United Kingdom, the Royal Statistical Society has published several guides (Royal Statistical Society 2010–2015), the Royal Society has also published a guide (The Royal Society and The Royal Society of Edinburgh 2020) and in the United States, the 'Reference Manual of Scientific Evidence' (Federal Judicial Center 2011). Universities offering degrees in forensic science or a related subject should ensure students fully understand these logical fallacies and how to avoid them. Forensic science providers should confirm such competence before allowing staff to give expert evidence. There is no excuse for a lack of awareness of these fallacies and their potential for contributing to a miscarriage of justice. Indeed, unless scientists, lawyers and judges can recognise and avoid these logical errors, miscarriages of justice will remain a risk.

The avoidance of the defence attorney's fallacy is perhaps the greater challenge, as defences may well utilise the fallacy to their advantage. Therefore, judicial authorities should ensure that judges can recognise the fallacy and reduce the risk of a miscarriage of justice.

Concluding Remarks

While these fallacies are well-characterised, there is much evidence that they remain extant in practice and can and have contributed to miscarriages of justice.

Bringing these fallacies to the attention of forensic scientists was an important step in the development of the probabilistic presentation of scientific evidence called for by Kirk in his Ontogeny paper, Chapter 3. The next stage of this development will be discussed in Chapter 6 on interpreting evidence.

Key Takeaways

This publication, building on the work of Tversky and Kahneman, demonstrates through experiments that human beings are ill-equipped to process statistical information and need guidance to do so.

In their paper, Thompson and Schumann introduce the terms 'Prosecutor's' and 'Defense Attorney's' fallacies.

The prosecutor's fallacy occurs when the probability of the evidence given guilt is incorrectly interpreted as the probability of guilt given the evidence.

The defence attorney's fallacy occurs when it is reported how many people with the matching characteristics are likely to be found in a defined population. This assumes that the accused is part of some arbitrarily large population and that there is no other information available.

If unrecognised, these logical errors can lead the fact-finder or jury to attach unwarranted weight to statistical evidence. In the case of the prosecutor's fallacy, which might unfairly strengthen the prosecution case, risking a wrongful conviction. Conversely, the defence fallacy might unfairly strengthen the defence case, risking a wrongful acquittal.

To reduce the risk, scientists, lawyers and judges must be aware of, understand and avoid these logical errors and ensure that the fact-finder or jury is properly instructed on how to weigh statistical evidence. This can only be achieved by appropriate training.

For forensic scientists giving statistical evidence, the greatest risk is from the prosecutor's fallacy and transposing the conditional; considering the probability of guilt IF the evidence is true ($pH|E$) rather than the probability of the evidence IF the accused is guilty ($pE|H$). It is the logical equivalent of deciding that because a cat has four legs, it must be a cow! ($pX|Y \neq pY|X$).

Transposing the conditional is avoided by remembering that interpretation is based on considering the probability of the evidence. This is the role of a forensic scientist acting as an expert witness and requires disciplined thinking.

Notes

1 Fact-finder is a more generic term than jury, a jury is the fact-finder in most criminal trials in common law jurisdictions such as those of the United States. However, there are jurisdictions where a justice will undertake the role of fact-finder, and in some instances that is also the case in common law jurisdictions.

2 The importance and impact of this paper can be measured by the number of times the paper has been cited; one source has 7369. Daniel Kahneman went on to write a book based on his work with Tversky called 'Thinking Fast and Slow'. It has been on many bestsellers' lists and is considered one of the most influential books of the twentieth century. It has sold over 10 million copies.

3 In a criminal trial the fact-finder, e.g. a jury, must consider all the evidence presented, some of which might be contradictory. As should be clear from earlier chapters, human testimony can be unreliable, so if eyewitness evidence is contradicted by physical evidence, the jury might attach more weight to the physical evidence.

4 The convention is to use H, hypothesis, with the subscript P for the prosecution and D for the defence; H is simply the case.

5 This term is used instead of 'innocence' as the fact-finder must initially presume innocence. The decision for the fact-finder is guilty or not guilty.

6 Social ecology is a social science that studies how people interact with their environment and how those interactions impact society and the environment.

7 Lucy Letby is a British nurse convicted of murdering babies (Rachel 2024). Also, see Times Radio podcast 'The Story' https://shows.acast.com/storiesofourtimes/episodes/why-some-experts-are-doubting-lucy-letbys-conviction.

8 This was one recognised weakness in the study, fact-finders/jurors deliberate and make decisions as a group and not as individuals.

Bibliography

Aitkin, Colin, Paul Roberts, and Graham Jackson. 2010. *Fundamentals of Probability and Statistical Evidence in Criminal Proceedings*. London: Royal Statistical Society.

Batty, David. 2005. "Timeline: Sir Roy Meadow." *The Guardian*, 15 July.

Edwards, W. 1968. "Conservatism in Human Information Processing." In *Formal Representation of Human Judgment*, edited by B. Kleinmuntz, 17–52. New York: John Wiley & Sons.

Evett, Ian. 1995. "Avoiding the Transposed Conditional." *Science and Justice* 35: 127–31.

Federal Judicial Center. 2011. *Reference Manual on Scientific Evidence 3rd Edition*. Washington, DC: National Academies Press.

Fenton, Norman, and Martin Neil. 2011. "Avoiding Probabilistic Reasoning Fallacies in Legal Practice Using Bayesian Networks." *Australian Journal of Legal Philosophy* 36: 114–51.

Gigerenzer, Gerd. 2003. "8 Wife Battering." In *Reckoning with Risk: Learning to Live with Uncertainty*, edited by Gerd Gigerenzer. Penguin.

Hicks, Tacha, John Buckleton, Vincent Castella, Ian Evett, and Graham Jackson. 2022. "A Logical Framework for Forensic DNA Interpretation." *Genes* 13: 1–26.

Kahneman, Daniel. 2012. *Thinking Fast and Slow*. Penguin.

Kaye, David H. 2010. *The Double Helix and the Law of Evidence*. Harvard University Press.

Kilberger, Kendall Brooke. 2023. "Something Doesn't Add Up: Solving DNA Forensic Science Statistical Fallacies in Trial Testimony." *Vanderbilt Journal of Entertainment and Technology Law* 25: 181–209.

Koehler, Jonathan J., Jennifer L. Mnookin, and Michael J. Saks. 2023. "The scientific reinvention of forensic science." *Proceedings of the National Academy of Sciences* 120 (41): 1–10.

R v Clark, Sally. 2003. Crim 1020 (EWCA, 11 April).

Rachel, Aviv. 2024. "A British Nurse Was Found Guilty of Killing Seven Babies. Did She Do It?" *The New Yorker*, 13 May.

Robertson, Bernard W., G. A. Vignaux, and Charles E. H. Berger. 2011. "Extending the Confusion About Bayes." *Modern Law Review* 74: 1–16.

Robertson, Bernard, G. A. Vignaux, and Charles E. H. Berger. 2016. "Transposing the Conditional." In *Interpreting Evidence: Evaluating Forensic Science in the Courtroom*, edited by Bernard Robertson, G. A. Vignaux and Charles E. H. Berger, 17. Chichester: John Wiley & Sons.

Royal Statistical Society – Statistics and the Law Section. 2022. "Statistics and the Law." *Royal Statistical Society*. September. Accessed November 21, 2024. https://rss.org.uk/RSS/media/

File-library/News/2022/Summary_Healthcare_serial_killer_or_coincidence_statistical_issues_in_investigation_of_suspected_medical_misconduct_September_2022_FINAL.pdf.

Royal Statistical Society. 2010–2015. *Statistical Guides*. Accessed November 11, 2024. https://rss.org.uk/news-publication/publications/law-guides/.

Semikhodskii, A. 2022. "Logical Errors and Fallacies in DNA Evidence Interpretation." In *Handbook of DNA Profiling*, edited by H. R. Dash, P. Shrivastava and J. A. Lorente, 799–820. Singapore: Springer.

Spellman, Barbara A., Heidi Eldridge, and Paul Bieber. 2022. "Challenges to Reasoning in Forensic Science Decisions." *Forensic Science International: Synergy* 4: 100200.

The Royal Society and The Royal Society of Edinburgh. 2020. *The Use of Statistics in Legal Proceedings: A Primer for Courts*. London: The Royal Society.

Tversky, Amos, and Daniel Kahneman. 1974. "Judgment Under Uncertainty: Heuristics and Biases." *Science* 185: 1124–31.

6

Interpreting Evidence – The Likelihood Ratio

Name of the Publication

The publication is titled *Interpreting Evidence: Evaluating Forensic Science in the Courtroom.* Bernard Robertson and G. A. Vignaux, John Wiley & Sons, 1995, Chichester, ISBN 0471 96026 8.

The publication has xxi and 240 pages.

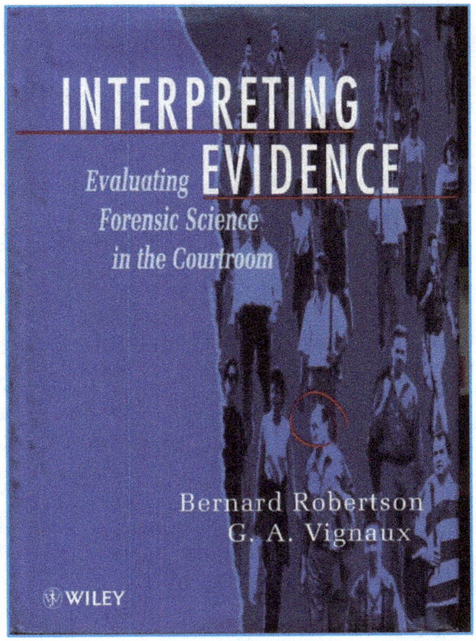

Image 6.1 Cover of the first edition 1995. Robertson et al. (1995)/with permission of John Wiley & Sons.

Introduction

The subject of this chapter is the first edition of the publication. A second edition was published in 66 (Robertson et al. 2016). For forensic scientists, lawyers and judges, this later edition is the one to study. It introduces some new concepts such as case assessment and interpretation (CAI), the hierarchy of propositions and the use of Bayesian networks to evaluate different types of evidence in combination[1]. The later edition has been restructured, making it an easier read and has deleted obsolete evidence types such as blood grouping and included the evaluation of DNA evidence. It also includes the discussion of some important judgements, particularly the controversial judgement of the England and Wales Appeal Court, *R v T* (R v T 2010).

However, from a historical perspective and in terms of the eventual impact on the development of forensic science, the first edition will be the subject of this chapter. It was the first codification or collective statement in one volume of the logical principles that had been developing for some time among pioneering statisticians and forensic scientists such as Ian Evett, John Buckleton, Colin Aitken, David Stoney, and Dennis Lindley (1923–2013)

A History of Forensic Science in 10 Publications: How They Established Current Practice, First Edition.
Sean Doyle.

as collected in the 1991 publication 'The Use of Statistics in Forensic Science' (Aitken and Stoney 1991). The fact that 'Interpreting Evidence' was written by a lawyer and a statistician, both New Zealanders, and not by European forensic scientists, gave it some added authority as a statement of good practice in interpreting scientific evidence.

The book is peppered with case examples that help to explain and support the principles introduced. Indeed, most of the text is devoted to these examples, which serve to drive home the principles promoted in the book.

For the non-specialist reader, this chapter may be a challenge. However, in the simplest of terms, it introduces, promotes and explains by way of examples the impacts and consequences of the likelihood ratio (LR), first mentioned in Chapter 5, and its effectiveness as a means of expressing the strength of evidence. As explained in Chapter 5, it is a ratio of conditional probabilities, i.e. probabilities including a condition identified by 'IF'. In a forensic context, these are generally the likelihood of a 'match' between two items IF they came from the same source and the likelihood of a 'match' between the same two items IF they came from different sources (these are also known as the two hypotheses, propositions or assertions). The IF is emphasised as it signals the condition. The LR is a measure of the strength of the scientific evidence and can be used to update previous or prior beliefs about the probability of an event (known as the prior probability) to form a new belief about the probability of the same event (known as the posterior probability).

Recalling the relationship from Chapter 5.

$$\text{Posterior Probability} = \text{LR} \times \text{Prior Probability}$$

Using a case example from the earlier chapter, the LR is the probability of a 'match' between a reference bullet (test fired from the alleged murder weapon) and the questioned bullet (that killed the victim) IF the gun is the murder weapon, divided by the probability of a 'match' IF it's not. As readers should now be aware, the LR is expressed mathematically in the following equation, where E is the evidence and H_p and H_d are the prosecution case and defence case, respectively.

$$\text{LR} = \frac{p(E|H_p)}{P(E|H_d)}$$

The publication demonstrates that using the LR to update the prior belief of the fact-finder or jury is logical, rational and conforms to the requirements of the law. It asserts that the LR and its verbal equivalent are the only evidence a forensic scientist can give.

A knowledge and understanding of the principles presented in this book and those derived later are perhaps the most important for the practising forensic scientists and lawyers engaged in litigating cases in which scientific evidence will play a part. For forensic scientists, this publication is effectively an instruction manual on how to present scientific evidence logically and rationally, to avoid misleading the court or other tribunal of fact and risking a miscarriage of justice. Conforming to those principles also ensures that the forensic scientist giving expert evidence does not usurp the role of the fact-finder or jury. It also reduces the risk of cognitive bias, the subject of Chapter 8 'Observer Effects', and prevents the expert from wandering outside his or her field of expertise. All essential requirements for a competent forensic scientist assisting a court in interpreting scientific evidence.

These requirements are met by adopting a likelihood ratio approach to interpretation. The publication introduces the concept of the likelihood ratio as a measure of the strength of evidence and explains its function and impact employing numerous examples. It is probably no exaggeration to state that the likelihood ratio is one of the most important concepts in forensic science and, indeed, tool available to the forensic scientist to help the court understand the strength of the scientific evidence. 'Interpreting Evidence' is a must read for forensic scientists who may act as expert witnesses.

In a sense, this publication picks up where Thompson and Schumann (Chapter 5) left off. The book covers the prosecutor's and defender's fallacies but in greater depth, giving real-world case examples. In addition, the scope is such as to include and promote a set of logical principles that, if adhered to, will ensure that forensic scientists, lawyers and judges will better serve justice.

Ian Evett, one of the pioneers mentioned earlier, a world-renowned expert in the field and a long-time advocate for a logical approach to interpreting evidence, is quoted as follows.

> *I am sure that this will become a standard work for all who need to understand the logic of evaluating evidence.*

Unfortunately for justice, the evidence is that it is yet, some 30 years later, to become a standard work and forensic scientists even today are failing justice by not understanding the logical principles set out in this publication and applying them. Equally disappointing, or even perhaps more so, is the lack of understanding by lawyers and judges, as evidenced in the latest edition of the publication (Robertson et al. 2016).

The most fundamental principle to be understood by all involved in the judicial process is that the correct interpretation of scientific evidence is best achieved by using the likelihood ratio to convey the strength of that evidence.

One reason for the slow progress may be that the approach is seemingly counterintuitive. The object of the court is to determine the probability of guilt given the evidence presented, in mathematical terms $p(H|E)$, whereas following the principles of the book the scientist giving expert evidence must only consider the probability of the evidence if the prosecution or defence case is true, $p(E|H)$.

For the non-specialist reader, the most important point to keep in mind is that the scientist must only consider the probability of the evidence $p(E)$ and never the probability of the prosecution or defence case $p(H)$.

Just to recap, adopting the likelihood ratio approach to interpretation has the following advantages.

- The scientific evidence is logical, rational and conforms to the requirements of the law.
- The expert does not usurp the role of the fact-finder.
- The risk of cognitive bias is reduced.
- The expert remains within his or her field of expertise.

According to the authors, the book began life as a project examining the applicability of logical and probabilistic reasoning to evidence. A survey of forensic science practice revealed an inconsistent approach to the interpretation of evidence, from fingerprint examiners' categorical opinions – include/exclude/inconclusive – to DNA experts conducting statistical analysis and reporting probabilistically – more likely to be the suspect than anyone else. The authors found the law to be equally inconsistent.

The remedy, as the authors saw it, was to apply a few basic logical principles to the interpretational issues identified, thus providing a coherent outcome that was independent of evidence type or jurisdiction.

Recognition by the authors, and many others, that current models of presenting evidence were illogical and misleading; something needed to be done. In addition, it was quite clear to the authors that communication between lawyers and scientists needed improvement, and so their book was designed to be read and understood by both parties.

In the text, the authors announce that their book is part of a movement to re-evaluate scientific evidence and is the first to codify the evaluative framework in a single volume. The authors also state an ambition that forensic science be considered the science of interpretation.

Biography of the Publication

The genesis of the publication is probably the 1975 paper by Dennis Lindley asserting the superiority and utility of Bayesian inference (Lindley 1975). Bayesian inference (or reasoning) was discussed in Chapter 5 and earlier in this chapter; essentially, it involves updating existing beliefs based on new evidence and, more broadly, reasoning under uncertainty.

The work of Lindley certainly influenced Ian Evett as he records in his essay in 'The Use of Statistics in Forensic Science' (Evett 1991). In fact, 'Interpreting Evidence' identifies Dr Evett as one of its progenitors.

In 1992, the authors wrote a paper based on a conference presentation on the law and logic. (Robertson and Vignaux 1992). In this paper, the authors discuss how expert evidence should be presented, evaluated and understood. They introduce Bayesian inference as a means of assessing the strength of evidence by assigning a likelihood ratio.

In 1993, Robertson and Vignaux made a further attempt to marry Bayesian inference and the law (Robertson and Vignaux 1993). The paper calls for Bayesian inference to underpin the evaluation of evidence and makes many of the points made in the publication.

Indeed, these two papers pretty much provide the raw material for 'Interpreting Evidence'. What began life as a project within 'New Evidence Scholarship'[2] is now in its second edition.

Professional Biography of the Authors

There is not much biographical detail about these authors publicly available.

At the time of publication, Bernard Robertson KC, a Barrister-at-Law, was a member of the Department of Business Law at Massey University, New Zealand and G A (Tony) Vignaux, a member of the Institute of Statistics and Operations Research at Victoria University of Wellington, New Zealand.

Mr Robertson is the former president of the Law and Economics Association of New Zealand (2009–2014).

According to a biography in the public domain and written by Mr Robertson in 1997, 'Bernard Robertson came to New Zealand in 1989 with a degree in law from Oxford and a Master's Degree in law from London. He is also qualified as a Barrister of the Inner Temple. Earlier, he had a career in the Metropolitan Police, which included attending the 12-month Special Course at the Police Staff College, Bramshill. In New Zealand, he has taught at the Victoria University of Wellington Faculty of Law and at the Department of Business Law at Massey University. Constitutional law has been one of Mr Robertson's specialities throughout. He has published numerous shorter articles and book reviews on public law matters and has recently published a paper on the Reserve Bank of New Zealand Act 1989 in the Oxford Journal of Legal Studies. Mr Robertson is now Editor of The New Zealand Law Journal and a freelance writer, researcher and teacher.'

Bernard Robertson KC now styles himself as a Barrister and Tony Vignaux as Professor Emeritus of Mathematics and Statistics at the University of Wellington, New Zealand.

Contexts

This publication stands out as the most isolated in this book from the broader scientific, historical, and social contexts of the time. It emerged from a small group of statisticians, scientists, and lawyers who collectively recognised the logical flaws in interpretational practice at the time. They then embarked on a concerted effort to alert forensic scientists and lawyers to the potential threat to justice posed by misleading evidence and to propose a logical and rational approach to interpretation.

One important context is the amount of pushback they originally received, and in some quarters, continue to do so. This pushback ranged from rejection of the fundamentals to the challenges of communication. However, the approach to evaluation advocated in this publication merely requires the forensic scientist giving expert evidence to state whether the probability of his or her findings is more likely if either the defence or prosecution case is true, in simpler terms, that the evidence is more supportive of either the prosecution or defence case.

However, applying the principles set out and promoted in the publication has certainly led to a major impact on science and the law, as will be discussed later in this chapter.

Structure of the Publication and Relevant Contents

The book has 240 pages and twelve chapters. It also includes a table of relevant cases and legislation, appendices and a selected bibliography.

The titles of the chapters are as follows.

Chapter 1 INTRODUCTION
Chapter 2 INTERPRETING SCIENTIFIC EVIDENCE
Chapter 3 THE ALTERNATIVE HYPOTHESIS

Chapter 4 EXPLAINING THE STRENGTH OF THE EVIDENCE
Chapter 5 THE CASE AS A WHOLE
Chapter 6 ERRORS IN THINKING
Chapter 7 CLASSICAL STATISTICS AND DATABASE MATCHING
Chapter 8 TRANSFER EVIDENCE
Chapter 9 BLOOD AND DNA EVIDENCE
Chapter 10 OTHER SCIENTIFIC EVIDENCE
Chapter 11 IMPLICATIONS FOR THE LEGAL SYSTEM
Chapter 12 CONCLUSIONS

Chapter 1 Introduction

This chapter is an introduction to the book, setting out what the authors consider to be the purpose of forensic science, which is to help establish the identity of criminals and reconstruct events. It then presents an ideal method of identifying criminals which DNA analysis may provide.

One important point is made: that in science, nothing is certain. This is a difficulty for the law as justice requires certainty to bring finality. The only conclusions available in a criminal trial are guilt or not guilt. This point leads to one of the main purposes of the book, which is to explain how 'uncertain' scientific evidence should be presented, to ensure the court (or other tribunal of fact) reaches a safe decision by a fair process.

Finally, the chapter documents the book's coverage.

- The fundamentals of logical reasoning will be explained.
- Fallacies will be discussed.
- It will be argued that the principles set out in the book apply to all types of scientific evidence, are universally applicable, giving examples in support.
- Legal aspects of the principles will be considered and recommendations made.

Chapter 2 Interpreting Scientific Evidence

This chapter considers how to interpret a single item of evidence. It first mentions two essential requirements for all evidence in common law jurisdictions: the evidence must be relevant to proving the facts in issue and must have probative value, i.e. be capable of helping to prove something. Only evidence that is relevant and has probative value can be admitted[3]. In the case of a shooting, the finding of gunshot residues on the hand of the alleged shooter would be both relevant to the question – did the suspect discharge a firearm? – and have probative value.

There follows an introduction to the concepts of probability and odds, which the authors acknowledge '*breaks the flow*' of the book but is considered so essential to their arguments that some '*revision*' is required.

Probability has been covered in the earlier chapter on fallacies, Chapter 5. A probability of one or 100% represents certainty (impossible in science!), and a probability of zero or 0% represents impossibility. Probabilities usually fall between these two extremes, e.g. based on the knowledge of weather patterns gained over a substantial period, a 50% chance of rain tomorrow is predicted.

Odds are explained as another means of expressing probabilities. This will be familiar to those who gamble. A 50% probability is described as 1 to 1 or 'evens' and is calculated thus:

$$\text{Odds} = \frac{0.5}{(1-0.5)} = \frac{0.5}{0.5} = \frac{5}{5} = \frac{1}{1}$$

The chapter then introduces the likelihood ratio and Bayes' Rule or Theorem. Again, these concepts have been well covered earlier in this chapter and Chapter 5. They are also explained in the section on Terms, Definitions and Explanations.

The likelihood ratio is introduced with an example of testing for alcohol in the breath. Probably a type of test familiar to many. Such testing devices usually provide a yes/no response to the question: Is the driver over the legal limit? The testing device has been calibrated and shown to have a 95% chance of returning a true positive result and a 5% chance of returning a false positive result.

Recalling that the equation for the LR is as follows:

$$LR = \frac{p(E|H_p)}{P(E|H_d)}$$

In this example, that is the probability of the evidence, a 'yes' result, IF the driver is over the limit, divided by the probability of a 'yes' result IF the driver is not over the limit, IF signalling the condition.

$$LR = \frac{\text{Probability of 'yes' if over the limit}}{\text{Probability of 'yes' if not over the limit}} = \frac{95}{0.5} = 190$$

The result is that the evidence is 190 times more likely if the driver is over the limit than not. This introduces the concept of the strength of evidence. LR is a measure of the strength of evidence.

It is very important to note that there are essentially only three outcomes from assigning a likelihood ratio.

1. LR > (is greater than) 1, the evidence supports the prosecution case; the driver is over the limit, or the gun is the murder weapon. The evidence is more likely if the prosecution case is true.
2. LR ≈ (close to) 1, the evidence is irrelevant, lacks probative value and should not be admitted.[4]
3. LR < (is less than) 1, the evidence supports the defence case; the driver is not over the limit; the gun is not the murder weapon. The evidence is more likely if the defence case is true.

The chapter then introduces Bayes' Rule or Theorem; again, this should now be familiar.

$$\text{Prior Probability} \times LR = \text{Posterior Probability}$$

The rule tells us how to update beliefs in the light of new information.

There is then a discussion on the effect of the prior probability. Here we get into difficult territory as mapping Bayes' rule onto the judicial process, the prior odds are the domain of the fact-finder or jury and not the forensic scientist. The jury will hear all the evidence and, as in the examples given in Chapter 5, it will apply the LR given by the expert witness to its current understanding of the case. As has been demonstrated, and is indeed the case, a strong prior may not be shifted by a high LR, in practical terms scientific evidence in support of the defence case might not shift the fact-finder's belief in the guilt of the defendant based on compelling evidence for the prosecution, e.g. a DNA 'match'. The effect of a strong prior was discussed in Chapter 5.

To be fair, the authors do go on to emphasise that all the forensic scientist giving expert evidence can present is the LR and that assessing the prior probability is '*... the job of the court*'.

> *... expert evidence should be restricted to the likelihood ratio given by the test or observation (or its components.)*

The chapter goes on to introduce one of the key fallacies: transposing the conditional, which is also known as the prosecutor's fallacy. This is one of the two fallacies discussed at length in Chapter 5, but in this publication, as is always the case, supporting examples are given. To recap, the fallacy, for example, equates the probability that an animal has four legs if it's a cow with the probability that an animal is a cow if it has four legs; those probabilities are not equal. The fallacy is graphically demonstrated in Figure 6.1.

Using the case example of a 'match' between the bullet that killed the victim and a bullet test fired from the suspect's gun, Table 6.1 should help identify the fallacy.

Transposing the conditional is termed the prosecutor's fallacy because, as explained in Chapter 5, it can unfairly strengthen evidence in favour of the prosecution. In the mind of the fact-finder, it is now the probability that the gun is the murder weapon that is now being considered. A high probability of a 'match' does not equate to a high probability that the gun is the murder weapon.

From a legal perspective, it favours the prosecution because it effectively shifts the burden of proof onto the defence.

What this chapter also reveals is that if an expert witness does give in evidence the probability of the hypothesis – the prosecution or defence case – i.e. $p(H|E)$ in logic, the expert

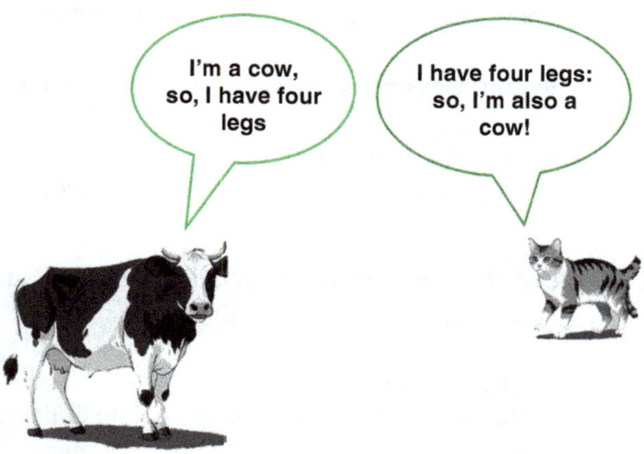
I'm a cow, so, I have four legs
I have four legs: so, I'm also a cow!

Figure 6.1 The logical fallacy of the transposed conditional.

Table 6.1 Identifying the transposed conditionals.

The Probability	The Conditional	
... of a 'match'	IF the gun is the murder weapon	✓
... that the gun is the murder weapon	IF there is a 'match'	×

must be assuming some prior and by doing so is usurping the role of the jury. So, in addition to being wrong in logic, having fallen into the trap of the prosecutor's fallacy and transposed the conditional, the expert is wrong in law.

Using the firearms example, the expert must not assess the probability of the hypothesis, how likely it is that the gun was the murder weapon, only how likely the evidence of a 'match' is IF the gun is the murder weapon.

The chapter then turns to the subject of the admissibility[5] and the relevance of evidence and emphasises the point that if the LR is close to one, then the evidence is not relevant and should be inadmissible. The greater the LR differs from one, the stronger the evidence is in support of one case or the other.

There follows a discussion on the significance of the numerical value of the LR and its relationship with probative value and, in turn, admissibility. At what point does the LR become irrelevant? LR's associated with DNA evidence can be in the billions. How does that compare in probative value with an LR of say 100? Some courts and commentators have considered LRs of less than 100 to reveal evidence with insufficient probative value, and some require a 'high probative value' without specifying what that might be in terms of an LR. The essential question is – what value of the LR equates to sufficient probative value to be admitted? Furthermore, some commentators have argued that the LR is not a measure of probative value, but only of the strength of evidence (Roberts 2018).

A helpful summary concludes the chapter. The scientist cannot assess the probability of the prosecution case; only the probability of the evidence if the prosecution case is true, and that LRs greater than or less than one mean that the evidence is relevant.

Chapter 3 The Alternative Hypothesis

The title and contents provide another example in forensic science of several terms meaning (almost) the same thing. Here, the term 'hypothesis' is introduced. It is synonymous with 'proposition', 'assertion', 'premise', essentially the prosecution or defence case concerning a certain piece of evidence.

The chapter opens with a paragraph warning against the forensic scientist acting as an expert witness doing anything other than reporting the likelihood ratio. The concepts covered are so important that the actual text is quoted as follows:

> *It is logically meaningless to suggest that any piece of evidence has any value in itself as support for any particular hypothesis* [in isolation]. *Its value depends entirely upon its ability to discriminate between one hypothesis and another.*

By convention, the first hypothesis will be the case that the prosecution has to prove (denoted as 'H_p'). This chapter addresses the question of what the defence hypothesis (denoted as 'H_d') is.

It makes the important point that the value of the evidence will be greater if both hypotheses are *'well formed, positive and specific'*.

However, finding an alternative hypothesis can be a challenge. In most cases, the burden of proof is on the prosecution – the defence is not required to prove anything. The defence case might just be silence, and that only leaves 'not H_p' as the alternative. If the defence does not offer a specific alternative hypothesis, one or more might be reasonably inferred from a plea of not guilty.

Also, there may be an innocent explanation for the evidence which defeats the prosecution case. Blood found on a suspect 'matches' that of the murder victim, and so H_p is that the suspect was the murderer. However, the truth is that the suspect went to the aid of a dying man. In a firearms case, the suspect was found to bear gunshot residues. However, the suspect did not discharge the firearm, but was close to the weapon when it was discharged. The important point is that hypotheses are determined by the case circumstances.

In many cases in which DNA evidence is presented, the alternative source of the DNA is someone else in the relevant population.

> *In the case of DNA evidence for example, the value of the denominator—the probability of obtaining a match between the crime scene profile and the defendant's profile, given the defendant's innocence—will differ considerably depending upon whether the defendant's proposition is (1) the perpetrator was some other unknown person; (2) it was someone else from within the defendant's ethnic community; (3) it was the defendant's brother (for whom a profile is unavailable) or (4) it was the defendant's evil identical twin. The probabilities may vary from, perhaps, one in a trillion, in the first case, to one in the last case.*
>
> *(Hamer 2012)*

One important condition is that the hypotheses must be exclusive, that is, if one is true, the other must be false.

The chapter addresses the issue of the forensic scientist being presented with novel circumstances while giving live evidence, which affects the LR. Doing so may be illogical and will not be subject to any quality checks, including peer review. In such circumstances, the proper response is to tell the court that if novel circumstances are presented, the scientist must go back to the lab and start again. All rational hypotheses to be considered at trial should ideally be known to the expert witness beforehand so that evaluation may be supported by a quality system including peer review.

As with all the chapters, it concludes with a summary of key points, on this occasion, the selection and effect of the alternative hypothesis. The key point is that evidence can only distinguish between the hypotheses of the prosecution and the defence. Those hypotheses must be exclusive; the defence may present no hypothesis or more than one, and those selected will be case-specific. The value of the evidence will depend on those hypotheses.

An example is given of the finding of an individual's DNA at a scene, which may have one of several explanations, including innocent explanations.

Chapter 4 Explaining the Strength of the Evidence

This chapter opens with an example of DNA expert evidence being presented as an LR.

> *I find the results I obtained were at least 12,450 times more likely to have occurred if the blood had originated from the accused than if it had originated from someone else.*

It is widely recognised that human beings have difficulty processing numerical information, and there is much research to support this. This is a major topic in Chapters 5 and 8. Therefore, presenting a number may not result in the jury or fact-finder properly understanding the strength of the evidence. To overcome this difficulty, the publication proposes a scale of verbal equivalents to the LR. The example given in the book is now outdated. Today's scales do vary in wording[6], but are similar to the one given in Table 6.2. It should be noted that the scale shown starts at 1 and increases. LRs less than one mean that the evidence is more likely if the defence hypothesis is true, in the case of the above example, that the blood is not that of the accused.

So, returning to the example given, '*the evidence provides very strong support for the hypothesis that the blood is that of the accused*'. A statement that a jury or fact-finder will find easier to understand than '*12,450 times more likely*'.

Using verbal equivalents is now common practice in several disciplines, but particularly when presenting DNA evidence, which lends itself to statistical analysis made possible by the databases that now exist in many jurisdictions.

The chapter then turns to issues with using the likelihood ratio approach to interpretation and the presentation of evidence. As stated above, DNA evidence is supported by databases and population statistics, which makes the assignment of an LR relatively straightforward. However, for evidence types such as handwriting and fingerprints, no such databases existed. However, there is nothing to prevent such feature-comparison examiners from expressing an opinion along the lines of the degree of resemblance found, supports/does not support a common source.

Table 6.2 Verbal equivalents for the LR.

Value of the LR	Verbal Equivalent
1	No support for either hypothesis
Greater than 1–9	Weak support for *Hp*
10–99	Moderate support
100–999	Moderately strong support
1000–9999	Strong support
10 000–999 999	Very strong support
Over 1000 000	Extremely strong support

The chapter is critical of the approach to interpretation in these so-called feature-comparison disciplines, a subject that will be further explored in the chapter on the 2009 NAS Report (Chapter 9). These disciplines usually report categorically; in the case of fingerprints, the categories are usually 'yes/no' or 'inconclusive'.

Suggestions are made as to how data could be generated to support the probabilistic reporting of, say, fingerprint evidence.

Often, the fingerprint expert will only report a 'match' to which absolute certainty can be attached. This could deny the court some probative evidence; the degree of resemblance found between the question and the reference fingerprints may be more likely if the prints are of the same person than if they are not. That very statement, borne of the fingerprint examiner's training and experience, would be of some probative value to the court. But because the examiner will only report categorically, the court is denied that evidence. As explained in Chapters 4 and 9, there is a lot wrong with fingerprint evidence, and even today, the transition from categorical reporting to probabilistic reporting of fingerprint evidence is not complete (Forensic Science Regulator 2021b).

The chapter takes issue with the term 'consistent' and the phrase 'practical certainty', arguing that neither should be used by forensic scientists. Essentially, 'consistent with' is simply the opposite of 'inconsistent with'. Also, the evidence might be 'consistent with' several explanations such as the finding of a suspect's DNA on an item of clothing worn by a victim at the time of an alleged assault is 'consistent with' transfer either: during the assault, through innocent social contact, through consensual activity, or contamination either at the scene or elsewhere. The evidence is 'consistent with' all those explanations, the important question is, which is the most likely?

If an LR approach is not used, then there is a risk that the term 'consistent with' will be used in connection with the prosecution hypothesis supporting guilt and other explanations not presented to, nor considered by, the fact-finder or jury, therefore putting justice at risk.

In addition, research has found that lawyers can interpret 'consistent with' as strongly supporting a particular hypothesis.

To be clear, a forensic scientist should never use the term 'consistent'. In addition, good practice should require the forensic scientist to list and consider all rational and reasonable explanations.

The argument against 'practical certainty' in support of an opinion of a common source is that, first, there was little or no data to support such certainty; it was little more than conjecture. In addition, the authors make the comparison with DNA evidence at the time, which could deliver an LR of a billion or more, where experts would not opine certainty with feature comparison evidence, which delivered lower LRs being afforded certainties.

This argument seems to have been won, and the phrase has fallen out of use. A similar phrase used in the United States, 'reasonable degree of scientific certainty' was outlawed by the US Department of Justice in 2018 (Weiss and LaPorte 2018).

Among other issues, the chapter discusses the forensic scientist, or any expert witness, usurping the role of the jury or fact-finder. The discussion is around the law, and strictly, an expert must not opine on a matter for the jury. However, for example, this might extend to a fingerprint examiner only being able to present the common features that led to the opinion and not the opinion itself, leaving the question of a common source to the fact-finder.

Legal arguments are presented to the effect that the fact-finder can, in any case, reject an expert opinion, and sometimes has.

One argument that the authors fail to make is that to express a categorical opinion (e.g. yes/no/inconclusive), some undeclared prior probability must be assumed by the expert. This prior can only be truly known by the fact-finder, and in this way, the expert is usurping the role of the jury and risks 'double counting'. 'Double counting' occurs when both the forensic scientist and fact-finder give weight to the same piece of evidence, unfairly giving it extra weight.

The most important point in this chapter is that forensic scientific evidence must be presented in the form 'this evidence is *n* times more likely if the prosecution hypothesis is true than if the defence hypothesis is true. This evidence therefore provides weak to extremely strong support for the prosecution hypothesis'. Remembering, of course, that an LR of less than one means that the evidence is more supportive of the defence hypothesis, and an LR close to one renders the evidence irrelevant and strictly inadmissible.

Chapter 5 The Case as a Whole

This chapter begins with a statistical approach to combining scientific evidence and a warning about the need to identify independent evidence, as that will determine how probabilities will be treated.

As the name implies, statistically independent evidence is such that the probability of the observation, measure or finding does not affect the probability of another observation, measure or finding. Or more simply, that the probability of one event occurring does not change the probability of the other occurring.

The simplest and clearest examples of independence evidence are of different types, such as DNA evidence of identity and gunshot residue as evidence of firearms involvement.

If the evidence is truly independent, then probabilities (and resultant LRs) can be multiplied. This is the discriminatory power of DNA evidence in that the STR (short tandem repeats of bases) sequence at a locus on one chromosome is independent of the sequence on another chromosome. Given that these STRs are highly variable from individual to individual, as discussed in Chapter 4 of this book, they produce very high probabilities, which are highly discriminating.

However, it is not always clear if the evidence is independent, and mistakes have resulted in several high-profile wrongful convictions. Perhaps some of the most infamous have involved the paediatrician Professor Sir Roy Meadow, to whom the aphorism 'Meadow's Law' is mistakenly attributed. However, he is on record as sanctioning it. The subject of the 'Law' is sudden infant death syndrome, sometimes known as cot-death.

> *One sudden infant death is a tragedy, two is suspicious, and three is murder, until proved otherwise.*

This line of reasoning helped to wrongly convict Sally Clark in 1999, Angela Canning in 2002, and Kathleen Folbigg in Australia in 2003 of murdering their infant children. In addition, Lucia De Berk in the Netherlands in 2003 was convicted of murdering infants in a hospital. The fundamental assumption being made is that the deaths of the children were independent events, and so the chance or probability of each death occurring by chance could be multiplied.

Meadow's evidence in the Sally Clark case was based on the ratio of births to cot deaths in affluent non-smoking families, which was about 8500 to 1. Meadow then squared that number to arrive at a 1 in 73 million chance of two deaths occurring by chance.

Statisticians later demonstrated that sudden infant deaths were not independent, i.e. having lost one infant child, the death of a second was more likely and so on.

Meadow's evidence in the Sally Clark case, in addition to the erroneous assumption that the events were independent, provides a catalogue of incompetence as an expert witness. This serves as a cautionary tale for all forensic scientists.

First, as a paediatrician, Meadow was not qualified to give statistical evidence, and his fundamental misunderstanding contributed to his incorrect assumption that the deaths were independent events. Second, by considering the probability of the hypothesis (murder) given the evidence (sudden infant death), he fell into the trap of the prosecutor's fallacy, thereby misleading the court and arguably usurping the role of the jury. In addition, a double murder is itself a rare event, and so the prior probability of Clark's innocence was not given enough weight. Third, and an oft-neglected factor, is that Meadow was the 'inventor' of Munchausen syndrome by proxy (MSBP), a controversial condition which would explain why a mother would harm or even kill her child. Therefore, any decision by a court or other tribunal of fact that a mother has harmed or abused her child would provide supporting evidence for his theory, MSBP. As a result, Meadow could not be considered an independent or unbiased witness and arguably should have been declared a partisan witness and prevented from giving evidence in such cases[7].

Most of the chapter is focused on combining evidence, how it should be done and what it can provide. A Bayesian model is promoted as the only logical approach. While this is no doubt true, even in 2024, courts, particularly in the common law jurisdictions, are cautious about weakening the role of the jury or fact-finder and strengthening the role of the expert. The adage is that experts should be 'on tap and not on top'. So, although this is a long chapter with many cases discussed, it is not considered that important in the development of forensic science from 1995 onwards.

There is then a long discussion about combining uncertain evidence, which is mainly from a legal perspective. It is then followed by an argument supporting the combining of evidence by forensic scientists, which in effect is an argument for Bayesian reasoning and interpretation at the activity level. Activity level is one of the propositions in the hierarchy of propositions discussed later in this chapter and in Chapter 8. Evaluating scientific evidence at the activity level is considered the ideal.

The chapter cautions against assuming prior probabilities and concludes by asserting again that Bayesian inference is the correct logical method for combining evidence.

Chapter 6 Errors in Thinking

These errors include the prosecutor's and defence attorney's fallacies covered in the earlier chapter on Thompson and Schumann's paper (Chapter 5), of which the authors give helpful and illustrative examples.

The chapter raises an intriguing issue: the initial prior belief of the lay fact-finder or jury, which should be neutral. Legal principles such as the presumption of innocence and the burden of proof usually favour the accused. However, the accused is on trial for a criminal offence, so it's hard to see the jury's prior belief being anything other than guilt. This puts the defence at a disadvantage. While this issue is interesting, it's beyond the scope of this book.

The chapter also discusses 'accuracy' by which the authors mean the discriminatory power of a particular test, an accurate test having a low false positive and false negative rate.

It then goes on to cover the need for 'honest reporting', ensuring that all relevant information, including that which may weaken the case, is disclosed. Many jurisdictions now have powerful rules about disclosure. Nondisclosure by the prosecution at trial may result in a conviction being overturned by Courts of Appeal.

Of greater significance for forensic science is incorporating the likelihood of laboratory or technical errors into the interpretation. With LRs now of the order of many powers of 10 (a million million or 10^{12} for example), the probability of laboratory error, however small, can have a significant effect on the LR.

Chapter 7 Classical Statistics and Database Matching

The major impact of this publication and the reason for its inclusion in this history is its introduction and promotion of the likelihood ratio approach to interpretation, which, as stated earlier, brings several important benefits, including avoiding logical errors such as transposing the conditional.

While the LR can stand alone, it is part of Bayes' rule, the basis of Bayesian reasoning.

$$\text{Posterior Probability} = \text{LR} \times \text{Prior Probability}$$

Scientists, particularly those in the analytical sciences, will be familiar with statistics such as the mean or average, its confidence intervals and significance tests such as the *t*-test and chi-square test. These can be termed 'classical' or frequentist statistics.

In this chapter, the authors make the case that frequentist statistics cannot be used to answer the question of interest to the court; only Bayesian reasoning can. The court wants to know '*by how much an item of evidence should cause it to change its belief in a hypothesis*'.

Fundamentally, the LR approach demands the consideration of alternative hypotheses and their evaluation, and that alternative ideally must be more than a 'match' by chance or the mere negation of the first hypothesis.

It may be of interest to the specialist reader to study this chapter and its excellent examples. However, the fact is that the LR approach has mostly been accepted as standard practice and, as a result, there is little but academic interest in why the frequentist approach is inappropriate.

Chapters 8–10

The next three chapters consider several different types of evidence and suggest methods of interpretation. Those evidence types are fingerprints, glass, fibres – including transfer and persistence, firearms, DNA and handwriting. These chapters make good primers for an understanding of these evidence types. The chapters highlight their strengths and weaknesses, clarify issues, and raise relevant questions contributing to the research agenda.

Chapter 11 Implications for the Legal System

This chapter assesses the value of expert witnesses to justice systems and identifies areas for improvement. In doing so asks some of the questions originally considered in Chapter 3 on the Ontogeny of Criminalistics and explored in depth in Chapter 10 on the Sydney Declaration. Those questions are: Is forensic science a science? Is it a profession? It also considers who qualifies as an expert, which, to some extent, is jurisdiction-specific.

Much of what is written is not unique to this publication. However, one important point made is worth recording here; it is trying to distinguish forensic science from other sciences and opines that,

> *Forensic scientists ... must try to assess the value as evidence of single, possibly non-replicable items of information about specific hypotheses referring to an individual event.*

And again,

> *Forensic science is a discipline in its own right concerned with assessing the value as evidence for competing hypotheses of single items of evidence.*

The publication urges forensic scientists in whatever field to consider themselves as experts in interpretation. Indeed, the authors argue that it is the interpretation method advocated in this publication that is the unifying characteristic of forensic science.

The book ends with five questions that should be asked of all scientific evidence.

1. What is the probability of this evidence if our story is true?
2. What are the appropriate alternative hypotheses?
3. Why are they the appropriate alternative hypotheses?
4. What is the probability of the evidence given the alternative hypotheses?
5. What is the value of the evidence?

Impact at the Time

The impact at the time of publication in 1995 was minimal. It is fair to say that the book is not an easy read; the golden nuggets of good practice in interpretation are sometimes hard to find among acres of case studies and examples. The logical principles require study to 'close the lid', as it were, and retain the knowledge.

There was initial resistance to the principles and practices advocated, and unfortunately, that resistance remains in some quarters. Common themes among opponents of the approach were 'fine for other disciplines but not ours' and a failure to see the many flaws in the old approach. Hence, the need arose to write and publish a second edition in 2016 to add momentum to the call for progress.

In addition, pioneers such as Ian Evett, Colin Aitkin and organisations such as the Forensic Science Service in England and Wales, ESR in New Zealand and the University of Lausanne in Switzerland kept up the pressure through publications, workshops and conference presentations.

Impact Today

It took some time for the principles set out in the publication to pass down from the ivory tower to reach practitioners. Perhaps the most significant step towards wider adoption was the publication of the so-called AFSP[8] Standards, much later in 2009 (AFSP 2009). These offered practical guidance in the application of the likelihood ratio approach to interpretation. The paper listed four guiding principles: logic, balance, transparency and robustness.

- Logic was, in effect, a restatement of the need to avoid transposing the conditional – to consider the probability of the evidence and not the hypothesis.
- Balance was a restatement of the need to consider mutually exclusive alternative hypotheses.
- Transparency – to report/document what was done.
- Robustness – ensure interpretation is supported by a body of knowledge.

The paper introduced the concept of an evaluative opinion, being one based on the likelihood ratio and distinguished between an investigative opinion and an evaluative opinion. An investigative opinion explains a finding or observation, e.g. the paint is from a particular car.

The AFSP paper also promoted the use of case assessment and interpretation (CAI), explained in Chapter 8, and refers to another paper introducing the hierarchy of hypotheses (Cook et al. 1998) commonly called the hierarchy of propositions (remember hypothesis, proposition, and assertion, etc., are all synonymous)

That hierarchy is as follows.

1. Offence – the accused murdered the victim.
2. Activity – the accused fired the gun.
3. Source – the blood on the accused's clothing is that of the victim.
4. Sub-source – the DNA recovered from the gun is that of the suspect.

Offence level hypotheses are a matter for the court and fact-finder, the forensic scientist can assist the court in evaluating the other hypotheses in the hierarchy.

The guidance in the AFSP paper states that changing hypotheses from activity to source level after the examination or results have been obtained must not be done. This means that once appropriate hypotheses have been selected and assigned a likelihood ratio, you can't go back and start again if you don't like the result.

In Europe, the European Network of Forensic Science Institutes (ENFSI) produced its own guidance based on the AFSP Standards (ENFSI 2015). Other regional organisations have produced similar guidance documents, as has the Forensic Science Regulator in England and Wales (Forensic Science Regulator 2021a).

Contribution to Current Practice

The codification of good practice in the evaluation of forensic scientific evidence in the courtroom in 1995 has eventually led to widely recognised standard practices, which ensure that the forensic scientist gives expert evidence that is logical, balanced, transparent and robust.

This all begins with selecting the appropriate hypothesis at the appropriate level and assigning a likelihood ratio as a measure of the strength of evidence.

There is much evidence that the most common mistake made by forensic scientists, especially when giving oral evidence, is the transposition of the conditional, i.e. considering the probability of the hypothesis rather than that of the evidence. At its most fundamental, the only role of the forensic scientist is to consider and report on the probability of the evidence. To guard against this unfair strengthening of the prosecution's case and better serve justice, the forensic scientist must be well-trained and demonstrably competent in interpretation.

Other elements of good practice are to know that priors are for the fact-finder, and so never assume a prior, and to try to evaluate at the activity level.

For today's forensic science practitioner, the ENFSI guide is probably the most comprehensive and easily understood, being replete with realistic casework examples.

Conforming to the principles and practices listed in this publication ensures that a forensic scientist giving evidence does so logically and that evidence is balanced, robust and transparent. Conformance also ensures that the forensic scientist giving expert evidence does not usurp the role of the fact-finder or jury. It also reduces the risk of cognitive bias and the expert wandering outside his or her field of expertise.

Concluding Remarks

Having rejected Paul Kirk's contention that forensic science is the science of individualisation (Chapter 3), there has been a slow movement towards forensic science being the science of interpretation, irrespective of 'discipline' as stated by Robertson and Vignaux almost 30 years ago.

Key Takeaways

'Interpreting Evidence' demonstrates that using the LR to update the prior beliefs of the fact-finder or jury is logical, rational and conforms to the requirements of the law.

The book:

- explains the fundamentals of logical reasoning and how it might be applied,
- discusses misleading and erroneous styles of presentation,
- argues that the principles enunciated apply to all forms of scientific evidence in all jurisdictions, and
- asserts that the LR is the only evidence a forensic scientist can give.

Using the LR approach to interpretation has some other benefits as follows.

- Avoids usurping the role of the jury or fact-finder.
- Keeps the expert from wandering outside his/her field of expertise.
- Reduces the risk of cognitive bias.
- According to the authors, forensic science is the science of interpretation.

'Interpreting Evidence' second edition is essential reading for forensic scientists who may act as expert witnesses. Its principles must be comprehended, and its requirements must be complied with in presenting scientific evidence.

Notes

1. These concepts are discussed later in this chapter. They are also explained in the section on Terms, Definitions and Explanations.
2. 'New evidence scholarship' refers to a movement in legal scholarship that analyses the process of proof and evidence, often drawing on insights from fields like logic, mathematics, psychology, and philosophy.
3. The admissibility of scientific evidence is a subject in its own right and is discussed in Chapter 8.
4. Admissibility is a matter for the court and the trend is to admit anything that might be relevant and have probative value, leaving weight to the fact-finder. However, an LR close to one means that the evidence is equally likely whether the prosecution or defence case is true, and therefore that evidence is irrelevant and has no probative value and should not be admitted.
5. As mentioned earlier, admissibility is a subject in its own right and is discussed further in Chapter 8.
6. A further example of the inconsistencies in forensic science that hinder development and communication.
7. The current case of the nurse Lucy Letby, convicted of the murder of neonatal infants, has echoes of the Meadows episodes.
8. The Association of Forensic Science Providers https://www.afsp.org.uk/, a group that included the Forensic Science Service and other major providers of forensic science within Great Britain and Ireland.

Bibliography

AFSP. 2009. "Standards for the formulation of evaluative forensic science expert opinion." *Science and Justice* 49: 161–64.

Aitken, Colin G. G. and David A. Stoney. 1991. *The Use of Statistics in Forensic Science.* Chichester, West Sussex: Ellis Horwood Ltd.

Cook, Roger, Ian W. Evett, Graham Jackson, P. L. Jones, and J. A. Lambert. 1998. "A Hierarchy of Propositions: Deciding Which Level to Address in Casework." *Science and Justice* 38: 231–39.

ENFSI. 2015. "ENFSI Guideline for Evaluative Reporting." *ENSI.* 8 March. Accessed March 21, 2024. https://www.google.com/search?q=enfsi+evaluative+reporting&rlz=1C5CHFA_enNZ948NZ948&oq=ENFSI+&gs_lcrp=EgZjaHJvbWUqDAgBECMYJxiABBiKBTIGCAAQRRg5MgwIARAjGCcYgAQYigUyBwgCEAAYgAQyBwgDEAAYgAQyBwgEEAAYgAQyBwgFEAAYgAQyBwgGEAAYgAQyBwgHEAAYgAQyBwgIEAAYgAQyBwgJEAAYg.

Evett, Ian W. 1991. "Interpretation: A Personal Odyssey." In *The Use of Statistics in Forensic Science*, edited by Colin G. G. Aitken and David A. Stoney, 9–22. Chichester, West Sussex: Ellis Horwood Ltd.

Forensic Science Regulator. 2021a. "Documents." *GOV.UK*. 11 February. Accessed March 21, 2024. https://assets.publishing.service.gov.uk/media/602407728fa8f5146f0769d9/FSR-C-118_Interpretation_Appendix_Issue_1__002_.pdf.

Forensic Science Regulator. 2021b. "FQSSG Fingerprint Interpretation Workshop Summary." *GOV.UK*. 21 October. Accessed March 20, 2024. https://assets.publishing.service.gov.uk/media/61faa3c5e90e0768a5adf2ab/FQSSG_write_up.pdf.

Hamer, David. 2012. "Probability, Anti-resilience, and the Weight of Expectation." *Law, Probability and Risk* 11 (2–3): 135–58.

Lindley, Dennis V. 1975. "The Future of Statistics: A Bayesian 21st Century." *Advances in Applied Probability* 7: 105–15.

R v T. 2010. 2439 (EWCA).

Roberts, Paul. 2018. "Making Sense of Forensic Science Evidence." In *Forensic Science Evidence and Expert Witness Testimony*, edited by Paul Roberts and Michael Stockdale, 66–67. Cheltenham: Edward Elgar.

Robertson, Bernard W., G. A. Vignaux, and Charles E. H. Berger. 2011. "Extending the Confusion About Bayes." *Modern Law Review* 74: 1–16.

Robertson, Bernard and G. A. Vignaux. 1992. "Expert Evidence: Law, Practice and Probability." *Oxford Journal of Legal Studies* 12 (3): 392–403.

Robertson, Bernard and G. A. Vignaux. 1993. "Probability—The Logic of the Law." *Oxford Journal of Legal Studies* 13 (4): 457–78.

Robertson, Bernard, G. A. Vignaux, and Charles E. H. Berger. 2016. *Interpreting Evidence: Evaluating Forensic Science in the Courtroom*. Chichester: John Wiley & Sons Ltd.

Weiss, Danielle and Gerald LaPorte. 2018. "Uncertainty Ahead: A Shift in How Federal Scientific Experts Can Testify." *National Institute of Justice*. 17 January. Accessed March 20, 2024. https://nij.ojp.gov/topics/articles/uncertainty-ahead-shift-how-federal-scientific-experts-can-testify.

7

ISO/IEC 17025:1999 – Demonstrating Competence and Validity

Image 7.1 ISO logo.

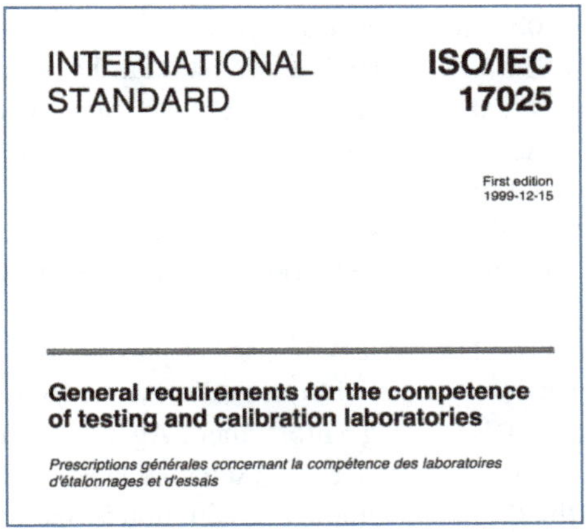
INTERNATIONAL STANDARD

ISO/IEC 17025

First edition 1999-12-15

General requirements for the competence of testing and calibration laboratories

Prescriptions générales concernant la compétence des laboratoires d'étalonnages et d'essais

Image 7.2 Part of the cover page of the standard. © 1999 ISO/IEC 17025:1999/ International Organization for Standardization.

Name of the Publication

ISO/IEC 17025:1999. The standard is titled *General requirements for the competence of testing and calibration laboratories.* The International Organization for Standardization (ISO) produced the standard, which had 28 pages. The standard is now in its third edition.

Introduction

This publication has no direct relationship with forensic science. Therefore, it will come as a surprise that of the publications included in this history of forensic science, ISO/IEC 17025 is arguably the one that has had the greatest impact on the practice of forensic science; certainly, in terms of regulation.

A raft of wrongful convictions that came to light in England in the late 1980s and early 1990s significantly undermined trust in forensic science and the criminal justice system.

A History of Forensic Science in 10 Publications: How They Established Current Practice, First Edition.
Sean Doyle.

Unreliable scientific evidence was found to have significantly contributed to some of these miscarriages of justice. The need to urgently restore confidence in forensic science saw providers look to quality standards as part of the response. That standard became ISO/IEC 17025, first adopted by forensic science laboratories in England and, in time, globally.

ISO/IEC 17025 is a quality standard; that is, a documented set of requirements that, if complied with, ensures the fitness for purpose of products, services and processes. In the context of a forensic science laboratory, conformance with ISO/IEC 17025 demonstrates the competence of the organisation and staff, the validity of its methods and the reliability of its results. Conformance enables stakeholders, collectively the criminal justice system, to have confidence in and place reliance on the scientific evidence produced by forensic science laboratories.

This chapter will explore the relationship between the international standard ISO/IEC 17025 and forensic science.

ISO/IEC 17025 is a joint standard of the International Organization for Standardization (ISO) and the International Electrotechnical Commission (IEC), hence the prefix ISO/IEC.

As its title implies, ISO/IEC 17025 applies to testing and calibration laboratories. So, it is not a standard that specifically applies to forensic science laboratories. Nevertheless, for reasons that will become clear, this standard has been adopted by almost every forensic science laboratory in the world. Regional organisations such as the European Network of Forensic Science Institutes (ENFSI) have made accreditation[1] to the standard a condition of membership (ENFSI 2023). The US Department of Justice requires its component agencies, the FBI (Federal Bureau of Investigation), ATF (Bureau of Alcohol, Tobacco, Firearms and Explosives) and DEA (Drug Enforcement Agency), to conform to the standard (Department of Justice 2015). Furthermore, to exchange DNA and fingerprint evidence within the jurisdictions of the European Union, accreditation is mandated (Council of the European Union 2009).

Given its global adoption, ISO/IEC 17025 is arguably the most impactful of all the publications included in this book.

The first edition of ISO/IEC 17025 was published in 1999. International standards are required to be reviewed every five years for continuing suitability. The standard was updated in 2005 and again in 2017. This third and latest edition differs from the 1999 edition in structure and content. It is the 1999 edition that is the subject of this chapter.

The 1999 edition was the first international standard to combine both technical and management requirements for testing laboratories in one document. Before the publication of ISO/IEC 17025, laboratories wishing to demonstrate competence and the reliability of scientific outputs had to conform to a quality management standard and a separate technical standard. In the United Kingdom, this was BS 5750 for quality management and M10 for technical competence. UK forensic science laboratories could be certified as conforming to BS 5750 and accredited to M10. In Europe, some forensic science laboratories were accredited to a European standard EN 45001:1989 'General criteria for the operation of testing laboratories' (Doyle 2019c).

As with other chapters, there will be a history of the publication itself, its genesis, and a look at its structure and contents. However, by far the most significant factor is the historical background to its adoption by forensic science laboratories in response to several high-profile miscarriages of justice in the United Kingdom in the late 1980s and early 1990s. The historical context will be discussed in some detail.

The profound impact of the standard on the practice, management and delivery of forensic science, both at the time of its adoption and its effect on the development of forensic science, will be discussed. Forensic science laboratories had to develop, document and conform to quality management systems, standard operating procedures and adapt to a very different culture. That culture is characterised by the requirement for an ethos of continuous improvement, an acceptance that there is always room for improvement. The practical outcome is proactively seeking opportunities for improvement.

As mentioned earlier, the standard had several impacts, including the eventual requirement by certain bodies for mandatory accreditation. This accreditation formed the basis of a regulatory framework.

Today, it would be exceptional for scientific evidence to be placed before a court of law unsupported by conformance to ISO/IEC 17025.

Before the introduction of ISO/IEC 17025 in 1999, no internationally accepted single standard for laboratories enabled a demonstration of both management and technical competence.

ISO/IEC 17025 began life as a revision of the ISO Guide 25:1990 'General requirements for the competence of calibration and testing laboratories'. The guide was a document drawn up by ISO in response to a request by the International Laboratory Accreditation Cooperation (ILAC) in October 1988. During a revision in the late 1990s, it was decided to convert the guide into a standard, providing a global basis for accreditation.

However, in the context of forensic science, what was of far greater significance than the development of the standard is the reason for the adoption of ISO/IEC 17025 by forensic science laboratories.

In the early 1970s, there was a series of terrorist bombings on the mainland of the United Kingdom, perpetrated by Irish republican terrorists. After due process, several people were convicted of those crimes. Forensic scientific evidence played a significant part in the prosecution case, seemingly establishing a link between the suspects and bomb-making. Concerns about the safety of those convictions grew over time, with the convictions eventually being overturned in the early 1990s. Perhaps the most famous case was that of the Birmingham 6, (Pallister 1991) released in 1991 after spending 16 years in prison for crimes they did not commit. The realisation that unreliable forensic scientific evidence had contributed to these wrongful convictions had a seismic effect on forensic science providers in the United Kingdom. With the encouragement of the UK House of Lords[2] (House of Lords 1993), these forensic science laboratories collectively decided to look to quality standards as a means of ensuring that scientific evidence was of sufficient quality to be relied upon by courts and reduce the risk of contributing to future miscarriages of justice. This initiative resulted in the accreditation to ISO/IEC 17025:1999 of the two forensic science laboratories at the heart of the scandal; other laboratories followed suit.

These miscarriages of justice, the reasons why unreliable scientific evidence was presented at trial, and the response of forensic science laboratories and the UK government are so important to the history of forensic science that the issues are explored in greater depth in the discussions on the scientific, social and historic contexts later in this chapter.

There is a lot of misunderstanding about the meaning of quality management terms. Although the terms are familiar, many differ from common everyday meanings. Quality is the degree to which a product or service is fit for its intended purpose. In the case of a forensic science laboratory, quality is the extent to which the test result it generates and interprets can be relied upon by a tribunal of fact, such as a court, to reach a safe decision or verdict by a fair process, i.e. justice. The scientific evidence produced by a forensic science laboratory does not have to be of the highest quality, although that should be the aim, but of sufficient quality to meet the needs of the justice system.

There is much confusion about the terms 'accreditation' and 'certification', sometimes used interchangeably and treated as synonyms. In quality management, they have specific meanings. An organisation that is accredited is technically a conformity assessment body (CAB) which certifies conformance with a set of requirements. So, an accredited forensic science laboratory effectively certifies the competence of its staff and the reliability of the scientific evidence it produces. A CAB that assesses conformance with the quality management standard ISO 9001 certifies conformance. That CAB will be accredited for providing that service.

Biography of the Publication

The origin of quality standards such as ISO/IEC 17025 can be traced back to the Second World War and the need for ammunition and armaments to comply with specified standards.

Post-war Japan is credited with a major advance in quality management under the influence of the American quality gurus Joseph Juran and W. Edwards Deming.

The formation and growth of what became the European Union also played a part in the development of quality standards. The single European market required the free movement of goods, services, capital and people. Ensuring that goods and services complied with common standards became essential to the successful operation of the single European market.

As stated earlier, before the introduction of ISO/IEC 17025 in 1999, no internationally accepted standard for laboratories demonstrated both management and technical competence and could provide a globally accepted basis for accreditation.

Its predecessor, ISO Guide 25 'General Requirements for the competence of calibration and testing laboratories' was published in 1988.

The guide had been used since 1990 as a generic criteria document for the competence of testing and calibration laboratories. The declared purpose of the guide was to establish the principle that '*third party certification systems* [for laboratories] *should, to the extent possible, be based on internationally agreed standards and procedures*'. ISO guides are intended to be used for the preparation of national standards. By this means, a high degree of compatibility between standards prepared in different countries might be achieved '*so as to facilitate bilateral and multilateral agreements*'. National and regional standards based on ISO Guide 25 would, therefore, be closely similar.

Among the standards based on ISO Guide 25 were the European standard EN45001:1989 'General criteria for the operation of testing laboratories' and in the United Kingdom, National Measurement Accreditation Service (NAMAS) standard M10 'General criteria of competence for calibration and testing laboratories'. To demonstrate technical competence, some continental European forensic science laboratories gained accreditation to EN45001:1989. In the United Kingdom, forensic science laboratories were accredited to M10. Although conformance was assessed against national standards, there was a considerable level of uniformity between the requirements expressed in these various standards due to their compliance with ISO Guide 25.

In order to demonstrate managerial competence and thus complete the quality management system, some UK forensic science laboratories were accredited to the NAMAS standard M10 for technical activities and certified to ISO 9001, the quality management standard, and its predecessor BS 5750, for their management system.

ISO Guide 25 stipulated that laboratories meeting the requirements of the guide also complied with the requirements of the quality management standard ISO 9001 when acting as suppliers producing calibration and test results. Some ISO 9001 Certification Bodies started auditing laboratories against ISO 9001 and issued compliance certificates to that effect. This created confusion in the minds of testing and calibration laboratory customers, raising the question as to whether a laboratory complying with ISO 9001 can also be technically competent. ISO Guide 25 was silent on this. This issue was resolved in the new standard ISO/IEC 17025:1999; a conforming organisation would be both managerially and technically competent.

ISO also decided that there should be as much compatibility as possible between ISO/IEC 17025 and ISO 9001, which was also under revision at the same time. The objective was to closely align the management requirements of ISO/IEC 17025 with ISO 9001, remembering that ISO/IEC 17025 includes both management and technical requirements. To be clear, the quality management system of an ISO/IEC 17025 accredited laboratory conforms to ISO 9001.

ISO/IEC 17025 was first published in 1999 and came into effective use after its adoption as a national standard (although the UK accreditation service, at the time NAMAS, accredited against ISO/IEC 17025 in 1998). The revised version of ISO 9001 was accepted in 2000.

Professional Biography of the Authors

ISO/IEC 17025 is one of a family of international standards jointly developed and published by the ISO and the IEC.

ISO is an independent, non-governmental international standards development and publication organisation composed of representatives from the national standards organisations of member countries. The US representative is the American National Standards Institute (ANSI), in the United Kingdom, it is the British Standards Institute (BSI), and in Australia, it is Standards Australia (SA). According to ISO, through its members, it brings together experts to share knowledge and develop voluntary, consensus-based, market-relevant international standards that support innovation and provide solutions to global challenges.

IEC is a similar organisation that develops and publishes international standards. However, those standards apply to electrical, electronic and related technologies.

Another important organisation in the story of ISO/IEC 17025 and its adoption by forensic science laboratories is ILAC (International Laboratory Accreditation Cooperation). ILAC is the international organisation for accreditation bodies operating in accordance with ISO/IEC 17011 'Conformity assessment – Requirements for accreditation bodies accrediting conformity assessment bodies'. This is the standard to which accrediting bodies such as UKAS (UK Accreditation Service) must conform. Conformance is evidenced by a mutual recognition agreement with ILAC, the aim being 'tested here accepted everywhere'; i.e. test results generated by a laboratory in England will be accepted by authorities in, say, Australia.

In addition to facilitating mutual recognition, ILAC also produces guidance documents, and one such guide was 'Guidance for Forensic Science Laboratories' issued in 2002 (ILAC 2002). As the title implies, this guide interpreted ISO/IEC 17025 for forensic science laboratories. For some time, this was the *de facto* standard against which forensic science laboratories were accredited.

Contexts

Scientific

In the early 1970s, the forensic application of analytical science was in its infancy; indeed, analytical science itself was at an early stage of development. Analytical science is essentially the separation, detection, identification, and quantification of the chemical components of substances.

In the late 1980s, the need for analytical methods that might produce comparable results, i.e. the amount of substance found by laboratory A might equal that found by laboratory B, which was increasingly recognised as essential. Work began developing so-called standard methods.

The following quote from a paper presented by the then UK Government Chemist provides some historical context.

> *Our files show that I started considering the need for a European organisation to provide a forum for discussing QA* [quality assurance] *matters in analytical chemistry soon after I was appointed the Government Chemist in July 1987. The Department of Trade and Industry (DTI), to which LGC* [the Laboratory of the Government Chemist, UK] *belonged, was preparing a White Paper* setting out its policy for the provision of the basic framework for ensuring the international comparability of measurements carried out in the UK. In the past, this policy had been mainly concerned with the provision of standards and measurement services for physical and engineering-based industries. We felt at LGC that analytical measurements were of at least equivalent importance.*
>
> *(Williams 1999).*

The point being that until this time, there was little concern for comparability of analytical chemical measurements, while it was considered essential to know how to accurately measure mass, length, time and other physical dimensions and know the uncertainty of the measurement, i.e. the +/– figure or margin of error. It was equally important that an analytical test, say measuring the amount of alcohol in a beverage, the constituents of drugs, the ingredients in foods, etc. or the amount of an additive in petrol, produced accurate results.

Initiatives taken to improve the quality of analytical chemical tests did not begin in earnest until the mid- to late 1990s. One example of this was the VAM (Valid Analytical Measurement) Initiative of the UK's Laboratory of the Government Chemist, which began in the mid-1990s.

The six VAM principles are a reasonably comprehensive statement of requirements for producing test results that are comparable and can be relied upon. The principles are as follows.

1. Analytical measurements should be made to satisfy an agreed requirement (i.e. to a defined objective).
2. Analytical measurements should be made using methods and equipment that have been tested to ensure they are fit for purpose.
3. Staff making analytical measurements should be both qualified and competent to undertake the task (and demonstrate that they can perform the analysis properly).
4. There should be a regular independent assessment of the technical performance of a laboratory.
5. Analytical measurements made in one location should be consistent with those made elsewhere.
6. Organisations making analytical measurements should have well-defined quality control and quality assurance procedures.

Forensic scientists practising in the 1970s would have had no knowledge of these yet-to-be-defined principles and the need to ensure that chemical tests were of sufficient quality to produce reliable results.

It may well be that the scientists at that time believed in their own minds that a positive test result was a true result, and near-absolute certainty could be attached. However, we now know that test results unsupported by evidence of reliability and a knowledge of uncertainty are worthless. To ensure the validity of methods and the consequent reliability of results, a framework of quality standards was required.

The emergence of this framework, ISO Guide 25, Good Laboratory Practice[3] and the VAM initiative coincided with the uncovering of the high-profile miscarriages of justice that prompted the adoption of quality standards by forensic science laboratories in response to the failings that came to light.

Encouraged by parliament, the need for standards was seized upon by United Kingdom forensic science laboratories rocked by scandals that helped send the innocent to jail and consequently allowed the guilty to walk free.

Historical

Wrongful Convictions

From 1968 until 1998, the British province of Ulster, also known as Northern Ireland, was engulfed in what effectively became a civil war between sectarian parties of republicans in favour of a united Ireland and unionists desiring to remain part of the United Kingdom; parties broadly aligned with Catholics and Protestants, respectively. This period is euphemistically known as the 'Troubles'[4]. Initially, the remainder of the United Kingdom was mostly unaware of the violence and cared little about the conflict. In an attempt to raise awareness of the conflict and underlying issues among the wider British people, a republican terrorist organisation known as the Provisional Irish Republican Army (PIRA), and similar republican terrorist organisations, conducted a bombing campaign on the UK mainland.

While there were many other atrocities during the Troubles, including violent deaths and serious injuries, four terrorist attacks stand out in infamy.

4th of February 1974, M62 coach bombing, killing 12 and injuring 38.

5th of October 1974, Guildford pub[5] bombings, Guildford Horse and Groom, Seven Stars and The Three Pigeons. Five were killed in the Horse and Groom; the Seven Stars was safely evacuated after an explosion, but a second bomb injured eight.

7th of November 1974, King Arms pub, Woolwich, one dead and one injured.

21st of November 1974, Birmingham pub bombings of the Mulberry Bush and Tavern in the Town pubs, 10 killed in the Mulberry Bush and 11 in the Tavern in the Town, and a combined total of 220 people were injured.

The targets of all these attacks were off-duty British servicemen and women, their families and loved ones.

It was (much) later accepted by most agencies that some of these attacks were conducted by a PIRA Active Service Unit (ASU) later to be identified as the 'Balcombe Street Gang'. Balcombe Street in London was the scene of their capture.

It is fair to state that from a justice and public safety perspective, quickly finding, arresting and, in due course, bringing to justice the perpetrators of these attacks were very high priorities for the UK government, its security agencies and police forces. Little effort was spared in speedily progressing the investigation. However, such circumstances increase the risk of inducing tunnel vision based on the 'preconceived theories' warned against in Hans Gross' Handbook (Chapter 1).

> *Preconceived theories are so much the more dangerous as it is precisely the most zealous Investigating Officer, the officer most interested in his work, who is the most exposed to them. ... An opinion is formed which cannot be got rid of.*

After due process, six men were convicted of the Birmingham bombings, and the group became known as the Birmingham 6. Eleven were convicted in relation to the Guildford and Woolwich bombings, known as the Guildford 4 and Maguire 7, and a single person, Judith Ward, was convicted of the M62 coach bombing. Apart from the Guildford 4, evidence of the alleged presence of explosive traces played a significant part in securing the conviction of all these people. A forced confession by one of the Guildford 4 included an assertion that the Maguire house was a bomb factory.

The explosives evidence was presented at trial by forensic scientists from separate forensic science laboratories. One was the Royal Armament Research Establishment (RARDE), located in Kent, which is now the Forensic Explosives Laboratory (FEL) part of Dstl (Defence Science and Technology Laboratory), an agency of the Ministry of Defence. The other was the Home Office's[6] Laboratory at Chorley in the county of Lancashire, England, later to become part of the Forensic Science Service (FSS). Notably, both were agencies of the UK government.

After numerous appeals, the conviction of the Guildford 4 was declared '*unsafe and unsatisfactory*' in 1989 (R v Richardson & Ors 1989). The convictions of the Maguire 7 were similarly declared in 1991 (R v Maguire & Ors 1992). And, perhaps most famously, the Birmingham 6 had their convictions quashed in 1991 (R v McIlkenny & Ors 1991). The conviction of Judith Ward was overturned in May 1993 (R v Ward 1992).

Birmingham Six Story The Birmingham 6 left the city shortly before the explosions on the 21st of November 1974. They were taken into custody at the port of Heysham, Lancashire, while travelling to Ireland by train and then ferry. Local Home Office forensic scientist Dr Frank Skuse was asked to examine their hands for traces of explosives. Skuse used positive Griess test[7] results of hand swabs to assert that two of the six had handled explosives. A more powerful technique, combining gas chromatography and mass spectrometry (GC-MS)[8], was later applied to the samples, and the results failed to confirm the earlier Griess test results. This failure to confirm the Griess test results was not disclosed to the defence and consequently not heard by the jury at trial.

Skuse's claim at trial that he was 99% certain that two of the six had explosive traces on their hands and had handled explosives was opposed by defence expert Dr Hugh Kenneth Black of the Royal Institute of Chemistry, and formerly Her Majesty's Chief Inspector of Explosives. The trial transcript clearly demonstrates that Skuse's evidence was preferred by the judge. The jury found the six men guilty of murder. On 15 August 1975, they were each sentenced to 21 life sentences.

Judith Ward Story On the 14th of February, 10 days after the M62 coach bombing, Judith Ward was taken into custody after being found sheltering in a shop doorway in Liverpool, England. The address on her Northern Ireland driver's license was found to be false; she claimed to be intending to travel to Ireland but seemed to have insufficient funds to pay for the journey. With Ward's consent, Dr Skuse took samples from her hands and claimed to have obtained a '*faint*' positive Griess test result, which was confirmed by another technique known as thin layer chromatography or TLC[9]. He also took samples from the caravan in which Ward was living and again obtained a positive result for a Griess test.

It is a salient fact that would have been known to Skuse, that the suspected explosive was nitroglycerine, which is highly volatile and therefore evaporates quickly. Consequently, the likelihood of any traces remaining on a bomber's hands after 10 days would be small; some might conclude that it was impossible. This should immediately have suggested to Skuse that an alternative explanation, other than handling explosives, should be considered. Nevertheless, Skuse's unreliable evidence was used by the prosecution to help convict Ward.

The RARDE scientists, Mr Douglas Higgs, Mr Walter Elliot, and Mr George Berryman, also conducted tests as part of the investigation of the M62 coach bombing and other bombings allegedly connected to Ward. They withheld from the trial the possibility that the positive results may have been false and that confirmatory tests were negative. This evidence would have weakened the prosecution case and supported the defence, and it was the prosecution's duty to disclose it. Ward was convicted and sentenced in 1974 to life imprisonment.

Reading the case history, admittedly with 20–20 hindsight, it is hard to understand how Ward could have been connected to the M62 coach bombing, let alone be convicted. Again, Gross's 'preconceived ideas' had perhaps fostered tunnel vision.

Maguire 7 Story The Maguire family shared a house. On the 3rd of December 1973, the house was raided by police following alleged admissions by two of the Guildford 4 that explosives were kept at that house. Scientific tests did not reveal any explosive traces at the premises, and no bomb-making paraphernalia was found in the house. Swabs were taken from the suspect's hands and the rubber gloves belonging to the mother, Ann Maguire, to test for explosive traces. The RARDE scientists conducted TLC tests and reported positive results for nitroglycerine for all male suspects but one, and positive results for Mrs Maguire's rubber gloves.

Again, the scientists failed to disclose the possibility of false positive results, and the existence of negative results obtained that would have weakened the prosecution case and supported the defence. In addition, Mr Higgs had misled the court when asked if the test applied could distinguish between the explosives nitroglycerine and another high explosive, PETN (pentaerythritoltetranitrate); the test could not.

The Maguire 7 were convicted in 1975 and sentenced to various terms of imprisonment from 4 to 14 years.

Appeals

Birmingham Six Appeal In 1991, the Court of Appeal stated that the Griess test should only be used as a gateway or preliminary test and that:

> *Dr Skuse's conclusion was wrong, and demonstrably wrong, judged even by the state of forensic science in 1974.* [§12]

Caustic soda (sodium hydroxide) is used to break down the molecule of nitroglycerine to produce nitrite ions. The concentration of caustic soda is crucial to the test. If Skuse had used a dilute solution, as he claimed, the test would have reacted positively only on hands '*dripping with nitroglycerine*', which was an absurdity. A stronger solution would react positively to any number of chemicals. Contaminants that might produce a positive result included laboratory detergents used to wash the test containers and some soaps and lacquers, as well as the nitrocellulose polymer used on playing cards.

Judith Ward Appeal Scientists had deliberately withheld information from the defence, which undermined the prosecution case.

In 1993, the Court of Appeal stated:

> *... there is...impressive...expert opinion...that Dr Skuse's tests...were of no value in establishing contact between the appellant and...explosives...* [§16]

Evidence demonstrated that the samples processed by Skuse were taken 57 hours after the bomb had exploded. Therefore, there could be no suggestion of explosives on Ward's hands. Skuse relied on one TLC test, which was not of the correct colour, causing the judges to question his handling of the Griess test as well.

The RARDE scientists had been found to have lied in claiming that a TLC test was exclusive for nitroglycerine (NG) and had failed to disclose exculpatory evidence of unreliable results.

The Maguire Appeal In addition to the non-disclosure of test results that would have weakened the prosecution case and strengthened the defence, evidence was given at trial that the results obtained could only be explained if the nitroglycerine-containing explosive had been 'kneaded'. Fresh evidence was presented that experiments had been conducted that demonstrated that kneading was not required to leave traces of NG under fingernails. Another piece of fresh evidence was the results of experiments in which a hand towel was found to be the source of innocent contamination spread among those using that towel.

Weaknesses Exposed

The weaknesses, quality failures and wrongdoing exposed by these wrongful convictions are as follows.

- Not being aware of the duties and responsibilities of an expert witness, particularly in the duty to the court to be impartial, on the contrary, seeing the role as helping the prosecuting agencies secure convictions to the extent of non-disclosure and lying.
- Usurping the role of the jury by considering the probability of the prosecution hypothesis that suspects had handled explosives, a matter strictly for the jury.
- Failing to interpret the findings according to the principles of balance, logic, transparency and robustness, discussed in Chapter 6.
  - Balance – a failure to consider or explore alternative explanations for findings, even when the prosecution hypothesis, that explosives had been handled, was clearly wrong.
  - Logic – transposing the conditional and thereby unfairly strengthening the prosecution case, as explained in Chapter 5 on the prosecutor's fallacy and Chapter 6. The focus of the forensic scientists should have been on the probability of a positive test result IF the suspects had handled explosives, which, given the several alternative explanations available and an inability to conclude that one is any more likely than another, robbed the explosives test results of any probative value; they were worthless.
  - Transparency – non-disclosure of relevant and probative evidence.
  - Robustness – employing methods that were not validated and not characterised, e.g. in terms of false positives.

Turning to organisational failings, in the early 1970s, the laboratories had no objective or independent assessment of the competence of the organisation or its forensic scientists, nor the validity of its methods and, consequently, the reliability of the scientific evidence.

While quality standards are no protection against forensic scientists who lie and/or fail to disclose significant evidence, seeing their role as helping to secure convictions, conforming to ISO/IEC 17025 will significantly reduce the risk of incompetence, the use of invalid methods and unreliable scientific evidence being presented at trial.

It is not too much of a stretch to argue that these cases saw a move away from a reliance on confession evidence (sadly, often obtained by unjust means, and certainly in these cases) and towards reliance on physical and scientific evidence of established reliability. Recalling the chapter on Hans Gross' Handbook, a principle established almost a century earlier and echoed in almost every chapter of this book.

It is worth a moment's reflection to be grateful that the death penalty was abolished in England in 1969 (except in the case of treason); otherwise, a dozen or more innocent persons may have lost their lives. Indeed, one appeal court judge wished some of those wrongly convicted had![10]

Responses

The response of the UK government was to establish a Royal Commission of Inquiry on criminal justice led by Viscount Runciman of Doxford, interestingly set up on the day the Birmingham 6 were released, the 14th of March 1991. Some commentators saw this as a damage limitation exercise with some justification (Bridges and McConville 1994). The inquiry report was published in 1993 (Runciman 1993). The main outcome was the establishment of the Criminal Cases Review Commission and a statutory requirement for the prosecution to disclose any evidence that might be of benefit to the defence, effectively all the evidence. Regarding forensic science, the commission proposed regulatory oversight by a Forensic Science Advisory Council, finally established in 2008, 15 years later. It also called for the registration of forensic scientists, which was met with the establishment of the Council for the Registration of Forensic Practitioners, CRFP, in 1999. Although the CRFP was closed by the government in 2009 on the grounds of financial viability, it produced a code of conduct which was incorporated into the quality management systems of some UK laboratories, which added a much-needed ethical dimension to the practice of forensic science. The successor of that code exists today in the code of the Forensic Science Regulator (FSR) of England and Wales (Forensic Science Regulator 2023).

Leaving the courtroom issues to the Royal Commission, the UK House of Lords conducted a parallel inquiry into laboratory practices in forensic science and the quality of scientific evidence. It recommended increasing engagement with the then-accrediting body NAMAS, a predecessor of UKAS (House of Lords 1993).

UK government pressure to acquire accreditation as a means of demonstrating the reliability of scientific evidence and the procrastination by some agencies in achieving that accreditation finally led to the appointment of a forensic science regulator in England & Wales in 2008 (House of Commons 2008), and giving the office statutory powers of enforcement in 2021 via the Forensic Science Regulator Act.

These and related historical events and their impacts are described in some detail in Section 4 of the book Quality Management in Forensic Science (Doyle 2019b).

Forensic Science Issues Arising

Skuse's 99% certainty that two of the Birmingham 6 suspects had handled the explosive nitroglycerine had no basis in science or logic. Nitrate ions have sources other than explosives, and so the Griess test is just a presumptive or screening test. A positive result must be confirmed using a more selective test. Therefore, the claimed 99% certainty was highly misleading and may have been decisive evidence in the minds of the members of the jury. In addition, as discussed earlier, Skuse had transposed the conditional by considering the probability of the prosecution hypothesis that explosives had been handled. He had not considered any alternative explanations for the test result he obtained. His evidence was fallacious and grossly misleading. However, it does seem that he merely lacked the necessary competencies and had not intended to mislead the court.

In the case of the Maguire 7 and Judith Ward, the actions of the RARDE scientists were deliberate. They succeeded in misleading the court by not disclosing scientific evidence, which would weaken the prosecution's case and had lied by suggesting that a test was exclusive for one type of explosive.

Social/Society

The reputation of the English system of justice was severely damaged by these high-profile miscarriages of justice. Gauging public opinion at the time was difficult. However, the reaction of the government was to act swiftly, taking several initiatives in an attempt to restore public confidence in the criminal justice system, initially establishing an inquiry followed by a Royal Commission on Criminal Justice. However, from a propaganda point of view and in the context of the Troubles, these miscarriages looked awful and gave ammunition to the republicans claiming that British justice was no justice at all. These wrongful convictions would have been a factor in the movement towards a settlement between the sectarian parties in Northern Ireland and the UK government known as the Good Friday or Belfast Agreement, signed on the 10th of April 1998.

There was even greater reputational damage to forensic science. With no standard that covered both managerial and technical standards, UK forensic science laboratories looked to BS 5750 for management and M10 for technical requirements.

On 1st April 1997, the Criminal Cases Review Commission took over responsibility for the review of alleged miscarriages of justice in England and Wales and Northern Ireland[11]. The Commission was set up following the recommendation of the Royal Commission on Criminal Justice – the Runciman Commission – which proposed that review of alleged miscarriages should be transferred from the Home Office to an independent non-departmental public body. The establishment of the Commission was warmly welcomed by organisations which had campaigned for such an independent body for many years.

Structure of the Publication

The 1999 edition of ISO/IEC 17025 has two major sections: the first specifying management requirements and the second the technical requirements. The management requirements were to establish a quality management system, document procedures and policies, and essentially ensure the competence of the laboratory and meet customer needs. The technical requirements cover the competence of the scientists, maintenance of equipment and facilities, the validity of the methods and the reporting of results, among other things.

The 1999 edition specifies general requirements for the competence to carry out tests and/or calibrations, including sampling. Those requirements cover testing and calibration performed using standard methods, non-standard methods, and laboratory-developed methods. The standard applies to all organisations performing tests and/or calibrations, regardless of the number of personnel or the scope of the testing and/or calibration. The standard can be used by laboratories in developing their quality, administrative and technical systems.

As stated earlier, ISO/IEC 17025 combined management and technical requirements into one standard and conformance to the standard demonstrated that the laboratory and its staff were competent, methods were valid, and test results could be relied upon.

ISO and IEC guard their copyright closely. However, the scope of the main sections of the 1999 edition was as follows.

- **Management requirements,** including the need for a quality system, capturing and meeting customer needs, and monitoring and improving performance.
- **Technical requirements,** including ensuring the competence of personnel, selection and validation of test methods, assuring the quality of test results and a whole series of requirements regarding the reporting of results.

Meeting the requirements set out in the standard is designed to ensure that laboratories demonstrate competence in producing reliable results, providing confidence to customers.

Copies of the latest edition of the standard can be purchased from ISO, and a preview of the standard, including the complete structure, can be found on the ISO website's online browsing platform (ISO n.d.).

Discussed later in the section under 'Impact at the Time', guidance on how a forensic science laboratory might conform to ISO/IEC 17025 is given. That discussion includes a more complete picture of the structure of the standard as it applies to forensic science laboratories.

Quality Standards Framework – Continuous Improvement

More important than knowing the structure of ISO/IEC 1025 is how it fits into the management, practice and delivery of forensic science. In many instances, forensic science laboratories are required to be accredited to the standard. As mentioned earlier, accreditation is a process whereby an independent third-party confirms the competence of the laboratory, its staff, the validity of its methods and the reliability of the results it reports.

In the English-speaking world, the major accrediting bodies are UKAS (UK Accreditation Service) based in the United Kingdom, ANAB (ANSI National Accreditation Board) and A2LA (American Association for Laboratory Accreditation) based in the United States and NATA (National Association of Testing Authorities) based in Australia. Forensic science laboratories in other countries can be accredited by these bodies, e.g. the New Zealand forensic science laboratory ESR (The Institute of Environmental Science and Research) is accredited by ANAB and laboratories in the United Arab Emirates are accredited by UKAS.

Gaining accreditation requires close familiarity with ISO/IEC 17025 and developing and documenting policies, systems, procedures, and guidance which conform. Once documented, the laboratory will need to operate for a period following what is now a conforming documented quality management system. Once satisfied that the laboratory conforms, the accrediting body is invited to audit against the standard. When the accrediting body is satisfied that the standard is being met, accreditation is granted. Thereafter, an internal quality auditing scheme will monitor conformance and identify opportunities for improvement. An annual surveillance by auditors of the accrediting body will also take place, and at the end of the accreditation cycle, usually four years, the laboratory, if still conforming to the standard, will be re-accredited.

The accrediting bodies must conform to ISO/IEC 17011 'Conformity assessment: Requirements for accreditation bodies accrediting conformity assessment bodies', which is formalised/recognised by entering into a mutual recognition agreement with ILAC and is intended to ensure that test results produced in one country or territory are accepted elsewhere.

This framework goes a long way towards promoting a culture of continuous improvement and assuring the quality of forensic scientific evidence produced by accredited forensic science laboratories. This acknowledgement of the potential for improvement emphasises that ISO/IEC 17025 should be regarded as a minimum standard.

Impact at the Time

For those forensic science laboratories that were already conforming to quality standards, the challenge of now conforming to ISO/IEC 17025 was less daunting than for those starting with a blank sheet of paper, as it were. It was also a challenge for accrediting bodies to interpret a generic standard applying to all types of testing laboratories in the context of forensic science and meet the needs of justice systems. There was much initial wondering and scratching of heads.

It was not until 2002 that ILAC, the International Laboratory Accreditation Cooperation organisation, issued a guidance document for accrediting forensic science laboratories to ISO/IEC 17025, and this became the *de facto* standard (ILAC 2002). The guide recognised in particular that reports for a court of law would be quite different from the outputs from a testing laboratory, and the format may be prescribed by legislation. It also documented the need for methods to be '*fully validated*' before being used in casework and the requirement for forensic scientists to have their performance monitored to ensure competence.

The management requirement emphasised by the ILAC guide was control of records. Forensic science laboratories were required to have documented procedures to ensure that a coordinated record relating to each case was maintained. The guiding principle was that records should be sufficiently detailed to allow another equally qualified scientist to determine what had been done and interpret the results, essentially to be able to repeat the process. Records would include instrument performance parameters, test results, calculations and photographs or diagrams. Each page of a case file should be uniquely identified by a date and page number and initialled by the examining scientist.

The ILAC guide required a case file review before issuing a report, which should include a '*critical findings*'[12] check.

Among the technical requirements interpreted by the ILAC guide for forensic science laboratories was the need to ensure the competence of scientists. This was to include documenting the necessary competencies[13] and the procedures for determining and maintaining competence.

The guide required each forensic scientist to have a training record listing academic and professional qualifications, external or internal courses attended, and relevant training received whilst working in the laboratory.

The guide drew attention to the need to maintain the integrity of items of evidence employing secure storage, the control of access and the prevention of deterioration. It suggested that operational areas might require environmental monitoring.

One of the most demanding requirements in terms of conformance and documentation related to the methods or analytical procedures used by a forensic science laboratory. These methods or procedures are often termed Standard Operating Procedures or SOPs. All SOPs had to be fully documented and fully validated before being used in casework. The guide also introduced the concept of verification, whereby a method developed elsewhere is checked for performance before use by the laboratory. This particularly applies to DNA analysis kits, which are purchased from external suppliers and must be performance-checked before use.

Validation involves providing evidence that an SOP is accurate, produces a true or almost true result[14]. The concept of full validation was developed to include inter-laboratory tests, where a method was checked for accuracy at several laboratories.

All chemical reagents were required to be adequately labelled to include the identity of the person who prepared the reagent and its expiry date.

All instruments required a documented maintenance schedule and a service record.

The guide also explained how the requirement for traceability might be met. Traceability is a highly technical requirement where any measurement must be traced through an 'unbroken chain' to an international standard such as the kilogram, meter or second or more commonly, a measure of concentration (moles per cubic meter mol/m^3). This is achieved in practice by comparison with reference materials.

The need for a chain-of-custody or continuity record was included. This records where an item of evidence is at any one time and who has responsibility for that item. That record should cover the entire history of the item, from recovery at the scene to disposal.

The requirement for quality control is explained, with examples of how the requirement might be met, such as control charts recording instrument performance.

Interestingly, the ILAC guide also required monitoring the performance of forensic scientists giving evidence in court. While such monitoring might seem essential, it is very difficult to achieve, and as yet, there is no adequate system in place for doing so. There are, however, mechanisms in some jurisdictions for capturing adverse comments made by a judge.

As stated earlier, the ILAC guide accepts that reports for court are often prescribed by legislation and may not meet the requirements of ISO/IEC 17025. It provides guidance on what form a report might take, including attaching technical annexes.

Initial conformance and obtaining accreditation to this new standard in 1999 was a challenging task requiring a major effort by forensic science laboratories and a culture change, accepting the need for continuous improvement. However, by conforming to ISO/IEC 17025, as interpreted by the ILAC guide, the risk of contributing to miscarriages of justice was greatly reduced.

The two UK forensic science laboratories that were at the heart of the scandal were among the first to be accredited to the new standard ISO/IEC 17025:1999.

A US Alternative - ASCLD/LAB

From 1998 onwards, major European forensic science laboratories were quick to adopt and conform to ISO/IEC 17025 as a means of independently demonstrating competence and the validity of their results. However, the journey towards the adoption of ISO/IEC 17025 by forensic science laboratories in the United States was very different and started from a different place.

In 1973, the directors of 47 forensic science laboratories (usually called crime labs) were invited by the then-director of the FBI to open lines of communication among US laboratories. In the United States, there are three federal law enforcement agencies of the US Department of Justice, the FBI, ATF and the DEA, each with their laboratories. So-called crime labs range in jurisdiction from state to local counties and often sit within police departments[15]. In response to the call for better communications, the American Society of Crime Lab Directors (ASCLD) was formed in 1974. Among the early objectives of the organisation was to address the quality of US forensic science services to criminal justice systems. 'Accreditation' was selected as the way forward. ASCLD developed a voluntary program of laboratory accreditation, and in 1981, the American Society of Crime Laboratory Directors/Laboratory Accreditation Board (ASCLD/LAB) was formed. Shortly afterwards, the first version of the ASCLD/LAB standards and program was released. As more laboratories became accredited, the financial stability of the accreditation program became established such that in 1988, ASCLD/LAB was incorporated as a not-for-profit corporation (Collins 2018) and had, as its stated mission, four objectives.

> *To improve the quality of laboratory services provided to the criminal justice system.*
> *To offer to the general public and to users of laboratory services a means of identifying throughout the nation those laboratory facilities which satisfy accreditation criteria.*
> *To develop and maintain criteria which can be used by a laboratory to assess its level of performance and strengthen its operation.*
> *To provide an independent, impartial and objective system by which laboratory facilities can benefit from a total organization review.*

As will be discussed shortly, the fourth objective was a challenge.

ASCLD/LAB's parent body, ASCLD, now seems keen to put clear blue water between it and the accreditation program (ASCLD 2023). However, the claim is that this was the first accreditation program in the world for forensic science laboratories. The ASCLD/LAB's standard was very much homegrown and was revised several times over its lifetime. It was a standard developed by crime lab directors for crime labs. It included a 'grading system'. The requirements of the standard were classified as 'essential', 'important' or 'desirable', akin to the 'shall', 'should', 'may' and 'can' of ISO standards, emphasising what must be done to conform. Accredited labs had to meet all the essential requirements and a specified proportion of the others. It also included the requirement for an 'accreditation ceremony' to celebrate and publicise the achievement. The standard included no reference to ISO Guide 25 in contemporary revisions, and it does not reflect the structure of the Guide. However, it is fair to state that most of the provisions of ISO/IEC 17025 are included. The claim to be the first depends on what is meant by the term 'accreditation'.

As stated earlier, accreditation is third-party or independent confirmation that an organisation conforms to a standard. ASCLD/LAB was a deeply conflicted organisation. Essentially, crime lab directors developed and documented the standard, were the auditors, assessing conformance, and the auditees. A common phrase to describe this degree of conflict is 'they were marking their own homework', and in this case also set the questions. It was the lack of independence that weakened the claim to be an accrediting body.

Consequently, none of the laboratories 'accredited' by ASCLD/LAB were accredited in the proper sense of the word.

This degree of conflict was heavily criticised by US commentators and may have contributed to the many quality failures that beset the ASCLD/LAB 'accredited' forensic science laboratories (Gabel 2014).

Perhaps as a result of the US attitude to regulation – the less the better, it was not until 2009 that ASCLD/LAB gained its ILAC mutual recognition agreement and began to accredit its members against ISO/IEC 17025, having first demonstrated conformance to ISO/IEC 17011. ASCLD/LAB continued to offer what was known as the 'legacy program', accreditation to its original non-ISO standard. ASCLD/LAB 'merged into' the US accrediting body ANAB in 2016 (ANAB 2016), and ASCLD/LAB ceased to operate.

Independence is demonstrated by having a separate development/publishing body and an independent accreditation body. Even having adopted ISO/IEC 17025, the residual lack of independence in the ASCLD/LAB program may have contributed to its demise.

Impact Today

There have now been three editions of ISO/IEC 17025; the latest 2017 edition is markedly different from the 1999 edition in structure and is far less prescriptive and broader in scope. As stated earlier, most forensic science laboratories in the world, certainly the developed world, are accredited to the standard.

Regional organisations require accreditation for membership, and legislation requiring the accreditation of forensic science providers sits on statute books across the developed world.

The central requirement for a culture of continuous improvement helps to guard against complacency, which can lead to false beliefs about performance and the quality of outputs. So, positively embraced as a means of continuously improving performance, accreditation to ISO/IEC 17025 has made a major contribution to improving the quality of scientific evidence and reducing the risk of miscarriages of justice.

However, even in accredited laboratories, mistakes still occur, and accreditation bodies can miss non-conformances, which puts justice at risk. In addition, accreditation is no protection against bad actors and fraud, such as 'dry labbing', where test results are fabricated. There are also noises from commentators claiming accreditation alone is not enough, in that it only applies to the analysis stage of the forensic science process (Ross and Neuteboom 2020). One model of the forensic science process is given by Figure 1 of the standard ISO 21043, which indicates where analysis sits in the forensic science process. The graphic given as Figure 7.1 is based on that process.

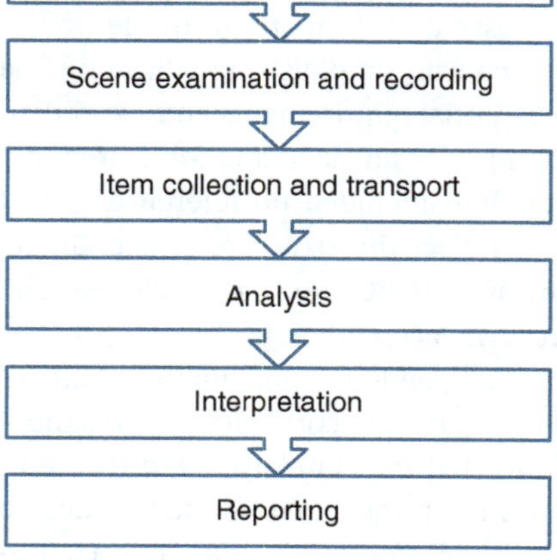

Figure 7.1 A forensic science process.

Crime scene activities properly fall under another standard, ISO/IEC 17020, and sampling (item collection and transport) is very much within the scope of ISO/IEC 17025, as is the reporting of opinions and interpretations. Incorporating into the accredited quality management system the requirement to comply with a standard for evaluative reporting[16], such as the AFSP Standards (AFSP 2009) or the ENFSI guide, (ENFSI 2015) would provide a reasonably comprehensive scope. Evaluative reporting is the subject of Chapter 6 'Interpreting Evidence'.

One real weakness of ISO/IEC 17025 is that it is the laboratory that effectively 'certifies' the competence of its scientists, and this lack of independent assessment does increase the risk of less-than-competent performance by individuals.

In England and Wales, the Forensic Science Regulator (FSR) has been given statutory powers to require providers of specified forensic disciplines to conform to ISO/IEC 17025 (HMG 2021). One legacy of the CRFP is the adoption of its code of conduct by the FSR, now enshrined in statute (Forensic Science Regulator 2023). The origin of this code can be traced back to UK forensic science laboratories (Gough 1997).

The latest edition of the standard includes a requirement for impartiality (§4.1). How this is maintained and demonstrated in a forensic science laboratory administered by a law enforcement or police agency is difficult to conceive. The risks associated with too close a relationship between law enforcement and forensic science provision are further explored in a later chapter on the 2009 NAS report (Chapter 9), the Sydney Declaration (Chapter 10) and in the WIREs article (Doyle 2019a).

Contribution to Current Practice

The contribution to current practice is pretty much covered in the earlier sections on impacts. Nevertheless, it is worth repeating that almost every forensic science laboratory in the world is now accredited to ISO/IEC 17025 and in many jurisdictions, accreditation is mandated for specified forensic science activities.

Accredited organisations must accept the need for continuous improvement and proactively seek opportunities for improvement. Embracing this need as a means of improving performance is a particular strength of quality management systems in ensuring forensic science meets stakeholder requirements.

One remaining weakness is that the certification of individual competence rests with the accredited organisation. An independent assessment of individual competence would be a significant improvement.

Concluding Remarks

In response to high-profile miscarriages of justice, UK forensic science laboratories adopted conformance to quality standards as a means of restoring public confidence, promoting a culture of continuous improvement and meeting the needs of the criminal justice system.

Accreditation is confirmation by an independent or third-party body that a forensic science laboratory conforms to the standard ensuring competence and validity.

Forensic science laboratories all over the world are now accredited to ISO/IEC 17025 by independent, third-party accreditation bodies.

Accreditation to ISO/IEC 17025 is sometimes mandated by relevant authorities and forms the basis of regulatory frameworks in some jurisdictions, such as England & Wales.

Conformance to ISO/IEC 17025 requires an ethos of continuous improvement, an acceptance by the accredited organisation that there is always room for improvement. Therefore, the standard should be considered a minimum.

There have been three editions of ISO/IEC 17025 since it was first published in 1999, and the latest 2017 edition differs in structure from earlier editions and is less prescriptive. However, the main requirements still fall into the categories of managerial and technical.

The latest edition includes a requirement for impartiality, which might be a challenge for some police based forensic science providers.

Of the publications covered in this history, ISO/IEC 17025 is perhaps the publication that has the greatest impact on the development of forensic science and its current practice.

Despite the adoption of quality standards, wrongful convictions and other quality failures in forensic science continue to this day, such as the scandal at the Queensland Health DNA Laboratory (Sofronoff 2022; Doyle 2024). So, there is room for improvement.

Unfortunately, quality failures demonstrate that forensic science is more reactive than proactive; progress is mostly driven by failures rather than success or striving for excellence, as some commentators claim.

Key Takeaways

A series of miscarriages of justice in England, which came to light in the early 1990s and to which forensic science was found to have contributed, resulted in UK forensic science laboratories adopting and conforming to the international standard ISO/IEC 17025:1999 'General requirements for the competence of testing and calibration laboratories'.

In 2002, ILAC published guidance for forensic science laboratories on conforming to ISO/IEC 17025, which, for a time, became the *de facto* standard against which forensic science laboratories were accredited.

Most forensic science laboratories in the developed world are accredited to the latest edition of this standard, and many authorities mandate accreditation.

Conformance is maintained by both internal audits and external independent checks, together with a culture of continuous improvement, proactively seeking opportunities for improvement.

The standard itself has been revised twice, and the latest edition differs in structure, is less prescriptive and broader in scope than the 1999 first edition.

Of all the publications included in this book, and despite having no direct relationship with forensic science, ISO/IEC 17025 is probably the one that has had the greatest impact on the development of forensic science and its current practice.

Notes

1 Accreditation is a process of verifying conformance to the standard by an independent third party such as the United Kingdom Accreditation Service (UKAS) and the US ANSI National Accreditation Board (ANAB).
2 The upper house of the bicameral UK parliament.
3 A quality system developed in the early 1970s for laboratories conducting non-clinical health and environmental safety studies.
4 During the Troubles, nearly 4000 people were killed and close to 50 000 injured.
5 'Pub' is a British term for a bar.
6 The UK Home Office is Britain's interior ministry, effectively the ministry of police.
7 A Griess test produces a pink colouration if a nitrate ion is present; nitrate ions are a component of many explosives including nitroglycerine.
8 Gas chromatology will separate the explosive from other components of the sample and the explosive will be detected by the mass spectrometer and produce a signal which is recorded.
9 Chromatography is a generic term for the separation of the chemical compounds of a sample; in TLC, this is achieved using a thin layer of silica on a supporting substrate such as glass or plastic.
10 One of the Lords of Appeal is quoted as stating 'We shouldn't have all these campaigns to get the Birmingham Six released if they'd been hanged. They'd have been forgotten and the whole community would have been satisfied'.
11 Scotland is a separate jurisdiction with a different justice system, a hybrid between an inquisitorial/civil law and an adversarial/common law approach.
12 Observations and results that have a significant impact on the conclusion reached and the interpretation and opinion provided.
13 Competencies are essentially the knowledge, skills and abilities required to perform the designated role.
14 Any measurement, such as the amount of alcohol in blood, has an uncertainty, a +/− figure, which must be reported as the true measurement will lie within the range given by the +/− figure.
15 The risks arising from the close relationship between forensic science laboratories and law enforcement agencies will be discussed in the chapter on the NAS Report.
16 Reporting the strength of evidence based on the assignment of a likelihood ratio, see Chapter 6 for details.

Bibliography

AFSP. 2009. "Standards for the Formulation of Evaluative Forensic Science Expert Opinion." *Science and Justice* 49: 161–64.

ANAB. 2016. "ANAB and ASCLD/LAB Merge Forensic Operations." *ANSI National Accreditaion Board*. 22 April. Accessed April 25, 2024. https://anab.ansi.org/anab-and-ascld-lab-merge-forensics-operations/.

ASCLD. 2023. "Our History." *The American Society of Crime Laboratory Directors*. Accessed April 23, 2024. https://www.ascld.org/our-history/.

Bridges, Lee, and Mike McConville. 1994. "Keeping Faith with Their Own Convictions: The Royal Commission on Criminal Justice." *The Modern Law Review* 57: 75–90.

Collins, John. 2018. "History of Forensic Laboratory Accreditation." In *HR Management in the Forensic Science Laboratory*, edited by John Collins, 457–75. London: Academic Press.

Council of the European Union. 2009. "Accrediation of Forensic Service Providers Carrying out Laboratory Activities." *Council Framework Decision 2009/905/JHA*. Brussels: Official Journal of the European Union, 30 November.

Department of Justice. 2015. "Justice Department Press Release." *Department of Justice*. 7 December. Accessed April 4, 2024. https://www.justice.gov/opa/pr/justice-department-announces-new-accreditation-policies-advance-forensic-science.

Doyle, Sean. 2019a. "A Review of the Current Quality Standards Framework Supporting Forensic Science: Risks and Opportunities." *WIRE's Forensic Science* 2: 1–23.

Doyle, Sean. 2019b. "Historical Perspective." In *Quality Management in Forensic Science*, edited by Sean Doyle, 155–71. London: Elsevier.

Doyle, Sean. 2019c. "The Development of Quality Standards." In *Quality Management in Forensic Science*, edited by Sean Doyle, 207–09. London: Elsevier.

Doyle, Sean. 2024. "QHFSS DNA Laboratory – ISO/IEC 17025 Conformance and Accreditation." *Forensic Science International: Synergy* 8: 1–15.

ENFSI. 2015. "ENFSI Guideline For Evaluative Reporting." *ENFSI*. 8 March. Accessed March 21, 2024. https://www.google.com/search?q=enfsi+evaluative+reporting&rlz=1C5CHFA_enNZ948NZ948&oq=ENFSI+&gs_lcrp=EgZjaHJvbWUqDAgBECMYJxiABBiKBTIGCAAQRRg5MgwIARAjGCcYgAQYigUyBwgCEAAYgAQyBwgDEAAYgAQyBwgEEAAYgAQyBwgFEAAYgAQyBwgGEAAYgAQyBwgHEAAYgAQyBwgIEAAYgAQyBwgJEAAYg.

—. 2023. "Policy on Accreditation." *ENFSI*. 10 May. Accessed April 4, 2024. https://enfsi.eu/wp-content/uploads/2023/08/BRD-ACR-001_Policy-on-Accreditation.pdf.

Forensic Science Regulator. 2023. *Code of Practice Ver 1*. Birmingham, UK: The Forensic Science Regulator, March.

Gabel, Jessica D. 2014. "Realizing Reliability in Forensic Science from the Ground Up (1973–), vol. 104, no. 2, 2014, pp." *The Journal of Criminal Law and Criminology* 104: 283–352.

Gough, Terry A. 1997. "Quality Assurance in Forensic Science: the UK Situation." *Accreditation and Quality Assurance* 2: 216–23.

HMG. 2021. *Forensic Science Regulator Act*. London, England: HMSO, 29 April.

House of Commons. 2008. "The Forensic Science Regulator and the Forensic Science Advisory Council." *UK Parliament Hansard*. 10 January. Accessed April 6, 2024. https://hansard.parliament.uk/commons/2008-01-10/debates/08011061000014/TheForensicScienceRegulatorAndTheForensicScienceAdvisoryCouncil.

House of Lords. 1993. "Forensic Science: Select Committee Report." *UK Parliament*. 15 April. Accessed April 6, 2024. https://hansard.parliament.uk/Lords/1993-04-15/debates/123d22f2-03b4-4f1d-a9ca-1e98cfeec88c/ForensicScienceSelectCommitteeReport.

ILAC. 2002. *Guidelines for Forensic Science Laboratories*. Guida, Silverwater NZW: ILAC.

ISO. n.d. *ISO/IEC 17025*. Accessed March 26, 2024. https://www.iso.org/obp/ui/en/#iso:std:iso-iec:17025:ed-3:v1:en.

Pallister, David. 1991. "News UK Northern Ireland." *The Guardian*. 15 March. Accessed March 28, 2024. https://www.theguardian.com/uk/1991/mar/15/northernireland.davidpallister.

R v Maguire & Ors. 1992. 133 (Cr.App.R.).

R v McIlkenny & Ors. 1991. 287 (Cr.App.R.).

R v Richardson & Ors. 1989. (EWCA Criminal Division, 19 October).

R v Ward. 1992. 96 (Cr.App.R.).

Ross, Alastair, and Wim Neuteboom. 2020. "ISO-Accreditation – Is That All There Is for Forensic Science?" *Australian Journal of Forensic Sciences* 54(1): 2–14.

Runciman, Viscount. 1993. *Royal Commission on Criminal Justice*. Royal Commission, London: HMSO.

Sippola, Erki, and Pekka Saukko. 2015. "History and Current Status of Forensic Science and Medicine in Finland." In *The Global Practice of Forensic Science*, edited by Douglas H. Ubelaker, 99. Chichester: John Woley & Sons Ltd.

Sofronoff, Walter. 2022. "Final Report Commission of Inquiry into Forensic DNA Testing in Queensland." Commission of Inquiry.

van Asten, Arian, Wim Neuteboom, Wiersma Sijtze, and Geradts Zeno. 2015. "The Netherlands." In *The Global Practice of Forensic Science*, edited by Douglas H. Ubelaker, 223. Chichester: John Wiley & Sons Ltd.

Williams, Alex. 1999. "History Booklet." *Eurachem*. June. Accessed April 2024. https://www.eurachem.org/images/stories/about/pdf/history-booklet.pdf.

8

Observer Effects – Cognitive Bias

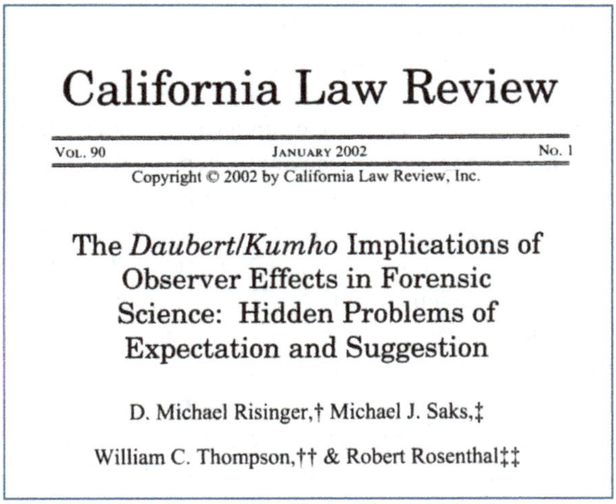

California Law Review

VOL. 90 JANUARY 2002 NO. 1

Copyright © 2002 by California Law Review, Inc.

The *Daubert/Kumho* Implications of Observer Effects in Forensic Science: Hidden Problems of Expectation and Suggestion

D. Michael Risinger,† Michael J. Saks,‡

William C. Thompson,†† & Robert Rosenthal‡‡

Image 8.1 The publication's header. With permission of California Law Review, Inc.

Name of Publication

The publication is titled *The Daubert/Kumho Implications of Observer Effects in Forensic Science: Hidden Problems of Expectation and Suggestion*.

D. Michael Risinger, Michael J. Saks, William C. Thompson and Robert Rosenthal

California Law Review

Vol. 90, No. 1 (Jan 2002), pp. 1–56 (56 pages)

Published By: California Law Review, Inc.

According to ResearchGate, this paper has been cited 243 times, and according to Harvard University, 644 times.

In this chapter, the title will be abbreviated to 'Observer Effects'.

A History of Forensic Science in 10 Publications: How They Established Current Practice, First Edition.
Sean Doyle.

Introduction

The publication is a response to a judgment of the US Supreme Court in the case of *Kumho Tire Co Ltd v Patrick Carmichael* (Kumho Tire Company, Ltd. v. Carmichael 1999), which clarified a trial judge's gatekeeping obligations as set out in Federal Rule of Evidence (FRE) 702 regarding expert testimony. The judgment made clear that the scope included all expert testimony, not just scientific testimony. FRE 702 refers to testimony by expert witnesses and requires the trial judge to ensure that only reliable expert testimony is admitted as evidence.[1]

The clarification required that '... *the testimony is the product of reliable principles and methods*' and concerned '*the task at hand*', which had the practical effect of emphasising that the gatekeeping role was case-specific.

> *Rule 702 grants the district court the discretionary authority ... to determine reliability in light of the particular facts and circumstances of the particular case.*

'Observer Effects' aims to demonstrate that '*certain factors*' can undermine the reliability of expert evidence, and FRE 702 requires such factors to be considered when deciding admissibility. Furthermore, feature comparison evidence, such as fingerprints and handwriting, is particularly affected by such factors, given its dependence on subjective judgement.

The reason this publication is included in this history is that in 2002, it was the first to raise the issue of bias in the context of forensic science. Here 'bias' means cognitive bias, errors in human reasoning that lead to poor decision-making.

The human brain has evolved to ensure that threats and opportunities are responded to quickly with as little effort as possible (both physical and mental) to ensure our survival as we roamed the savannah hunting and gathering. However, when we are not responding to threats or opportunities, we can think more carefully, or more slowly, as Daniel Kahneman describes in his book *Thinking Fast and Slow* (Kahneman 2012). As a result of our innate laziness, humans can overly rely on the hardwired response to threats and opportunities when considering more complex matters, and this manifests itself as cognitive bias, resulting in poor decision-making. We prefer to address simple questions rather than more difficult ones; comforting lies are often preferred to uncomfortable truths.

Cognitive bias is the main subject of the publication and is what the authors term observer effects, which are the many biases that infect human judgement (The Decision Lab 2024). Biases in human thinking and decision-making can lead to erroneous or fallacious outcomes. The existence and effect of bias were recognised as long ago as the seventeenth century (Bacon 1620) and possibly earlier. The basis of our current understanding of human biases is the Nobel Prize-winning work of Daniel Kahneman and Amos Tversky (Tversky and Kahneman 1974).

The primary objective of this publication was to raise awareness of observer effects, or cognitive bias, within forensic science. By doing so, the authors argue that the risk of bias should be considered when determining the admissibility of expert evidence. Trial judges exercising their gatekeeping duties, as required by FRE 702, should check that measures for reducing the risk of cognitive bias are in place before admitting scientific evidence.

The publication catalogues the forms bias might take, describes how it might affect scientific evidence, how it might be recognised and what can be done to minimise its effects.

This publication was the first to raise the issue of bias in the context of forensic science. It should also be acknowledged that the work of Itiel Dror, discussed later in this chapter, did much to raise awareness among forensic scientists.

The main remedy set out in 'Observer Effects' is to shield the examining forensic scientist from information outside his or her field of expertise, which might bias opinions and conclusions and result in misleading evidence being presented at trial, thereby putting justice at risk.

The publication is very well researched, drawing on a great deal of related scientific, legal and psychological scholarship, and sources from Julius Caesar to Daniel Kahneman. It includes many examples that help the reader to understand the points made. It begins with a historical perspective of one of the most common and, in forensic science, one of the most pernicious cognitive biases, and that is the so-called confirmation bias. This bias arises where, once a hypothesis or proposition is adopted, only supporting evidence is recognised and anything to the contrary is ignored. As well as being recognised by historical natural philosophers such as Francis Bacon and studied by later figures such as Daniel Kahneman, this is also the bias at the heart of the 'preconceived theory' of Hans Gross's nineteenth-century Handbook, the subject of Chapter 1.

The authors use the term 'observer effects' rather than bias, meaning the results of observation depend upon the state of the observer as well as the thing being observed. It is interesting to note in passing that the influence of the state of the observer is a factor that finds echoes in quantum mechanics through Heisenberg's uncertainty principle and in Einstein's theory of relativity.

Following an extensive historical sketch and before getting into the meat of the subject, the authors make clear what the publication is not about: forensic fraudsters manufacturing results. However, in this early section, the main risk is introduced: that the information given to forensic scientists might influence their conclusions and opinions. And it chillingly states the following.

> *... observer effects can lead competent and honest forensic scientists, using well-validated techniques, to offer sincere conclusions that are, nevertheless, distorted and inaccurate.*

The publication is in four parts plus a general introduction. Those parts are as follows:

1. Observer Effects
2. Observer Effects in Forensic Science
3. Minimising Observer Effects in Forensic Science
4. Observer Effects and Admissibility Under [US] Federal Rule of Evidence 702

Part 1 General Observer Effects

In Part 1, the publication demonstrates some visual or optical observer effects in support of arguments for the existence of bias or observer effects in general. It then goes on to describe some specific types of bias, including confirmation bias, only accepting evidence that supports a held belief and rejecting that which does not. The need to clearly distinguish between signal and noise is emphasised; failure to do so may lead to false results. Anchoring bias is also described in which conclusions are overly reliant on starting points, which could affect subjective probability estimates of the rarity of certain characteristics of an evidence type, e.g. in handwriting examination.

Of particular relevance is conformity bias, where the opinion of a senior scientist influences the opinion of a junior colleague conducting a review of the senior colleague's work. In the Scottish Fingerprint Inquiry, the influence of senior fingerprint examiners on their more junior colleagues was found to be a contributory factor to the misidentification of a fingerprint found at a murder scene (Campbell 2011) (see recommendation 33, p. 744). Indeed, the inquiry, prompted by a wrongful conviction, is a case study of how many cognitive biases combined that led forensic scientists in the wrong direction. This suggests that there should be a requirement in a blind review that the reviewer should not know the identity of the original examiner to guard against conformity bias.

There is also the risk of bias arising from the working environment. Culture and ethos may affect outcomes. Another inquiry readily supports this point (Sofronoff 2022). A bad actor instilled a culture, which resulted in numerous miscarriages of justice over many years.

Bias resulting from motivation should also be recognised. A forensic scientist examining evidence of a horrific crime may make a greater effort to find evidence in support of a specific hypothesis, particularly if a prime suspect has been identified and is known to the examining scientist. As will be discussed later under the Biography of the Publication, this is another risk of motivational bias when a forensic scientist is asked to conduct further tests or experiments in support of a previously drawn conclusion.

This erudite study of biases that lead to poor decisions concludes by examining the relationship between information, conclusion accuracy, and confidence. While more information can increase confidence, it doesn't necessarily improve the accuracy of the evidence. This is particularly concerning in disciplines like handwriting or tool marks, where subjective probability estimates are made. For example, if a forensic scientist relies on extraneous information to increase confidence in a 'suspect probably signed the document' conclusion, the true probability remains unchanged. The key is to protect the forensic scientist from biasing irrelevant information.

Part 2 Observer Effects in Forensic Science

Part 2 starts with a claim that subjective judgment has a major role in forensic science to add to the inculpatory expectation[2] of the examining scientist. It also draws attention to the contemporary lack of awareness and consequent lack of recognition, together with the absence of measures that might reduce the risk and impact of bias arising from this expectation.

Part 2 then goes on to describe a number of these observer effects and how they affect forensic science.

However, the publication begins by specifying the proper role of a forensic scientist, which is to answer questions appropriate to the discipline and not,

> *... to give an answer, even an honest and accurate answer, by any other means.*

The authors warn that a forensic scientist who relies on or is even exposed to information outside the discipline abuses their role. The publication demands that only information derived from the discipline must be relied on in reaching conclusions and offering opinions in expert testimony.

An extreme example is offered to make the point. A forensic odontologist considering bitemark evidence[3] concludes that there is sufficient evidence to support the contention that the bite mark was made by the suspect; however, he is not certain. Learning that the suspect's DNA was found in the region of the bitemark, he now concludes with confidence that the mark was made by the suspect. This also raises another issue, which is double counting.[4] The odontologist relied on the supporting DNA evidence to arrive at his conclusion, which was not warranted on the bite mark evidence alone. The jury will also rely on the DNA evidence in reaching its verdict, and so that DNA evidence is counted twice, it has double the impact it might otherwise have had.

The publication then sets out a scenario in which a police 'hunch' infects the independence of several evidence types pointing to a suspect. This has been the pattern in many wrongful convictions, such as those discussed in Chapter 7 on ISO/IEC 17025. The publication then offers the following quote (Campbell 1994).

> *Insofar as systematic biases have been observed, they are overwhelmingly ... a tendency to contaminate one's reports in the direction of agreement with what others are reporting and thus fail to report what is uniquely available from one's own perspective. In addition, the agreement achieved represents pseudo-confirmation. The tremendous literature on conformity and suggestion shows how strong and persuasive this effect is. It could scarcely fail to operate among teams of scientists.*

The publication draws attention to the risks of such informational contamination, weakening strong evidence and strengthening weak evidence. In either case, the evidence becomes misleading.

The publication goes on to describe the situation in 2002. It reports that the protective measure of shielding the examining scientist from potentially biasing non-essential information is not included in any standards or guidance at the time, nor in any forensic science textbooks. In fact, it records that one textbook advises that as much circumstantial information as possible should be acquired before conducting an examination. It also makes the point that no research on the influence of bias is or has been conducted. It reports that standard police practice involves potentially biasing case information being made available to examining scientists as a matter of routine. Examples are then given of where biasing information has resulted in misleading evidence.

The overall point being made is that the potential effect of bias on the reliability of scientific evidence was not recognised, and therefore nothing was being done to protect the forensic scientist from its influence, putting justice at risk.

The hope is expressed, and the recommendation made that the case of *Kumho* might spur the development of suitable standards to shield the examining scientist from potentially biasing information and that conforming to such standards might be a condition of admissibility. As discussed later under Contexts, this hope has been fulfilled by the work of Itiel Dror (Dror n.d.) and colleagues and the response of regulatory authorities (Forensic Science Regulator 2014).

Current outcomes that are the result of exposing forensic scientists to potentially biasing information are then discussed. These include examples of the effect of information from the submitting authority, usually the police, where even details of other evidence are included. Accounts are given of how forensic scientists became invested in cases and effectively became members of the investigation team. Finally, it discusses revising findings in light of information outside the field of expertise and selective re-examination at the request of law enforcement to try to achieve a more favourable result. This introduces selection bias as the original favourable result remains in place and is not subjected to re-examination.

In a footnote, the publication raises the matter of review by another scientist. It distinguishes between a blind review and an administrative or process check to ensure that all procedures have been properly followed and that the report adequately explains findings and conclusions. A blind review is an independent check by a reviewer 'uncontaminated' by the original examination.

This part of the publication has a word or two about pathologists. A distinction should be made between forensic science and medicine. The fundamental reason is medical practitioners' over-reliance on the inferential method of abduction – the educated guess – and less on the other methods, deduction and induction[5]. The main body of forensic medicine practitioners is pathologists, specifically called upon to determine the cause and time of a suspicious death. Interestingly, the publication draws attention to another weakness – exposure to numerous cognitive biases. Their way of working exposes pathologists to many biases.

Following is a quote from a footnote from the publication on page 34:

> *Finally, forensic pathologists apparently consider absolutely any information to be within their domain. Consider the following passage from Dominick J. Di Maio & Vincent J. M. Di Maio, Forensic Pathology (1989):*
>
> *How does a medical examiner* [forensic pathologist] *approach a case? He or she approaches it just like any other physician approaches a patient. In medical school, one is taught that to make a correct diagnosis, one has to take a history, perform a physical examination, and order relevant laboratory tests. Based on this, a diagnosis is made. The forensic pathologist performs all these functions but with some variance. Thus, the history is not obtained from the patient, but is an account of the events leading up to and surrounding the death obtained from witnesses, relatives of the deceased, police agencies, treating physicians, and/or records (medical, nonmedical, police, governmental, etc.).*

This exposure to so many potential biasing effects risks increasing the confidence in the evidence while reducing its accuracy. A good example of how this might result in wrongful convictions is the cases of Sally Clarke (R v Sally Clark 2003) and other mothers wrongly convicted of infanticide.

Part 3 Minimising Observer Effects in Forensic Science

Part 3 begins with a remarkable statement borne of the success of the Innocence Project[6], which relies on DNA evidence to expose wrongful convictions secured, in part, with unreliable scientific evidence.

> *... it is beginning to appear that forensic science contributes more to convicting the innocent than anyone previously suspected.*

The publication then imagines an ideal forensic science laboratory, separate from law enforcement and prosecuting authorities, staffed by scientists with no previous law enforcement association, trained to see their role as one of integrity and ensuring accuracy, and having procedures in place to shield examining scientists from extraneous, potentially biasing information. This is pretty much the opposite of the then-current model, which the publication argues exists only for historical reasons. It also argues that to move from the current model to that envisaged would be nigh on impossible and certainly was in 2002.

Restating the main aim of the publication, raising awareness of bias, it then goes on to argue that awareness is not enough, action is required and suggests some remedies. The first is blind testing, shielding the examining scientist from all information that is not relevant to the task at hand. To quote the publication.

> *The simplest, most powerful, and most useful procedure to protect against the distorting effects of unstated assumptions, collateral information, and improper expectations and motivations is blind testing.*

Therefore, there needs to be an individual responsible for controlling the information given to the examining scientist and the process documented. This individual would be the coordination scientist (however named) within the laboratory, allocating work and acting as the point of contact between the laboratory and commissioning authority, usually law enforcement or the police.

Reference is made to the then Forensic Science Service in England, which developed a process known as Case Assessment and Interpretation (CAI). CAI can be an important tool in reducing the risk of cognitive bias, and so a detailed description follows.

Case Assessment and Interpretation

CAI is an approach to decision-making in an operational forensic science laboratory based on a model embodying the principles of Bayesian inference. A paper describing the model was published in 1998 by a team working at the Forensic Science Service for the following stated purpose (Cook et al. 1998).

> *To enable decisions to be made which will deliver a value for money service meeting the needs of our direct customers and the Criminal Justice System.*

It has six basic steps:

1. Define customer requirement
2. Asses how forensic science can help
3. Agree on a case forensic examination strategy
4. Carry out examination
5. Interpret the results
6. Communicate the test results and opinion

CAI is not a rigidly defined process, but it can guide workflow so that resources are directed towards the issues and items expected to produce the most valuable information. In steps 2 and 3, CAI involves developing an efficient and effective examination strategy relying on Bayesian reasoning, identifying which evidence types best progress the investigation.

(Continued)

(Continued)

A forensic scientist would be involved at an early stage to help decide based on an assignment of a likelihood ratio for each potential evidence type. A practical example would be if a particular scenario is proposed that might result in the transfer of fibres from say a carpet to the perpetrator, then fibre examination would be a priority.

While such a scheme is theoretically optimal, applying CAI in a fast-moving investigation of a major crime may seem cumbersome and impracticable. In addition, in today's world, most investigations rely on DNA, CCTV (closed circuit TV – facial recognition) and mobile phones. However, a strong argument can be made that CAI is essential in identifying which evidence types are important in a particular investigation. Non-application can lead to important evidence being missed (Doyle and Doyle 2011).

The publication then turns to what may be an intractable problem, which the publication terms '*Assumed Base Rates of Inculpation*'. This refers to the fact that evidence is submitted to a forensic science laboratory because the police (or other law enforcement agency) believe that it will advance their investigation, particularly if that evidence links a suspect with a crime. Evidence falls into two broad categories: exculpatory, pointing away from the suspect and inculpatory, associating the suspect with the crime. Because the police do not select suspects at random, there is a strong expectation that the evidence submitted will be inculpatory; this is the inculpatory expectation referred to earlier. The publication acknowledges that blind testing will not remove this inculpatory expectation and may bias the examining scientist.

To give a simple, practical example. A bullet is being examined for association with a gun that was used in a murder. The firearms examiner knows that the only reason he is being asked to examine the bullet is that the police believe that it might have been fired by the murder weapon. Not only that, but as a firearms examiner, he has reported far more positive associations than negative ones. These factors result in this inculpatory base rate, an expectation that there will be a positive association between the bullet and the gun before the examination begins.

The suggested remedy is 'evidence lineups', akin to eyewitness lineups where the suspect is included among other individuals and the eyewitness is asked to select the suspect. To use the example above, the firearms examiner, in addition to the questioned bullet, would be presented with several bullets known not to be from the murder weapon.

There is no doubt that this procedure would reduce the risk of bias in forensic science. Since the publication of 'Observer Effects' in 2002, research has demonstrated the effectiveness of 'evidence lineups' and academics have called for its inclusion in standard practice, currently to no avail, perhaps because of the cost of doing so (Kukucka et al. 2020).

This part of the publication ends by considering likely objections to the recommendations made earlier.

The first is that it might be difficult to decide what information is essential for examining scientists to do their job well. This would be addressed by CAI, a coordinating and non-testifying scientist, and using the likelihood ratio approach to both identify evidence types of potential probative value and the interpretation of results as described in Chapter 6 on Interpreting Evidence.

The next objection is that through their education and training, forensic scientists are immune from bias, which today seems laughable. All relevant authorities recognise the existence and risks of bias.

Finally, there is the objection based on cost. The creation of the role of coordinating scientist will be an increased cost. However, one of the motivations for CAI was to reduce costs by identifying early on which evidence types were more likely to advance the investigation and not waste resources on those that would not. Not only that, but the quality and reliability of the scientific evidence would be improved by such a measure. In addition, the financial cost of a miscarriage of justice may well be of the order of millions of dollars. Furthermore, to add to the misery inflicted on those wrongly convicted, their families and loved ones, the guilty party goes free, justice is not delivered to the victims, and the reputation of the justice system suffers. On the matter of cost, in the United Kingdom, the compensation paid to someone who has been wrongly convicted can be around £1 million, and in a recent case, the compensation was estimated to be more than £1 billion (Taaffe-Maguire 2024).

Part 4 Observer Effects and Admissibility Under FRE 702

In the final part, and of less importance to this book, it looks at bias and admissibility under FRE 702 that expert evidence contaminated by bias should be considered unreliable and not be admitted. The hope being expressed that this judgment will prompt courts to recognise the risk of expert evidence being contaminated by bias and potentially contributing to a miscarriage of justice.

And so, the main conclusion drawn is that forensic scientists can be influenced by information outside their field of expertise, that information can bias their opinions resulting in misleading evidence being admitted and heard by the fact-finder, the jury, thereby putting justice at risk.

Recommendations are made to reduce that risk, and these include and are related to shielding the examining scientist from all but essential information to complete the task at hand, to effectivity do his/her duty.

One wonders how the requirement for impartiality in the latest edition of the international standard ISO/IEC 17025 is being met by accredited forensic science providers. ISO/IEC 17025 is the subject of Chapter 7.

Biography of the Publication

The US case of *Daubert* (Daubert v. Merrell Dow Pharmaceuticals, Inc. 1993) led to a significant revision of US Federal Rule of Evidence 702[7] in 1993 to impose a gatekeeping role on the trial judge to ensure that expert testimony is based on reliable science. The judgement included a set of criteria for the admissibility of scientific evidence, which became known as the Daubert Criteria and are as follows.

- Whether the theory or technique in question can be and has been tested,
- whether it has been subjected to peer review and publication,
- its known or potential error rate,

- the existence and maintenance of standards controlling its operation, and
- whether it is widely accepted in the relevant scientific community.

In the judgement, the court set out four factors that the trial judge should consider in determining if evidence should be admitted: such as a theory's 'testability', whether it 'has been a subject of peer review or publication', the 'known or potential rate of error', and the 'degree of acceptance ... within the relevant scientific community'. The Daubert court stressed that this analysis was intended to be flexible, with the trial judge determining how and whether the factors applied in each case.

At this point it is important to say a little about the admissibility and weight of evidence and in doing so introduce the requirements of FRE 702 based on the Daubert judgement. As the name implies, admissibility concerns whether scientific evidence can be admitted and presented to the court, fact-finder, or jury. The requirements for the admission of expert evidence set out in FRE 702 are as follows.

- The forensic scientist must be qualified as an expert.
- The expert's scientific knowledge will help the fact-finder to understand the evidence or to determine a disputed fact.
- The evidence is based on sufficient facts and data.
- The evidence is the product of reliable principles and methods, and
- The expert has reliably applied the principles and methods to the facts of the case.

If the trial judge decides that those requirements are met, then the evidence is deemed reliable and is admitted.

Weight is essentially the weight given to the evidence by the fact-finder or jury. The scientific evidence is admitted. However, if other evidence weakens it or it is tested in cross-examination and found to be less reliable than scientific evidence presented by the other party then the fact-finder will give the evidence less weight.

It is fair to argue that in most common law jurisdictions, scientific evidence of questionable reliability is admitted and left to the adversarial process and the fact-finder to determine weight. However, so-called Daubert Hearings are often called for by the defence when scientific evidence based on novel methods or techniques is a major plank in the prosecution case. In that case, a formal hearing is held to consider whether the scientific evidence meets FRE 702 and decide on admissibility. The introduction of evidence based on the analysis of stable isotopes is an example of the mechanisms of a Daubert hearing in which that evidence was challenged (Doyle et al. 2023).

As this is a history, it is perhaps important to note that the Daubert judgement in 1993 superseded an earlier criterion for admissibility, the Frye test, a general acceptance test in the relevant scientific community (Frye v United States 1923). The weakness of this now century-old test was that it might exclude novel but sound and reliable scientific evidence that might be of assistance to the factfinder.

As explained earlier, the *Kumho* case looks at whether the Daubert criteria may also be applied to non-scientific expert testimony.

At the original *Kumho* trial, the judge had applied the Daubert criteria and found that the expert evidence was unsound and unscientific and therefore was not admitted. An appeal was lodged and was successful. The (lower) appeal court found that the trial judge had erred by applying the Daubert criteria to non-scientific evidence and sent the case back to the trial court with instructions to re-evaluate the expert testimony without using the Daubert criteria. The unsuccessful party then appealed to the US Supreme Court. That court found that it was not an error for the trial judge to use the Daubert criteria to evaluate the expert testimony. So, in effect, *Kumho* is a clarification of *Daubert*, which did not seem to apply to non-scientific expert evidence; the US Supreme Court decided that it did.

A careful reading of the Supreme Court's judgement makes clear that the determination of the admissibility of expert evidence should be case-specific. Expert evidence must be relevant to the '*task at hand*'. This is the starting point for the publication, the need for the trial judge to be aware of the potential effects of cognitive bias when considering admissibility. The judge should ensure that satisfactory measures are in place to reduce the risk of cognitive bias, which may render scientific evidence unreliable.

After *Daubert* and before *Kumho*, FRE 702 was as follows.

> *If scientific, technical or other specialized knowledge will assist the trier of fact to understand the evidence or to determine a fact in issue, a witness qualified as an expert by knowledge, skill, experience, training, or education, may testify thereto in the form of an opinion or otherwise.*

After *Kumho* FRE 702 was amended by adding the following text.

> *... the testimony is the product of reliable principles and methods.*

Again, emphasising the task-specific approach required of the trial judge exercising the gatekeeper role.

It is important to note that the judgment of the lower court when hearing the original appeal introduced a fifth criterion which arose from a concern about motivational bias; a self-serving bias, resulting from being invested in a specific outcome.

The lower and initial court of appeal when deciding the case added a criterion that takes into consideration whether the expert's opinion was developed independently of the case or strictly with the intent to testify as an expert, as the lower court put it.

> *One very significant fact to be considered is whether the experts are proposing to testify about matters growing naturally and directly out of research they have conducted independent of the litigation, or whether they have developed their opinions expressly for purposes of testifying.*

The point is that research conducted in response to a specific case is at risk of another cognitive bias, motivational bias. The expert is invested in a particular outcome. This bias' risk is reduced by relying on independent research conducted separately from any specific case.

A practical example of where motivational bias might infect scientific evidence is further testing or experimentation conducted by an expert instructed by the prosecution in response to a report by an expert instructed by the defence. The prosecution expert is already heavily invested in a particular outcome, a bias against which little can be done other than recognising that the bias might render the test result and its interpretation unreliable.

Professional Biography of the Authors

At the time of its publication, the authors were undoubtedly the most highly qualified and distinguished of those included in this history. They continue to be regarded as 'stars' in their respective fields. Sadly, Robert Rosenthal, the psychologist, passed away recently.

D. Michael Risinger

Professor of Law, Seton Hall University School of Law, B.A., Yale University, 1966, J.D., Harvard University, 1969.

The following is a current quote from the Seton Hall Law School website.

'Professor Risinger holds a B.A., magna cum laude, from Yale University, and a J.D., cum laude, from Harvard Law School. He clerked for the Honorable Clarence C. Newcomer of the United States District Court for the Eastern District of Pennsylvania. He is a past chair of the Association of American Law Schools (AALS) Section on Civil Procedure, the immediate past chair of the AALS Section on Evidence, and a life member of the American Law Institute. He was also a member of the New Jersey Supreme Court Committee on Evidence for 25 years, which was responsible for the current version of the New Jersey Rules of Evidence. Professor Risinger came to Seton Hall Law School in 1973. He served as a visiting senior fellow on the law faculty of the National University of Singapore from 1985 to 1986. Professor Risinger has published in the areas of evidence and civil procedure. He is the co-author of Trial Evidence, A Continuing Legal Education Casebook and the author of two chapters in Faigman, Kaye, Saks and Sanders, Modern Scientific Evidence ("Handwriting Identification" and "A Proposed Taxonomy of Expertise"). Professor Risinger was selected as one of Seton Hall's two inaugural Dean's Research Fellows (2002–2004) and was named the John J. Gibbons Professor of Law in May 2008. His scholarship has recently concentrated on wrongful convictions as well as expert evidence issues'.

Professor Risinger is also a life member of the American Law Institute. He was a member of the Human Factors Subcommittee of the US National Commission on Forensic Science, discussed in Chapter 9 on the 2009 report of the US National Academies.

Michael J. Saks

Professor of Law and Professor of Psychology, Arizona State University, B.A., B.S., Pennsylvania State University, 1969, M.A., Ohio State University, 1972, Ph.D., Ohio State University, 1975, M.S.L. (Master of Studies in Law), Yale University, 1989.

The following is a current quote from the Arizona State University website.

'Michael Saks is a Regents Professor in the Sandra Day O'Connor College of Law and Department of Psychology at Arizona State University (ASU). He is also a faculty fellow with the Center for Law, Science and Innovation at ASU.

Professor Saks' research interests focus on empirical studies of law and the legal system, especially decision-making in the legal process, evidence law, the law's use of science, the behaviour of the litigation system, and legal policy affecting medical patient safety.

He has served as editor of the journals Law & Human Behavior and Jurimetrics, as president of the American Psychology-Law Society and chair of the Section on Law and Social

Science of the AALS. Among his approximately 250 publications (including 11 books): He has been co-editor/co-author of "Modern Scientific Evidence" (five volumes) and the "Annotated Reference Manual on Scientific Evidence," and co-author of "The Psychological Foundations of Evidence Law" (2016). His article on The Behavior of the Tort Litigation System, 140 U. Pa. L. Rev. 1147 (1992), has been the most-cited tort law article in the past 25 years. His work has earned numerous awards and been cited in a number of judicial opinions, including by the US Supreme Court.'

Before coming to ASU in 2000, Saks was the Edward F. Howrey Professor of Law and professor of psychology at the University of Iowa, after starting his academic career at Boston College and serving on the staff of the National Center for State Courts. Courses he has taught include criminal law, evidence, law and science, and torts. He has also taught courses in scientific evidence to appellate judges in the University of Virginia Law School's LL.M. program for appellate judges and in Duke Law School's "Judging Science" program, as well as to law faculty at the Georgetown University Law Center and the Ohio State University'.

Professor Saks is also an affiliated faculty member at the University of Haifa, Israel. He has taught courses in scientific evidence to appellate judges in the University of Virginia Law School's LL.M. program and Duke's 'Judging Science' program, as well as to law faculty at Georgetown University and the Ohio State University. Saks's work is among the most-cited research in the 2009 National Academies report, the subject of Chapter 9. Among over 230 other publications, he has been co-editor/co-author of Modern Scientific Evidence (five volumes), the Annotated Reference Manual on Scientific Evidence, Second, and The Psychological Foundations of Evidence Law. His work has earned several awards, and he has been cited in various judicial opinions, including several by the United States Supreme Court.

William C. Thompson

William C. Thompson is the joint author with Edward L. Schumann of the publication discussed in Chapter 5, which identified the phenomena of the prosecutor's and defence attorneys' fallacies. His biographical details can be found in that chapter.

Robert Rosenthal (1933–2024)

Distinguished Professor of Psychology, University of California at Riverside (UCR), and Edgar

Pierce Professor of Psychology, Emeritus, Harvard University, Ph.D., U.C.L.A., 1956.

This is a current quote from the UCR website, which is Rosenthal's obituary.

'Robert Rosenthal, a father of meta-analysis who was named one of the 20th century's top 100 psychologists, died Jan. 5 2024, at 90'.

Twenty-five years ago, following his retirement from Harvard University, Rosenthal joined the UC Riverside faculty. He was named a University Professor in 2008 by the University of California system, a distinction shared by only 40 professors in UC's history.

He retired from his full-time UCR professorship in spring 2018 but continued teaching part-time in UCR's Graduate Division through the fall quarter of 2023.

Unlike the other authors, Rosenthal gained recognition in popular culture. He achieved worldwide notoriety in 1968 with the publication of his book 'Pygmalion in the Classroom'. It concluded that academic achievement in school was predetermined by teacher expectations. 'The Pygmalion Effect', also called 'The Rosenthal Effect', became part of the vocabulary of the time. He made the front page of The New York Times and was interviewed on the US Today Show by Barbara Walters.

The fame and controversy his book generated were uncomfortable for Rosenthal, who preferred the quiet life of an academic.

With statistician Gene Glass, he co-founded modern meta-analysis, which transformed scientific research by combining studies to compound probability. He is also among the fathers of psychological principles, including experimenter bias and interpersonal expectations.

In 2002, 'The 100 Most Eminent Psychologists of the 20th Century' was published in the Review of General Psychology. Rosenthal is No. 84 on that list, which includes the likes of Sigmund Freud, B.F. Skinner, Ivan Pavlov, and Carl Jung (impressive company!).

He was chosen for tenure at Harvard over Stanley Milgram, and he inherited the Harvard office of the disgraced Timothy Leary (an advocate for the use of psychedelic drugs).

For all his professional accolades, colleagues emphasise Rosenthal's gentle nature.

'It transformed our department to have someone here who was not only a legendary authority but also about the kindest, least pretentious person you'd ever meet', said David Funder, who first taught with Rosenthal at Harvard in the 1980s, then at UCR. 'What a role model, in a field (academia) not exactly known for humility or self-effacement among its luminaries'.

'He is the most consistent person I've ever met, both in his temperament and the way he treated people', Funder said. 'If an undergraduate poked their head into his office, or the president of the university happened to stop by, they would both find themselves treated exactly the same way – with kindness, respect, and genuine interest'.

Peter Blanck was Rosenthal's friend and colleague since 1979. Blanck is a University Professor at Syracuse University who collaborated with Rosenthal on many research papers, including 'The Appearance of Justice', in 1985, which parlayed (transform something into something greater or more valuable) the Pygmalion classroom dynamic to the courtroom.

'The word that comes to mind is "mensch"; if there ever was a mensch, it was Bob', Blanck said, referring to the Yiddish word meaning 'person of noble character'. 'He was a giant, but you would never know his stature from talking to him'.

Contexts

General

The relevant historical, legal, and psychological contexts are detailed in the publication itself. The clarification of FRE 702 in the light of *Kumho* provides the authors with the opportunity to raise awareness of bias, demonstrate how it might affect the reliability of scientific evidence and suggest safeguards. In addition, it asks US trial judges, when exercising their gatekeeping role to consider cognitive bias when assessing admissibility.

This publication was ahead of its time in that it drew attention to issues in forensic science that were not widely recognised until Itiel Dror and colleagues at University College London began studying the effect of bias on fingerprint evidence in 2006 (Dror et al. 2006; Dror and Charlton 2006). Furthermore, it was not until 2014 that the bias avoidance measures recommended in the publication, as augmented by the work of Dr Dror, began to be incorporated into standard practice (Forensic Science Regulator 2014).

Scientific

Beginning in the 1940s and certainly by the late 1990s, medical research had recognised that bias avoidance measures were essential to ensure the accuracy of clinical trials (Bhatt 2010; EMA 1998). However, until this publication, essentially by and for lawyers, there was little or no recognition of the dangers of cognitive bias among forensic scientists, and, as recorded above, it took around a decade after the publication in 2002 for the risk of bias to be taken seriously.

This ignorance or naivete on the part of forensic science perhaps lay in its non-scientific and law enforcement origins and in jurisdictions where law enforcement agents/police directed criminal investigations (Saks and Faigman 2008). This issue is further explored in Chapter 9 on the 2009 National Academies report.

Cognitive bias as it relates to forensic science is more a matter of psychology than science, so there was little going on in the world of mainstream science and forensic science that was relevant to this issue. The mapping of the human genome was completed in 2003. In forensic science, national DNA databases were being developed and automated fingerprint information systems (AFIS) were being introduced. As recorded earlier, the publication itself had little impact on the practice of forensic science at the time.

However, as argued in Chapter 4 on DNA 'fingerprinting', the advent of DNA analysis in 1987 indirectly and in due course brought to the attention of forensic science the risk of bias, its effects and how that risk might be reduced.

Up until the forensic exploitation of the DNA molecule, fingerprints were the only 'scientific' means of identification. Fingerprint evidence had rarely, if ever, been contested in court, and the examiner's claims to infallibility came to be accepted without challenge. As DNA analysis developed and, more importantly, its reliability was aggressively challenged (Doyle 2019c), unfavourable comparisons began to be made with fingerprints and the stark differences began to come to light. DNA's scientific and statistical foundations were initially challenged, as were the analysis and interpretation of DNA results. In time, DNA evidence developed to address these concerns and met the challenges.

However, the challenges faced by DNA prompted the question: why doesn't fingerprint evidence have to clear these hurdles? The question highlighted the fact that there was little or no scientific or statistical foundation for fingerprint evidence, and there was no standard procedure for examination or interpretation. In addition, there was no satisfactory proficiency test to measure performance and reliability. Fingerprint evidence lacked the underpinning scientific and statistical foundations that were demanded of DNA evidence. In comparison with DNA, fingerprint evidence was inherently unreliable and, in those jurisdictions that have not yet adopted good practice, still is (Edmond 2020).

The lack of a scientific and statistical basis for fingerprint evidence (and other subjective feature-comparison disciplines such as handwriting and tool marks) manifested itself in a marked difference in practice. Even though DNA evidence of 'a match' was able to be expressed with a very high probability, forensic scientists would not attribute certainty, always allowing the possibility that a 'matching' DNA profile of two unrelated people might be found. In contrast, a fingerprint examiner would report a positive result with absolute certainty, a fingerprint 'match' identified a person to the exclusion of all others. As discussed in Chapter 3 on the Ontogeny of Criminalistics, this outcome was also known as 'individualisation'. While this might have been believed by the fingerprint examiner, 'individualisation', as discussed in Chapter 3, was not supported by logic or a body of research. There was no way of finding out deductively that the fingerprints of no two individuals 'matched'. Claims that, in all the fingerprint examinations ever undertaken, it was never found that the prints of different people 'matched' may have been true, but there was no way of establishing the truth of that claim. In logic, the possibility could not be excluded that among the population now living and those who have died, two individuals shared the same fingerprint.

This acceptance of uncertainty when presenting DNA evidence and the absence of uncertainty regarding fingerprint evidence was a troubling contrast (Mnookin 2003).

The highly subjective 'method' of fingerprint examination and the resultant susceptibility to human biases drew the attention of those making a serious study of bias and the effect of information given to the examiner before the examination. This research was principally led by Itiel Dror at University College London. His studies clearly established the biasing effect of what he termed domain-irrelevant information in fingerprint examination (Dror and Charlton 2006; Dror et al. 2006).

Initially, there was a great deal of pushback from fingerprint examiners, mostly police based, and some authorities thought bias did not exist[8]. Many fingerprint examiners claim infallibility and, in support of their opinion, offer 'because I say so', 'I have been trained in this discipline and have the requisite experience'. This *ipse dixit* or 'I say so' approach ignores one of the basic duties of an expert witness as expressed in the case of *Davie v Edinburgh Magistrates* (Davie v Magistrates of Edinburgh 1953).

> *Expert witnesses, however skilled or eminent, can give no more than evidence. They cannot usurp the functions of the jury or the Judge sitting as a jury ... Their duty is to furnish the Judge or jury with the necessary scientific criteria for testing the accuracy of their conclusions, so as to enable the Judge or jury to form their own independent judgment by the application of these criteria to the facts proved in evidence. ...In particular, the bare ipse dixit of a scientist, however eminent ... will normally carry little weight.*

In everyday terms, according to this judgment, such 'I say so' evidence may be worthless.

The lack of challenge to fingerprint evidence introduces another potential weakness, and that is the risk of 'validation by verdict', a form of confirmation bias. The evidence given is that the fingerprint found at the scene of the crime is that of the subject. In truth, it is the fingerprint of the suspect, and in truth, he or she was guilty as charged and rightly convicted. For the sake of this example, assume that the fingerprint examiner was less than fully competent and did a poor job, as in truth there was insufficient resemblance between the questioned and reference prints to justify a conclusion of 'individualisation'. As the suspect was convicted (on the preponderance of other evidence), the examiner incorrectly believes that the conclusion was justified, 'validated by verdict'. Given the exposure of fingerprint examiners to irrelevant case information and the general lack of bias avoidance measures in their examination process, one wonders how many times such 'validations by verdict' have occurred and perhaps contributed to miscarriages of justice.

Fingerprint evidence in its methods and presentation is, in many jurisdictions, fundamentally flawed and should be vigorously challenged whenever presented.

In contrast with limited opportunities for bias to affect the results of DNA analysis, fingerprint examinations, and similar feature-comparison disciplines are highly subjective, providing many opportunities to bias results.

Historical

At the time of publication in 2002, most forensic scientists in the West were in some way or other engaged in the 'war against terrorism'. The '9/11' terrorist atrocity took place the year before publication. The attack against the World Trade Center in New York took the lives of 2977 people and sent out huge geopolitical shock waves which have largely shaped the world as it is today, many would argue not for the better.

On the other side of the Atlantic, there were also the terrorist bombings in Madrid in 2004[9] and London in 2005. As forensic science is in part a servant of the law, it is directed to a significant extent by the needs of law enforcement. Therefore, the 'war against terrorism' was given priority over other potential developments in forensic science. Huge amounts of effort were directed at the analysis and detection of explosives recovered from scenes and at transport hubs. Novel explosive materials like TATP[10] required novel approaches to detection to be developed. Also, the detection and defeat of improvised explosive devices (bombs) and suicide bombers were the principal objectives in which forensic science was jointly engaged. So, there was little effort devoted to reducing the risk of cognitive bias, which, as mentioned earlier, the existence of which was denied by some authorities until 2014. Figure 8.1 shows the timeline between the publication and the acceptance of the existence of cognitive bias by relevant authorities.

It is of interest to contrast this progress with the use of a likelihood ratio (LR) approach to the evaluation of scientific evidence. This approach was pioneered by Ian Evett (Evett 1986, 1991), fully documented in 'Interpretation Evidence', first published in 1995, the subject of Chapter 6. The LR was incorporated into the CAI process in 1998, the AFSP Standard in 2009 (AFSP 2009) and now in 2025, almost three decades later, there is still some resistance to this logical and balanced approach to the interpretation of evidence, particularly in the feature comparison fields.

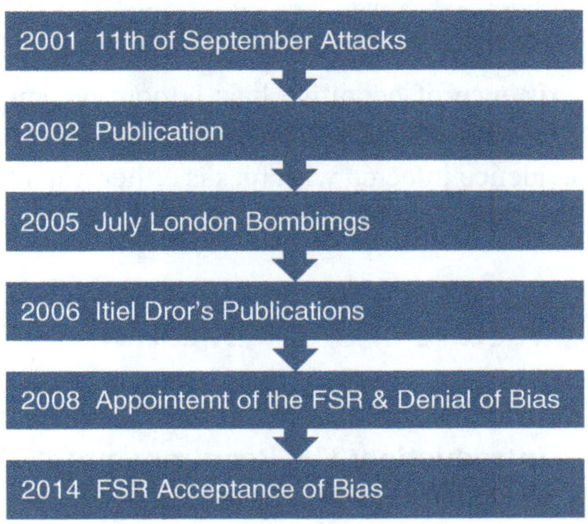

Figure 8.1 Timeline of the acceptance of cognitive bias in forensic science.

Social/Society

The societal impact of the lack of recognition of cognitive bias is the multitude of wrongful convictions to which bias has contributed (Meterko 2021; Shiyuan 2018; Moles 2024). As these mount, lawyers are becoming increasingly aware of the potential impact of bias and are exposing its presence. However, this is usually post-conviction. Once biased evidence reaches a court of law or another tribunal, there is little that can be done. A court of law is ill-equipped to recognise biased evidence once deemed admissible. That was one of the main issues the publication was trying to address. In the United States, the trial judge must act as a gatekeeper, ensuring only reliable scientific evidence is admitted. To be effective, the judge must ensure that the evidence is not infected by bias, only admitting evidence generated with bias avoidance measures in place. The main one is shielding the examining scientist from irrelevant and potentially biasing information.

This test is rarely applied, and there is still some way to go for all criminal justice system stakeholders to take bias seriously and promote and foster an optimal model including CAI, a coordinating non-testifying[11] scientist, linear sequential unmasking[12] and a likelihood ratio approach to evaluation. Adherence to this model should be taken into account when considering the admissibility of scientific evidence. Failures to do so have contributed to many of the multitude of wrongful convictions uncovered.

Artificial Intelligence should, in time, be able to significantly reduce the risk of bias and increase the reliability of feature comparison evidence such as fingerprints.

It is of interest to note that at the time of writing [2024], an inquiry is being held in England regarding wrongful convictions secured by the British Post Office (PO) of hundreds of its franchisees for theft and false accounting. Many have been given prison sentences, their lives and reputations ruined, suffered financial hardship, loss of their homes and in one case loss of life (Espiner and Smith 2024). It has been called the biggest miscarriage of justice in British history. The PO investigators, many of the PO lawyers and those acting on behalf of the PO began with a presumption of guilt, Hans Gross's 'preconceived theory', and then proceeded with tunnel vision, two obvious precursors of a miscarriage of justice. The investigation was infected with confirmation bias with a twist: the investigators and prosecuting authorities didn't ignore evidence to the contrary; they just decided not to look for any.

Through the efforts of Itiel Dror and his colleagues at University College London, the existence of cognitive bias is now recognised by many criminal justice stakeholders in many jurisdictions (Dror n.d.). However, there is still work to do to ensure that scientific evidence infected with bias is either not admitted or, if it is, the justice system is equipped to expose that bias during the trial process.

Structure of the Publication

What follows is taken from the table of contents of the publication.

Introduction: The Requirements of Kumho Tire Co. v. Carmichael.
Part 1 Observer Effects.

A. Evolution of the Awareness of Observer Effects.
B. What This Article Is Not About (Honesty and Observer Effects).

C. The Psychology of Observer Effects.
  1. In General.
  2. Observer Effects and Decision Thresholds.
  3. Anchoring Effects.
  4. Role Effects.
  5. Conformity Effects.
  6. Experimenter Effects.

D. The Pervasiveness of Observer Effects.
E. The Enhancement of Observer Effects by Desire and Motivation.
F. The Lack of Linkage Among Confidence, Accuracy, and Amount of Information

Part 2 Observer Effects in Forensic Science.

A. Proper and Improper Information in the Forensic Science Practice.
B. Improper Information Contamination in Forensic Science Practice.
C. Specific Sources of Induced Observer Error in Forensic Science Practice.
  1. Direct Communication Between Investigators and Examiners.
  2. Revision of Findings in Light of New Test-Irrelevant Information.
  3. Selective Re-examination of Evidence.

Part 3 Minimizing Observer Effects in Forensic Science: Conclusions and Recommendations.

A. Preventing Distortions Due to Expectation and Suggestion: Blind Testing.
B. Preventing Distortions Due to Assumed Base Rates of Inculpation: Evidence Lineups.
C. Likely Objections to the Recommendations.

Part 4 Observer Effects and Admissibility Under Federal Rule of Evidence 702.

Impact at the Time

Written by eminent academic lawyers and psychologists, published in an American law journal and primarily aimed at lawyers and judges, prompted by an appeal court judgment, the publication had little traction with forensic scientists, even in the United States. However, its place in this book is partly due to the early recognition/documentation of the potential effects of bias and the extensive scholarship it represents.

As has been concluded elsewhere in this book, forensic science is very much a responsive science and responds best to failure. Certainly, among examiners comparing features, there was no sense of 'failure' in 2002. Unfortunately, there are pockets of practice where that is still the case.

Impact Today

It was not until 2006 that research started to be published on the effects of bias in forensic science. This was very much led by Itiel Dror. The first discipline to come under the spotlight was fingerprints (Dror et al. 2006; Dror and Charlton 2006). A recognition of bias and avoidance procedures is now incorporated in the Codes of the FSR (Forensic Science Regulator 2020).

A significant procedural development in the examination and comparison of questioned and reference material is the logic of examining and characterising questioned material first. This process has been termed linear sequential unmasking (LSU).

Linear Sequential Unmasking (LSU)

Ensuring the information provided to the examining scientist is revealed in such a way as to minimise the risk of bias. Research has demonstrated that the order or sequence in which information is presented plays a critical role in decision-making processes and outcomes (Dror and Kukucka 2021)

A simple example of how sequence might influence decisions is demonstrated as follows.

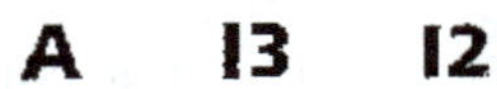

If the observer begins with the number 12 and reads from right to left, then the middle character is the number 13. If the observer begins with the letter A and reads from left to right, then the middle character must be the letter B.

In forensic science, one important step in linear sequential unmasking is to fully characterise questioned material before looking at any reference material. This shields the examining scientist from a potentially powerful bias. Having determined the significant features in the reference material, the examiner's mind turns to trying to find resemblances in the questioned materials. According to Itiel Dror (Dror 2024) this sequence is akin to firing an arrow at a tree and then painting the target around it. That way, every arrow hits the target. This step applies mostly to feature comparison disciplines such as fingerprints and handwriting, which rely largely on subjective judgement. Being familiar with the characteristics of reference material, such as handwriting, potentially biases the examiner. Instead of 'matching' features of the questioned writing with the reference writing, which is the purpose of the examination, the examiner, by characterising the reference writing before looking at the questioned writing, is biased in favour of those features and is trying to match features of the reference writing with the questioned writing.

This backward sequence involves not having the actual evidence guide the comparison, seeing if the evidence matches the reference, but, rather, going the wrong way, looking for the reference material in the evidence. Therefore, the questioned material must be examined and characterised first.

Contribution to Current Practice

As set out earlier, in practice, the only arrangement that protects the examining scientist from potentially biasing information and ensures that he/she has sufficient information to properly evaluate evidence is having both a coordinating and an examining scientist. The coordinating scientist liaises with law enforcement agents and prosecuting authorities, participates in the

CAI process and acts as the point of contact for the forensic science laboratory. The coordinating scientist then has the responsibility of properly instructing the examining scientist and ensuring that she or he is shielded from potentially biasing information by implementing linear sequential unmasking. Ideally, the coordinating scientists should be non-testifying as she or he will have been exposed to much potentially biasing information. The conclusion should be independently reviewed by a second scientist blinded to both the initial conclusion and the identity of the examining scientist. The procedure should be documented and be part of the accredited quality management system of the forensic science laboratory. Such a model is presented in 'Quality Management in Forensic Science' (Doyle 2019b), and the FSR has suggested this model be employed in certain cases where it is practicable to do so (Forensic Science Regulator 2020)

There is also a duty on the forensic scientist to resist tunnel vision by always keeping an open mind and not allowing confirmation bias to influence their role. These requirements are documented in the codes of the forensic science regulator (Forensic Science Regulator 2023)[13] and implied in the requirement for impartiality in ISO/IEC 17025:2017 (the first edition of this standard is the subject of Chapter 7). However, the separation of forensic science provision and law enforcement remains a challenge. This separation is recommended in the 2009 National Academies report, which will be further discussed in Chapter 9. On the other hand, the Sydney Declaration, the subject of Chapter 10, argues for a closer relationship between forensic science and law enforcement.

Slowly, some would say glacially, but surely, that optimal model is emerging. The main elements are CAI; bias avoidance measures, such as a non-testifying coordinating scientist and linear sequential unmasking; a likelihood ratio approach to interpretation; independent blind review, and the requirement for impartiality in the latest edition of ISO/IEC 17025.

Concluding Remarks

Published in 2002, 'Observer Effects' was the first publication to bring to the attention of lawyers and judges in the United States the existence of cognitive bias in forensic science, to detail the many biases that might infect scientific evidence, provide examples and suggest risk reduction measures.

However, it was not until Harvard psychologist Itiel Dror turned his attention to forensic science at University College London that the existence and impact of bias in the field began to be recognised. Through research led by Dror, risk reduction measures were incorporated into regulations and procedures.

Key Takeaways

Forensic science is conducted by human beings prone to a whole raft of cognitive biases, which can result in poor decision-making, thereby putting justice at risk.

These biases may arise from the working environment, the culture and ethos of the organisation, relationships with colleagues, the influence of irrelevant information and the absence of independent blind review.

All criminal justice stakeholders must recognise the risk of cognitive bias and ensure that it is effectively managed by raising awareness and putting in place measures to reduce the risk. Failing to do so may render the scientific evidence unreliable and misleading.

Risk reduction measures include the following.

- Shielding the examining scientists from potentially biasing information.
- Characterising questioned material before examining reference material.
- Employing a likelihood ratio approach to evaluation.
- Conducting an independent, double-blind review.
- Relying on independent research unconnected with the facts at issue.

A forensic scientist who takes account of potentially biasing extraneous information abuses their role, may be overconfident and risks the 'double counting' of evidence.

Expert evidence given by medical practitioners is particularly prone to bias, as is 'feature comparison' evidence, such as fingerprints and handwriting, due to its subjectivity.

Trial judges should take account of bias avoidance measures when considering the issue of admissibility.

Although 'Observer Effects' was the first to document the issue of bias, its potential effects and the remedy of shielding the examining scientist from irrelevant information, it was Itiel Dror and colleagues who first produced empirical evidence of bias in forensic science, leading to its recognition and action by regulators (Dror n.d.).

Notes

1 The criteria for admission are (i) the expert is qualified to provide opinion testimony on the issue at hand; (ii) the expert's testimony will help the factfinder (jury) understand the evidence or determine a fact at issue; and (iii) the expert used a reliable methodology to support his or her opinions.

2 The forensic scientist knows that the item would not have been submitted for examination unless it was potentially supportive of guilt. Therefore, the forensic scientist expects the evidence examined to be inculpatory.

3 Now known to be an inherently unreliable evidence type (Saks et al. 2016).

4 The LR approach to the interpretation of evidence as discussed in Chapter 6on Interpreting Evidence avoids the risk of double counting in that the focus of the forensic scientist is on assigning a likelihood ratio.

5 These methods are discussed in the section on Terms, Definitions and Explanations.

6 Now an international organisation dedicated to helping those wrongly convicted, which relies heavily on DNA analysis to expose the unreliable scientific evidence that supported the conviction.

7 'If scientific, technical, or other specialized knowledge will assist the trier of fact to understand the evidence or to determine a fact in issue, a witness qualified as an expert by knowledge, skill, experience, training, or education, may testify thereto in the form of an opinion or otherwise'.

8 Professor Dror tells of a meeting with the first Forensic Science Regulator (FSR) in England & Wales who denied the existence of bias. But now the Regulator not only accepts its existence but also publishes guidance on risk reduction (Forensic Science Regulator 2020).

9 The investigation of this attack resulted in one of the most famous fingerprint misidentifications. The FBI concluded that a fingerprint found on a bag containing explosive devices 'matched' that of a lawyer in the US State of Oregon who was taken into custody. A review concluded that a whole raft of biases together with poor practice led to the misidentification (Office of the Inspector General 2006).

10 Tri-acetone tri-peroxide, an extremely sensitive primary high explosive, manufactured by terrorists for use in their bombs.

11 Of course, anyone involved in a criminal investigation may be called to give evidence at trial. However, the coordinating scientist could only give evidence on procedure and techniques as he or she would have been exposed to much potentially biasing information.

12 Decision-making processes and outcomes (Dror and Kukucka 2021). One important step is to fully characterise questioned material before looking at any reference material.

13 It is of interest to note that the requirement to consider alternative hypotheses/explanations which was explicitly stated in the Required Competencies of the now defunct Council for the Registration of Forensic Practitioners (Doyle 2019a) is absent from the 'Standards of Conduct' in the code of the Forensic Science Regulator of England and Wales (Forensic Science Regulator 2023).

Bibliography

AFSP. 2009. "Standards for the Formulation of Evaluative Forensic Science Expert Opinion." *Science and Justice* 49: 161–64.

Bacon, Francis. 1620. *Novum Organum (New Tools)*. London: Joannem Billium.

Bhatt, Arun. 2010. "Evolution of Clinical Research: A History Before and Beyond James Lind." *Perspectives in Clinical Research* 1: 6–10.

Campbell, Anthony. 2011. *The Fingerprint Inquiry Report*. Inquiry Report, Edinburgh: APS Group.

Campbell, Donald T. 1994. "Systematic Errors to be Expected of the Social Scientist on the Basis of a General Psychology of Cognitive Bias." In *Interpersonal Expectations: Theory, Research, and Applications*, edited by Peter David Blanck, 25–44. Cambridge: Cambridge University Press.

Cook, Roger, Ian W. Evett, Graham Jackson, P. J. Jones, and Jim A. Lambert. 1998. "A Model for Case Assessment and Interpretation." *Science and Justice* 38 (3): 151–56.

Daubert v. Merrell Dow Pharmaceuticals, Inc. 1993. 509 U.S. 579 (US Supreme Court, 28 June).

Davie v Magistrates of Edinburgh. 1953. SC 34 (Court of Session (Scotland)).

Doyle, Sean. 2019a. "4.3.4 Psychology and Performance." In *Quality Management in Forensic Science*, edited by Sean Doyle. London: Academic Press.

Doyle, Sean. 2019b. "Appendix G." In *Quality Management in Forensic Science*, edited by Sean Doyle, 361. London: Academic Press.

Doyle, Sean. 2019c. "The Forensic Exploitation of DNA and Its Development as an Evidence Type: Legal Challenges." In *Quality Management in Forensic Science*, edited by Sean Doyle, 197–99. London: Academic Press.

Doyle, Sean and Dianne Doyle. 2011. "The AFSP Standard – A Lesson for Law Enforcement Agencies." *Science and Justice* 52: 17–19.

Doyle, Sean, Thuan Chau, and John Howa. 2023. "IRMS Based Evidence Passes the Test." *Science & Justice* 63 (6): 743–46.

Dror, Itiel. n.d. "Dr Itiel Dror's Website." *University College London*. Accessed May 8, 2024. https://www.ucl.ac.uk/~ucjtidr/.

—. 2024. "Private Communication."

Dror, Itiel and David Charlton. 2006. "Why Experts Make Errors." *Journal of Forensic Identification* 56 (4): 600–16.

Dror, Itiel and Jeff Kukucka. 2021. "Linear Sequential Unmasking–Expanded (LSU-E): A General Approach for Improving Decision Making as well as Minimizing Noise and Bias." *Forensic Science International: Synergy* 3: 1–5.

Dror, Itiel, David Charlton, and Ailsa E. Péron. 2006. "Contextual Information Renders Experts Vulnerable to Making Erroneous Identifications." *Forensic Science International* 156: 74–78.

Edmond, Gary. 2020. "Fingerprint Evidence in New Zealand's Courts: The Oversight of Overstatement." *New Zealand Universities Law Review* 29: 1–24.

EMA. 1998. "Statistical Principles for Clinical Trials." *European Medicines Agency*. September. Accessed May 10, 2024. https://www.ema.europa.eu/en/documents/scientific-guideline/ich-e-9-statistical-principles-clinical-trials-step-5_en.pdf.

Espiner, Tom and Oliver Smith. 2024. "Post Office Paid Widow in Instalments for Silence." *BBC News*. 27 April. Accessed May 8, 2024. https://www.bbc.com/news/articles/c88z431n2v5o.

Evett, Ian. 1986. "Bayesian Inference and Forensic Science." *The Statistician* 36: 99–105.

Evett, Ian. 1991. "Interpretation: A Personal Odyssey." In *The Use of Statistics in Forensic Science*, edited by C. G. G. Aitkin and D. A. Stoney, 9–22. New York: Ellis Horwood.

Forensic Science Regulator. 2014. *Draft Guidance: Cognitive Bias Effects Relevant to Forensic Science Examinations*. Guidance, Birmingham UK: The Forensic Science Regulator, 58.

Forensic Science Regulator. 2020. "Cognitive Bias Effects Relevant to Forensic Science Examinations." In *Forensic Science Regulator Guidance*, 9. Birmingham: The Forensic Science Regulator.

Forensic Science Regulator. 2023. *Code of Practice*. Birmingham: The Forensic Science Regulator, 362.

Frye v United States. 1923. 3968 (Court of Appeals of District of Columbia, 3 December).

Kahneman, Daniel. 2012. *Thinking Fast and Slow*. Penguin.

Kukucka, Jeff, Itiel E. Dror, Melissa Yu, Lisa Hall, and Ruth M. Morgan. 2020. "The Impact of Evidence Lineups on Fingerprint Expert Decisions." *Applied Cognitive Psychology* 34 (5): 1143–53.

Kumho Tire Company, Ltd. v. Carmichael. 1999. 97-1709 (United States Court of Appeals for the Eleventh Circuit, 23 March).

Meterko, Vanessa. 2021. "What Is Cognitive Bias and How Does It Contribute to Wrongful Conviction." *Innocence Project*. 19 August. Accessed May 14, 2024. https://innocenceproject.org/what-is-cognitive-bias-how-it-contributes-to-wrongful-conviction/.

Mnookin, Jennifer L. 2003. "Fingerprints: Not a Gold Standard." *Issues in Science and Technology* 20 (1): 47–54.

Moles, Robert N. 2024. *Networked Knowledge*. Accessed May 14, 2024. http://netk.net.au/.

Office of the Inspector General. 2006. *A Review of the FBI's Handling of the Brandon Mayfield Case*. Review, Oversight and Review Division, US Department of Justice, US Department of Justice, 330.

R v Sally Clark. 2003. Crim 1020 (EWCA, 11 April).

Saks, Michael J., Thomas Albright, Thomas L. Bohan, Barbara E. Bierer, C. Michael Bowers, Mary A. Bush, Peter J. Bush, Arturo Casadevall, Simon A. Cole, M. Bonner Denton, Shari Seidman Diamond, Rachel Dioso-Villa, Jules Epstein, David Faigman, Lisa Faigman, Stephen E. Fienberg, Brandon L. Garrett, Paul C. Giannelli, Henry T. Greely, Edward Imwinkelried, Allan Jamieson, Karen Kafadar, Jerome P. Kassirer, Jonathan 'Jay' Koehler, David Korn, Jennifer Mnookin, Alan B. Morrison, Erin Murphy, Nizam Peerwani, Joseph L. Peterson, D. Michael Risinger, George F. Sensabaugh, Clifford Spiegelman, Hal Stern, William C. Thompson, James L. Wayman, Sandy Zabell, and Ross E. Zumwalt. 2016. "Forensic Bitemark Identification: Weak Foundations, Exaggerated Claims." *Journal of Law and the Biosciences* 3: 538–75.

Saks, Michael J. and David L. Faigman. 2008. "How Forensic Science Lost Its Way and How It Might Yet Find It." *Annual Review of Law and Social Science* 8 (July): 149–71.

Shiyuan, Huang. 2018. "Cognitive Biases That Lead to Wrongful Convictions: Illustrated by Twenty-Three Erroneous Chinese Cases." *California Western Law Review*: 54 (1): 103–36.

Sofronoff, Walter. 2022. "Final Report Commission of Inquiry into Forensic DNA Testing in Queensland." Commission of Inquiry.

Taaffe-Maguire, Sarah. 2024. "Business." *Sky News*. 27 February. Accessed April 26, 2024. https://news.sky.com/story/post-office-scandal-bill-to-compensate-victims-will-be-more-than-1bn-as-no-financial-talks-with-fujitsu-under-way-13082044.

The Decision Lab. 2024. "Cognitive Biases." *thedecisionlab.com*. Accessed April 12, 2024. https://thedecisionlab.com/biases.

Tversky, Amos and Daniel Kahneman. 1974. "Judgment Under Uncertainty: Heuristics and Biases." *Science* 185 (4157): 1124–31.

9

The 2009 NAS Report – Strengthening Forensic Science

Name of the Publication

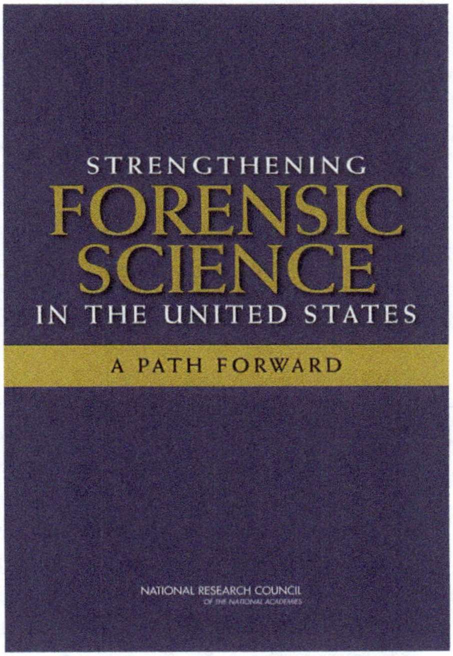

Image 9.1 The cover of the 2009 NAS Report.

The publication is titled **Strengthening Forensic Science in the United States: A Path Forward.** Committee on Identifying the Needs of the Forensic Sciences Community, National Research Council 2009.

It is sometimes referred to as 'NAS, NRC, Committee on Identifying the Needs of the Forensic Science Community'. In this chapter and elsewhere in this book, it is referred to as the NAS Report.

According to ResearchGate on 23rd of December 2022, it had been cited 131 times; according to the NRC, it has been cited 1362 times.

Introduction

It is generally accepted by the entire forensic science community that the publication of this report (the 2009 NAS Report) was a watershed moment in the history of forensic science. The NAS Report set a reform agenda in both research and practice for forensic science, including more and better research and higher practice standards. The response to the NAS Report, though initially slow to develop, has continued over many years. It is often used as a starting point for conversation about reform, and its impact continues to this day.

The NAS Report comprised 254/350 (PDF copy) pages and included 11 recommendations relating directly to forensic science and encompassed all aspects of forensic science. It certainly has the widest scope and is the most comprehensive of all the publications that

A History of Forensic Science in 10 Publications: How They Established Current Practice, First Edition.
Sean Doyle.

are the subject of this book. It is a publication that sparked much debate and controversy at the time of publication in 2009 and is still having an impact a decade and a half later.

One principal aim of assembling the NAS Committee, which collectively wrote the report, was to establish the requirements for improving the quality and reliability of scientific evidence, particularly for evidence types other than DNA. DNA analysis at that time was considered the 'gold standard' and the standard to which other evidence types were to be held. As discussed in Chapter 4, DNA analysis had set the standard for others to meet.

The NAS Report called into question the validity of many forensic methods and consequently the reliability of many evidence types, drawing attention to the absence of a scientific basis. Indeed, the publication went so far as to conclude that, except for nuclear DNA[1] (nDNA) analysis, many forensic techniques had not established their validity, i.e. the ability to produce accurate results and evidence that a court might rely on to reach a safe verdict by a fair process.

The NAS Report concluded that there was a,

> *... notable dearth of peer-reviewed, published studies establishing the scientific bases and validity of many forensic methods.*

The NAS Report also concludes that apart from nDNA.

> *... no forensic method has been rigorously shown to have the capacity to consistently, and with a high degree of certainty, demonstrate a connection between evidence and a specific individual or source.*

The NAS Report found that these weaknesses were systemic outside the field of DNA analysis and particularly prevalent in so-called feature-comparison disciplines such as fingerprints and handwriting. These disciplines are subjective, relying on the skills and knowledge of the examiner and thus prone to the cognitive biases discussed in Chapter 8. At the time, false-positive and false-negative rates were unknown for these disciplines, and no research studied the frequency of occurrence of features used in comparisons, effectively their relative rarity. Essentially, there was little or no research that supported the claims made by examiners in these comparison disciplines.

In addition, the NAS Report concluded that the relationship with law enforcement needed to be less close, identified the need for greater oversight of forensic science, and found that proficiency testing, competence assessment and performance monitoring were inadequate.

Finally, to progress and deliver the reforms needed, the NAS Report recommended the creation of a new federal agency, the National Institute of Forensic Science (NIFS).

The NAS Report echoed the point made in Chapter 4 that, indirectly, it was the advent of DNA evidence and the challenges that the evidence type faced in the early years that prompted scrutiny of fingerprints. It questioned the validity of many feature-comparison methods. As recorded in Chapter 4, a fingerprint 'match' declaration was held to be unassailable. When an examiner concluded that the fingerprints 'matched', it was with 100% certainty. The NAS Committee forensically undermined that claim, which led to some soul-searching among these 'traditional' forensic disciplines.

So, the NAS Report responding to the concerns of the day, critically assessed forensic science and set out the position in 2009. It then made recommendations, some of which have been acted on and taken root. However, others had a short life, and still others gather dust. Therefore, even today, miscarriages of justice continue to occur as a result of poor-quality forensic evidence being adduced, even with accreditation, regulation and admissibility criteria such as Daubert discussed in Chapter 8.

A careful reading of the report also provides a detailed explanation of the complexities of the US legal system, including its separation of federal and state jurisdictions and the variations in the rules of evidence from state to state. This fragmentation is exacerbated by forensic science provision at local, county, state and federal levels, which hinders the efficient and effective provision of forensic science in the United States.

Summary

The NAS Report contains an assessment of the strengths, weaknesses, current and future needs of forensic disciplines, and makes recommendations for improving the use of forensic technologies and techniques.

The scope of the report is both broad and deep. Thus, in this report, the term 'forensic science' covers a broad array of activities, with the recognition that some of these activities might not have a well-developed research base, are not informed by scientific knowledge, or are not developed within the culture of science.

The outcome of the NAS Report was a set of recommendations, 13 in all, which are explored in greater detail later in this chapter, but the most important and relevant may be summarised as follows:

- Research that would assess the validity and reliability of methods used in feature-comparison disciplines such as fingerprint examination.
- Further research into the issues of cognitive bias and its effects on decision-making.
- Standardisation of laboratory reports and a definition of terms, especially those expressing the association between an item of evidence and a possible source.
- Mandatory accreditation of all forensic science laboratories and mandatory certification of all forensic scientists.
- A mandatory code of ethics, which is enforced with sanctions for breach.

Motivation for Writing

The NAS Report was a response to concerns about miscarriages of justice in the United States, many uncovered by the Innocence Project (The Innocence Project 2023).[2] In 2005, the US Congress authorised the National Academy of Sciences (NAS) to conduct a study on forensic science. The premise for the study was that the US Senate had concluded that the requirements of DNA analysis were well-known; in contrast, for disciplines other than DNA, little was known of their requirements.

There were also concerns about standards and oversight. In 1989, the molecular biologist and later co-chair of the US President's Council of Advisors on Science and Technology (PCAST), the 2016 report of which is discussed later in this chapter, Eric Lander, was quoted as follows.

> *At present forensic science is virtually unregulated – with the paradoxical result that clinical laboratories must meet higher standards to diagnose strep throat than forensic labs must meet to put a defendant on death row.*

There were also societal impacts from miscarriages of justice. These included a loss of public confidence in criminal justice and, where scientific evidence might have contributed to the miscarriage, a loss of confidence in forensic science. Furthermore, the wrongful conviction of the innocent meant that the guilty were free, and if the crime was violent, public safety was put at risk.

The US Senate had set the terms of reference (TOR) for the Forensic Science Committee assembled by NAS as follows.

1. Assess the present and future resource needs of the forensic science community.[3]
2. Make recommendations for maximising the use of forensic technologies and techniques.
3. Identify potential scientific advances.
4. Make recommendations for programs that will increase the number of qualified forensic scientists.
5. Disseminate best practices and guidelines.
6. Examine the interoperability of AFIS (Automatic Fingerprint Information Systems), i.e. the sharing of fingerprint data across internal borders.

There were other TOR concerning US homeland security and medical examination/pathology, but they lie outside the scope of this book, which focuses on forensic science.

The committee assembled by NAS was multidisciplinary and included most stakeholders, scientists, lawyers, judges and policymakers. Although, as will be discussed later, skewed towards academia.

Terms

So, what are feature-comparison disciplines? Except for bloodstain pattern analysis, what feature-comparison disciplines have in common is that they attempt to determine whether or not a particular pattern or impression – be it a shoeprint, a tyre tread, a fingerprint, or a bullet – can be associated with a particular source.

Feature-comparison disciplines can include the following evidence types.

- Bite marks
- Bloodstain patterns
- Fabrics
- Fibres
- Fingerprints
- Firearms and ammunition (spent and unspent)
- Footwear
- Glass
- Hair
- Handwriting

- Inks/Paint
- Papers
- Plant material
- Soil
- Tire marks
- Tool marks (marks made by a harder material on a softer material, which includes firearm barrel marks on lead bullets)

Biography of the Publication

According to the NAS website.

> *The National Academy of Sciences (NAS) is a private, non-profit society of distinguished scholars. Established by an Act of Congress, signed by President Abraham Lincoln in 1863, the NAS is charged with providing independent, objective advice to the nation on matters related to science and technology.*

As mentioned earlier, in 2005, the US Congress directed the NAS to conduct a comprehensive study to assess the current state of forensic science and make recommendations for improvement. The NAS Committee was established in 2006 to identify the needs of the forensic science community. The Committee met on eight occasions between January 2007 and November 2008. During these meetings, the Committee heard expert testimony and considered the information it heard and received. Between meetings, the Committee reviewed numerous publications related to the forensic science disciplines, engaged in independent research on the subject, and drafted the report.

The NAS Committee reached a consensus on the most important issues faced by the forensic science community and agreed on 13 specific recommendations to address these issues.

Following this extensive review by a multidisciplinary committee assembled for the purpose, the NAS Report was first issued in February 2009.

Professional Biography of the Authors

The Report was written by the Forensic Science Committee established by the NAS to address the terms of reference given by the US Senate. Represented on that committee were members of the forensic science community, members of the legal community and a 'diverse' group of scientists.

The committee co-chairs were then US appeal court Judge Harry T Edwards and Constantine Gatsonis, then a professor of biostatistics at Brown University, Rhode Island and founding director of the Centre for Statistical Sciences. A detailed biography of Professor Gatsonis can be found at the Brown University website (Brown University 2017). A detailed biography of Professor Edwards can be found on the New York University website (NYU School of Law 2024).

There are extensive biographies of all the NAS Committee members in Appendix A of the Report.

The affiliations of the other Committee members are given later in the section discussing the structure of the publication.

Contexts

Scientific

While DNA had an indirect causative effect on the recognition of bias as discussed in Chapter 4, it also had a direct effect on the NAS Report. DNA had to overcome many initial challenges and became the standard to which other evidence types were held. In addition, DNA had been used by the Innocence Project to uncover miscarriages of justice, exposing weaknesses in other evidence types, for example, microscopic hair comparison (FBI 2015). Therefore, the NAS Report begins by excluding DNA from its scope as it is the 'gold standard'. It concluded that other evidence types, particularly those relying on comparison, should be required to meet the same standards as DNA analysis.

However, in 2007, DNA evidence faced a new challenge. In England, in the late 1990s and early 2000s, the Forensic Science Service (FSS) pioneered a more sensitive nuclear DNA analysis technique, essentially by running the amplification reaction for a few more cycles.[4] This significantly increased the amount of DNA available for analysis, making the technique much more sensitive, and obtaining more information from less material. The FSS called this low copy number (as in not much to start with) DNA, abbreviated as LCN DNA. A more generic name is low template DNA, abbreviated as LT DNA.

In 2007, the validity of the FSS method was questioned by the judge at the trial of a person charged with several terrorist-related offences, including the 1998 bombing in Omagh, Northern Ireland, in which 29 people were killed and around 300 injured. LCN DNA-based evidence allegedly linking the accused to the terrorist incidents was a major plank in the prosecution case. However, because of poor practice, particularly in terms of inadequate contamination avoidance given the extreme sensitivity of the LCN technique, the judge excluded that evidence (R v Hoey 2007). The defence attacked the LCN DNA evidence, alleging that it was not fully validated. Again, DNA met the challenge and the LCN DNA technique was subsequently declared valid with some caveats (Caddy et al. 2008).

However, because of the challenge of interpretation resulting from the increased risk of contamination, mixed profiles, random effects caused by the increased amplification, and lingering controversy, some providers shied away from its use. At that time, LCN was not taken up by the US Federal Bureau of Investigation (FBI)

A milestone in the regulation and oversight of forensic science, to be called for in the NAS Report, was the appointment in 2008 of the Forensic Science Regulator in England and Wales. Uniquely (and some would argue, foolishly (Roberts 1996), a forensic science market had been created in the jurisdiction and an authority was required to regulate that market and ensure a 'level playing field', for all forensic science providers. In maintaining that level playing field, the Regulator was also tasked with ensuring minimum standards were in place in support of the criminal justice system (Doyle 2019a-e).

On a less positive note, the body responsible for assessing individual competence established in the wake of the miscarriages of justice, discussed in Chapter 7 on ISO/IEC 17025, the Council for the Registration of Forensic Practitioners (CRFP), incorporated in 1999, was closed in 2009 by the government of the United Kingdom. The closure ended the independent assessment of the competence of the individual in the United Kingdom. In contrast, the United States has responded to the call in the NAS Report for mandating certification of individuals by accrediting certification bodies to the international standard ISO/IEC 17024 'Conformity assessment – General requirements for bodies operating certification of persons', which is discussed later in this chapter.

Also, during the period of the NAS Committee's work, so-called Next-Generation Sequencing (NGS) was developed, enabling rapid and cost-effective sequencing of entire genomes. A genome is the complete set of genetic information in an organism. It consists of nucleotide sequences, abbreviated as A, C, G and T, discussed in Chapter 4. NGS is now the basis for forensic genomics. It allows forensic scientists to generate data that spans the entire human genome and address a wider range of questions in a single, targeted analysis.

Outside of forensic science and more technological than scientific, 2007 saw the launch of the iPhone, which, besides being the death knell for the BlackBerry, has had a profound effect on society.

The Large Hadron Collider was completed in 2008 to smash subatomic particles and acquire new knowledge about the origin of the universe. In 2012, it found the Higgs boson or 'God particle', which helped explain why some elementary particles have mass. Without the Higgs boson, there would be no atomic elements, stars or universe. Any further detail is beyond the scope of this book and the knowledge of its author!

Historical

Perhaps the greatest upheaval during the period in question, certainly in the 'West', was the 2008 global financial crisis. Governments had to borrow heavily and curb spending to stabilise economies. The crisis ushered in a period of austerity, so, as ever, the poorest in society took the biggest hit.

The United States was engaged in conflicts in Afghanistan, a direct result of the 9/11 atrocity, and in Iraq, with the consequent drain on the public purse.

While there is little or no scholarship on the impact of the financial crisis on forensic science, the pressure on government spending of this, and the conflicts must have had some, if only in terms of slowing development and limiting capital expenditure. It may partly explain the slow response to the NAS Report and the recommended creation of a National Institute of Forensic Science being a non-starter.

In 2008, Barack Obama was elected the 44th President of the United States, and his administration began in January 2009. This fact is important to the NAS Report's outcomes and the implementation of its recommendations. It is fair to say that the reforms recommended by the NAS Committee were looked on more favourably by US Democrats. In 2017, the incoming Republican administration under Donald Trump had signalled that the body established to progress the recommendations made in the NAS Report, the National Commission on Forensic Science (NCFS), would be wound up if and when the administration changed, and it was (Hsu 2017). The PCAST Report, discussed later in this Chapter, published in September 2016, was one of the last acts of the Obama administration in trying to advance the NAS Report's reform agenda and continue to support the strengthening of forensic science in the United States.

Social/Society

One of the motivations for assembling the NAS Committee in 2005, which published the NAS Report in 2009, was wrongful convictions uncovered by the Innocence Project.

The Innocence Project was founded in 1992 by the lawyers Peter Neufeld and Barry Scheck. Since then, the Innocence Project has been at the forefront of criminal justice reform in the United States, using DNA and other scientific advancements to identify and overturn wrongful convictions. However, there is a broader societal impact of wrongful convictions; they are miscarriages of justice.

In addition to the wrongful conviction and the damaging effects on those individuals and their loved ones, the truly guilty party goes free, the crime is not 'solved', and victims of crime are denied justice. If the crime was violent, then public safety is put at risk. Additional effects are a loss of confidence in the criminal justice system and, if scientific evidence played a part, then confidence in forensic science may be undermined; one of the motivations for setting up the NAS Committee.

There is also a financial cost, which can run into millions of dollars. In the United Kingdom, the cost of bringing justice to those falsely convicted based on unreliable evidence in the so-called Post Office Scandal could reach one billion pounds (Baker 2024).

For the reasons recorded above, all criminal justice stakeholders, particularly lawmakers, lawyers and judges, should do all in their power to reduce the risk of a miscarriage of justice.

Hopefully, it is not too controversial to argue that US Republicans are not in favour of any initiative that might make it more difficult to secure the conviction of those truly guilty of crime. Certainly, the reforms and developments post-NAS are counter to that objective. This view is supported by the changes made when the Republicans took office in 2017, such as the non-renewal of the NCFS charter in 2017, referred to earlier.

There is much talk of balance in common law/adversarial criminal justice systems, such as in the United States, together with an equality of arms and a presumption of innocence. There is also Blackstone's adage or ratio, that 10 guilty persons should go free rather than one innocent person being falsely convicted. Again, the reality is quite different. The accused faces the full strength and resources of the state, which normally far outweigh those of the accused. This inequality of arms is sometimes seen in cases where the assumption is that the scientific evidence is so powerful that the accused is pressured into entering a guilty plea or plea bargain and pleading guilty to a lesser charge. In the United Kingdom, the Post Office scandal has exposed this practice (Willis 2021). However, it is recognised that plea bargaining is part of the US justice system – whether that is in the interests of justice is a question beyond the scope of this book. Plea bargaining and a lazy defence have and will continue to contribute to many miscarriages of justice. Furthermore, the strength of the prosecution's scientific evidence is believed to be such that the accused is often advised not to, or even prevented from, instructing an expert to review that evidence critically.[5] The position is clear; anyone facing a charge that is supported by scientific evidence should, as a matter of course and of right, have that evidence independently reviewed, especially if that is subjective, feature-comparison evidence, such as fingerprints, the weaknesses of which were exposed by the NAS Report and others.

While the presumption of innocence might be a revered legal principle. The reality is that the accused would not be on trial if there were not a strong case to answer. Even lay fact-finders (juries), seeing the accused in the 'dock', cannot start from a neutral position. The initial belief of the jury is discussed in some detail in Chapter 6 'Interpreting Evidence'.

Most states, or at least the public, would prefer the reverse of Blackstone's ratio, one innocent person falsely convicted rather than 10 guilty persons going free. The state would readily accept a false conviction or two as the price of ensuring all truly guilty parties are convicted and the public is kept safe. The number of miscarriages of justice that continue to be uncovered seems to support this conclusion.

With these contributory factors in play, it is understandable why the system lacks balance, which, in turn, leads to miscarriages of justice.

To repeat the point made earlier, all criminal justice stakeholders, particularly lawmakers, lawyers and judges should do all in their power to reduce the risk of a miscarriage of justice, which was one of the high-level aims of the NAS Report – a report prompted by the exposure of miscarriages of justice to which poor quality scientific evidence had contributed.

Structure of the Publication

The report begins with a series of chapters describing forensic science as currently practised in the United States, the use of forensic science and its disciplines. It then sets out areas in need of improvement and how those improvements might be realised through standards, good practice, education and training.

Contents

The report has 11 sections, a preface, a summary which includes 13 recommendations, two appendices and an index. Sections 9 and 11 are not particularly relevant to this book, and the two recommendations made in those sections lie outside the scope. The PDF copy of the Report, which is available online (National Academy of Sciences 2009), has 350 pages. The sections are as follows.

1. Introduction
2. The Forensic Science Community and the Need for Integrated Governance
3. The Admission of Forensic Science Evidence in Litigation, Law and Science
4. The Principles of Science and Interpreting Scientific Data
5. Descriptions of Some Forensic Science Disciplines
6. Improving Methods, Practice, and Performance in Forensic Science
7. Strengthening Oversight of Forensic Science Practice
8. Education and Training in Forensic Science
9. Medical Examiner and Coroner Systems: Current and Future Needs
10. Automated Fingerprint Identification Systems
11. Homeland Security and the Forensic Science Disciplines

Appendices

A. Biographical Information of the Committee and Staff
B. Committee Meeting Agendas

The NAS Report begins with a sizable quantity of what is known as 'front matter', which includes a description of the composition of the National Academies' 'Advisers to the Nation of Science, Engineering and Medicine', which comprises:

- National Academy of Sciences (NAS)
- National Academy of Engineering (NAE)
- Institute of Medicine (IOM)
- National Research Council (NRC)

There is then a list of members of the multi-disciplinary Committee assembled for the stated purpose of '*Identifying the Needs of the Forensic Science Community*'.

Harry T. Edwards co-chaired the Committee, an appeal court judge for the District of Columbia and Constantine Gatsonis, Director of the Centre for Statistical Sciences, Brown University. A further 15 members of the committee were named and listed with their affiliations. They were in alphabetical order.

1. Margaret A. Berger. A member of the National Academies Committee on Science, Technology, and Law, on the Committee on Science, Engineering, and Public Policy, and on the Committee on Ensuring the Utility and the Integrity of Research Data.
2. Joe S. Cecil. Senior Research Associate and Project Director in the Division of Research at the Federal Judicial Centre.
3. M. Bonner Denton. Professor of Chemistry and a Professor of Geosciences at the University of Arizona.
4. Marcella F. Fierro. Former Chief Medical Examiner for the Commonwealth of Virginia, and Professor of Pathology and Professor and Chair of the Department of Legal Medicine at Virginia Commonwealth University.
5. Karen Kafadar. Rudy Professor of Statistics and Physics at Indiana University.
6. Peter M. Marone. Executive Director of the Virginia Department of Forensic Sciences.
7. Geoffrey S. Mearns. Dean of the Cleveland-Marshall College of Law at Cleveland State University.
8. Randall S. Murch. Associate Director, Research Program Development, Research Division, National Capital Region, Virginia Tech.
9. Channing Robertson. Director of the Stanford-National Institutes of Health Graduate Training Program in Biotechnology.
10. Marvin E. Schechter. A solo practitioner, specialising in criminal defence matters.
11. Robert Shaler. Professor and Director of the Forensic and Investigative Sciences Program at Indiana University Purdue University, Indianapolis.
12. Jay A. Siegel. Professor and Director of the Forensic and Investigative Sciences Program at Indiana University Purdue University, Indianapolis.
13. Sargur Srihari. State University of New York, Distinguished Professor at the University at Buffalo in the Department of Computer Science and Engineering.
14. Sheldon M. Wiederhorn. A Senior Fellow at NIST.
15. Ross E. Zumwalt. Chief Medical Investigator of the State of New Mexico.

The academic/university sector has the greatest representation and consequently the loudest voice.

The (sub)committee assembled on science, technology and law is then listed. It was co-chaired by Donald Kennedy (NAS/IOM), President Emeritus and Bing Professor of Environmental Science Emeritus, Stanford University; Emeritus Editor-in-Chief, Science and Richard A. Merrill (IOM), Daniel Caplin Professor of Law Emeritus, University of Virginia Law School. Other members of this committee are listed with their affiliations. This committee had 26 members in total.

Next, the committee on applied and theoretical statistics is listed. It was chaired by Karen Kafadar. Other members of this committee are named and listed with their affiliations. This committee had nine members.

There is an acknowledgment of experts who made presentations to the committees; it is a long list. There follows an acknowledgement of reviewers, a shorter list.

Then there's the list of contents, on page Roman 15 (XV) beginning with a preface. The preface introduces some of the challenges facing forensic science, e.g. lack of adequate resources, sound policies and national support. The NAS Committee aimed to chart a development agenda to deliver the necessary improvements in forensic science. The agenda included standardisation and good practice. The Committee stated that the recommendations made were '*inexorably interconnected*' and required a national/federal response. Unfortunately, as will become clear, the two recommendations that would have most efficiently and effectively delivered that response were not implemented.

The main body of the NAS Report begins with a helpful 33-page summary including the main findings and recommendations; the general reader of the Report needs to progress no further.

Summary

The NAS Report proper begins with a helpful summary given in Section 1, Introduction.

The summary starts with the origin story, as it were, an explanation as to the reason for the establishment of the NAS Forensic Science Committee and its main terms of reference (TOR) developed from those given earlier and are summarised as follows.

- Assess the present and future resource needs of the forensic science community.
- Make recommendations for maximising the use of forensic technologies and techniques.
- Identify potential scientific advances that may assist law enforcement in using forensic technologies and techniques.
- Make recommendations for programs that will increase the number of qualified forensic scientists.
- Disseminate best practices and guidelines concerning the collection and analysis of forensic evidence to help ensure quality and consistency in the use of forensic technologies and techniques.

The overall focus of the TOR was to.

> *... solve crimes, investigate deaths and protect the public ...*

There is then a section giving the background to the Committee, its warrant from the US Senate, its make-up of members of the forensic science community, together with members of the legal community, and a diverse group of scientists. The NAS Report also records the working practices of the Committee. But as stated earlier, the Committee had a heavy academic/university bias.

The summary then lists the issues covered, which included applying the scientific method to the practice of forensic science. Here, the scientific method is defined as.

> ... *hypothesis generation and testing, falsifiability and replication, and peer review* ....

Also included in the scope were:

- An assessment of methods and technologies used in forensic science, in particular, the accuracy of the results obtained and the reliability of their interpretation.
- Identifying research, training and education needs.
- The operation of forensic science laboratories and the resources needed.
- The accreditation of providers and the certification of practitioners.

The report goes on to place forensic scientific evidence into three categories, which is helpful.

1. Pattern/experience evidence, such as fingerprints, handwriting and bloodstain pattern analysis.
2. Analytical evidence, such as the analysis of DNA, drugs of abuse and explosives.
3. Digital evidence, extracting information from mobile phones and computers.

While forensic science activities are being categorised, it is important to note that the NAS Report also recognised the importance of crime scene processing and that it can require scientific knowledge and judgement; errors introduced at the scene are difficult to rectify later in the forensic process. However, it reports that forensic scientists are not often involved at the crime scene. That is not true in the case of some serious crimes, such as crimes of violence and terrorist attacks. The issue of scientists at the crime scene is discussed often in this book, and particularly in Chapter 10 on the Sydney Declaration.

The scope of the NAS Report also included the examination of the use of forensic science in criminal litigation, to look at the practice of forensic science providers at the local, state and federal level. The last in the list of tasks was to consider the forensic science community in the United Kingdom.

The introduction then turns to the challenges perceived to be facing the forensic science community. The report repeats the point made earlier and in Chapter 4 of this book that the advent of DNA analysis led to uncovering weaknesses in some forensic disciplines, and these weaknesses had, in turn, contributed to wrongful convictions. To identify the issues facing forensic science and make recommendations, the Committee realised that it had to gain an understanding of the disciplines, their strengths and weaknesses, and the relevant stakeholder community.

It lists some of the problems facing forensic science. The first is the disparity between the resources available to providers at the federal, state and local levels. The NAS Report concludes that this has resulted in fragmentation or disconnection and inconsistent practices.

The Committee concluded that the lack of standard practices, the certification of practitioners as competent and the accreditation of providers were major threats to the quality and reliability of scientific evidence.

The broad range of forensic scientific disciplines was also identified as an issue, some laboratory-based, some at the scene. The practitioners also varied from those with higher degrees in the natural sciences to technicians and law enforcement officers who examine and compare patterns, such as fingerprints.

Interpretation is the next issue raised. The NAS Report mentions '*individualisation*' and initially seems to suggest that the word is synonymous with 'matching'. We know from Chapter 3 that individualisation, attributing evidence to a source to the exclusion of all others, is not supported by science or logic. The report then draws attention to perhaps the greatest weakness at the time: not all interpretation in forensic science has a valid basis. To quote the report.

> *... there is a notable dearth of peer-reviewed, published studies establishing the scientific basis and validity of many forensic methods.*

Expert evidence had been given for many decades and accepted by courts of law on the assumption that the evidence was based on valid methods when no such basis existed.

The urgent requirement for research in support of subjective, feature-comparison disciplines was recognised, as was the potential for cognitive bias, errors in thinking, to affect decision-making, which is the subject of Chapter 8. It concluded that research was required to measure performance and determine the limits. The NAS Committee concluded that individualisation, attributing an item of evidence to a source to the exclusion of all others, is not possible. However, it accepted that placing evidence in a particular general class may assist an investigation.

The introduction then turns to admissibility, which is extensively discussed in Chapter 8. However, the NAS Report's focus is the contribution of science to a particular discipline.

> *... the question of whether – and to what extent – there is science*[6] *in any given forensic science discipline.*

There is much wisdom contained in this part of the introduction. The requirement for reliable scientific evidence drawn from valid methods, employed by competent scientists working in competent organisations, is restated together with the risks to reliability; those being error, bias, unvalidated methods and poor performance standards. The NAS Report laments the fact that these requirements are not always demanded by the trial judge when considering admissibility, in the United States under Daubert and Federal Rule of Evidence 702 (FRE 702 is discussed in Chapter 8). The Report highlights the latitude the Supreme Court under FRE 702 granted to the trial judge. The lax application of Daubert/FRE 702 risks the admission of unreliable scientific evidence. If unreliable evidence is admitted, then the US Supreme Court relies on the adversarial system to weed it out using the tools of '*vigorous*' cross-examination and presenting contrary evidence. However, the authors of the NAS Report do not consider the adversarial system of justice suited to the task of finding '*scientific truth*'. The Report records the concern that Daubert/FRE 702 effectively makes the trial judge the 'gatekeeper' and not the scientific community, which is the competent authority.

One of the nuggets of wisdom is a statement of a fundamental distinction between Science and the Law, which has the two always in tension.

> *Scientific conclusions are subject to perpetual revision. Law, on the other hand, must resolve disputes finally and quickly.*

Whether legal disputes, criminal or civil, proceed quickly is a matter of debate, but the law does require finality. Science will never be 'final', it is always a work in progress.

The NAS Report states a requirement that to reduce the risk of unreliable evidence being admitted, the trial judge should determine whether methods are supported by research and have been validated by the relevant scientific community. However, the authors recognise that some judges appear to be reluctant to insist on such supporting research and offer an example of a court admitting fingerprint evidence in the absence of supporting research. This highlights another distinction between the Law and Science. In common law jurisdictions, such as those of the United States, the Law relies on precedent and is unlikely to question the validity of methods used to produce evidence over many decades.

Given the hit-and-miss approach of the judiciary to the admissibility of scientific evidence and its lack of competence in scientific matters, the NAS Report places the responsibility for ensuring that scientific evidence is of sufficient quality as to be reliable on the forensic science community itself. Whether the community has or has not accepted and exercised that responsibility is the high-level question addressed in this book.

The introduction then recaps the requirements necessary to ensure that quality.

- More and better educational programs.
- Accredited laboratories.
- Certified forensic practitioners.
- Valid methods.
- Research to establish limits and measures of performance for each discipline.

The NAS Report concludes that the current situation, i.e. in 2009, is '*seriously wanting*'.

The introduction concludes by acknowledging the political hurdles faced in the United States, although a sovereign nation, it is also a federation of states, each a separate jurisdiction with its own law enforcement agencies. The NAS Report, in making its recommendations, is less prescriptive than it otherwise might be and recognised that putting the recommendations into practice would require time and creativity, not to mention money.

Findings and Recommendations

The Summary then turns to findings and recommendations. The NAS Report makes 13 recommendations.

Recommendation 1: The Establishment of a National Institute of Forensic Science (NIFS) The NAS Report sets out the evidence in support of creating this new federal agency. It recorded the fragmentary nature of the US justice system, and the consequent variety of support provided and capability offered by forensic science providers at local, state and federal levels.

It found forensic science provision to be under-resourced, had poor links with academia, and suffered from inadequate training and education. In response, it recommended the adoption of good practice, mandatory accreditation of forensic science providers and the certification of practitioners. The overall requirement was for harmony, standardisation, and a strong independent governance structure.

The Report reviewed existing agencies and, after due consideration, concluded that none were suitable. The reasons can be summarised as the need for independence and a fresh start. The new agency should focus on the needs of the forensic science community and be separate from law enforcement. It concluded that the new agency should be federal, have a science-based culture and be well-connected to all justice stakeholders.

The new federal agency, the National Institute of Forensic Science (NIFS), should, among other things, prioritise:

- establishing standards and enforcing conformance,
- promoting research, and
- provide financial support for disciplines other than DNA analysis.

The NAS Report then goes on to set out the benefits to the justice system of such an institute, essentially improving the quality and reliability of scientific evidence.

The Report acknowledges the political and budgetary challenges in establishing a new federal agency and accepts that this recommendation, although foundational to the improvements sought, may be politically too difficult to implement.

Many of the subsequent recommendations are contingent on the creation of NIFS for their implementation. As will be discussed later, NIFS was not created; the responsibility for implementation fell to existing federal agencies, and this affected those dependent recommendations.

Recommendation 2: Standardised Terminology and Reporting The NAS Report raises the issue of varying and therefore confusing terminology, a long-running and current issue in forensic science. Examples given are *'match', 'consistent with', 'identical', 'similar in all respects tested'*, and *'cannot be excluded'*. The NAS Report calls for a standard vocabulary in forensic science. Inconsistent and confusing terminology in forensic science is a constant theme in this book.

Regarding reports, it requires reports to contain all the information necessary to support conclusions, including methods and raw results. Furthermore, conforming to model laboratory reports should be a requirement of certification and accreditation.

Recommendation 3: More and Better Research Recalling the observation that some forensic science disciplines lack the support of validating research, the NAS Report calls for research that will address the issues of accuracy and validity of scientific methods and the reliability of the results obtained. This research should be funded by NIFS. It should encompass the development of methods to determine the reliability and accuracy of analyses and distinguish between the reliability and accuracy of the method itself and the practitioner employing the method. This distinction is one of the subjects of the President's Council of Advisors on Science and Technology (PCAST) Report, which is discussed later in this Chapter.

Recommendation 4: Best Practice and Standards The NAS Report notes the lack of regulatory oversight and conformance with operating standards, ethics, certification and accreditation. It recommends that forensic science should be independent of law enforcement, a recommendation made several times in the Report. It specifically recommends removing all forensic science laboratories from the administrative control of law enforcement agencies or prosecution authorities. To quote the report:

> *The best science is conducted in a scientific setting as opposed to a law enforcement setting.*

It is one of the conclusions in this book that many of the major advances in forensic science and contributors to current practice have been external, unrelated to forensic science.

Recommendation 5: Minimise the Effects of Cognitive Bias Bias was covered extensively in Chapter 8. The NAS Report calls for further studies on the effect of cognitive bias in forensic practice and to develop procedures that will minimise its effect.

Recommendation 6: NIFS to collaborate with the US National Institute of Standards and Technology (NIST) The NAS Report calls on NIFS to work with NIST, together with government laboratories, universities and the existing Scientific Working Groups[7] to develop tools such as interlaboratory comparison exercises to monitor performance and establish standard operating procedures.

Recommendation 7: Mandatory Laboratory Accreditation and the Certification of Individual Practitioners The need for an ethos or culture of continuous improvement is mentioned. As discussed in Chapter 7, such an ethos is required for conformance to ISO/IEC 17025. Regarding the certification of individual practitioners, it mandates that no individual should be allowed to practice or give evidence unless certified. The NAS Report goes on to spell out some minimum requirements that might demonstrate competence; these are listed as follows:

- Written examinations
- Supervised practice
- Proficiency testing
- Continuing education
- Recertification
- Adherence to a code of ethics

The timetable for accreditation and certification was to be determined by NIFS.

Recommendation 8: Forensic laboratories should establish routine quality assurance and quality control procedures to ensure the accuracy of forensic analyses and the work of forensic practitioners While conforming to ISO/IEC 17025 (the subject of Chapter 7) should meet most of the specified requirements, the NAS Report includes a requirement to address fraud, which is difficult to guard against.

Recommendation 9: Establish a national code of ethics and a means of enforcement The NAS Report places reliance for implementing this recommendation on NIFS which the authors hope to be created. Ethics remains a live issue. Several organisations, particularly professional bodies such as the American Academy of Forensic Sciences and the California Association of Criminalists, have a code of practice in place, but a means of effectively policing codes remains elusive. Enforcement through certification is a mechanism suggested.

Recommendation 10: Congress to financially support appropriate postgraduate courses via NIFS Again, the recommendation relies on the creation of NIFS to develop suitable education programs with funding provided by the federal government. The NAS Report requires forensic scientists to be well-versed in the scientific method in addition to the scientific basis of the discipline. The educational phase should precede any period of 'apprenticeship', which the authors consider has a secondary role.

Recognising that lawyers and judges might not have a sufficient grasp of science to properly exercise their roles in cases involving scientific testimony, the NAS Report calls for a closer relationship between forensic science and the law, and some appropriate scientific training and awareness.

Recommendation 11: This relates to forensic medicine, specifically forensic pathology and is therefore beyond the scope of this book.

Recommendation 12: Relates to the Automated Fingerprint Identification Systems (AFIS) The authors highlight the difficulties in exchanging fingerprint data between agencies and jurisdictions. Different systems are used by different agencies, and there are jurisdictional issues with access to different fingerprint databases. A harmonised system with common standards to facilitate the exchange of data among agencies is needed.

The thirteenth and final recommendation relates to the security of the USA. The NAS Report calls on all relevant agencies coordinated by NIFS to aim for maximum evidential value to be gained with due regard to the health and safety of those involved.

This concludes the summary, which sets out the issues, identifies areas of weakness and makes recommendations to address those weaknesses and 'strengthen' forensic science.

As a postscript to this section on the summary of the findings and recommendations of the NAS Report, it is important to emphasise that the highest-level recommendation was the creation/establishment of a National Institute of Forensic Science (NIFS) as an agency to implement many of the other recommendations. However, it is a fact that NIFS was not created and is unlikely to be so created in the foreseeable future. Other routes to implementation have been opened, while some of the recommendations have fallen on deaf ears. As will be discussed later in this Chapter, politics has also had an effect, unsurprisingly.

Impact at the Time

American Academy of Forensic Sciences (AAFS)

In September 2009, the AAFS issued a statement (AAFS 2009) broadly supporting the recommendations made in the NAS Report, translating them into seven principles which the AAFS endorsed and promoted. Those principles are as follows.

1. All forensic science disciplines must have a strong scientific foundation.
2. All forensic science laboratories should be accredited.
3. All forensic scientists should be certified.
4. Forensic science terminology should be standardised.
5. Forensic scientists should be assiduously held to the Codes of Ethics.
6. Existing forensic science professional entities should participate in governmental oversight of the field.
7. Attorneys and judges who work with forensic scientists and forensic science evidence should have a strong awareness and knowledge of the scientific method and forensic science disciplines.

The AAFS proposed taking the following actions in support of those principles.

- To establish a committee to consider concerns raised regarding the scientific basis and validity of a method, and after due process, issue a report to a relevant authority.
- Consider whether the AAFS can contribute to the standardisation of terminology.
- Assist in improving the knowledge of lawyers and judges concerning forensic science and scientific evidence by developing a curriculum covering all forensic science disciplines.

Early Responses from the Disciplines

The NAS Report was met with some controversy and was not universally well-received, particularly among forensic scientists engaged in subjective feature-comparison disciplines. That being said, the day after the NAS Report was published, the president of the International Association of Identification (IAI), an international professional body representing fingerprint examiners, wrote to the membership 'suggesting' ...

> *... that members not assert 100% infallibility (zero error rate) when addressing the reliability of fingerprint comparisons.*
>
> *(Mnookin et al. 2011)*

That was followed by a softening of the situation regarding the mandatory[8] use of only one of the three categorical conclusions: 'match', no match or inconclusive. The IAI opened the possibility of a probabilistic approach that is opinions expressing the likelihood of a 'match' (International Association for Identification 2010).

The next step in rolling back on the claim to the infallibility of fingerprint examiners was the removal of the concept of 'individualisation', identification to the exclusion of all others. This should have been the end of 'individualisation'[9]. To sustain that conclusion, the fingerprints of everyone who was alive at the time and who had ever lived would have had to have been examined and characterised!

The then chairman of the Scientific Working Group on Friction Ridge Analysis, Study and Technology (SWGFAST), a standard development organisation for fingerprint examination, issued a '*clarification*' asserting that the phrase '*to the exclusion of all others*' is likely to be removed from its Friction Ridge Examination Methodology materials (Mnookin et al. 2011).

However, despite these apparent concessions, the feature-comparison disciplines were defensive.

> *There is an extensive body of research, extending back over one hundred years, which establishes the accuracy, reliability, and validity of conclusions rendered in the field of firearm and toolmark identification.*
>
> *(Association of Firearm and Toolmark Examiners 2009)*

> *Study, research, and experimentation have led to and supported fingerprints as a means of individualization and a forensic tool of incalculable value. The research and practical knowledge accumulated over the course of many centuries well support the science*
>
> *(Barnes 2010)*

According to a memorandum from Robert J. Garrett, then president of the IAI, to members dated 19th of February 2009, perhaps pre-empting the publication of the NAS Report in August,

> *There is no research to suggest that properly trained and professionally guided examiners cannot reliably identify whole or partial fingerprint impressions to the person from whom they originated.*
>
> *(Mnookin et al. 2011)*

According to the Scientific Working Group for Firearms and Toolmarks (SWGGUN).

> *The reliability of the science has been demonstrated and supported through proficiency tests and validity studies over many decades.*
>
> *(SWGGUN 2010)*

The Forensic Science Community

Shortly after the publication, a major international conference was held in Glasgow, Scotland, of the European Academy of Forensic Science (EAFS); EAFS 2009, 8–11 September. Although it has the word European in the title, it is international in scope, both in terms of presenters and delegates.

At the conference, the NAS Report was the subject of some of the presentations. One given by Professor David H. Kaye, a leading figure, provided an excellent appraisal of the NAS Report with some interesting insights (Kaye 2010).

Regarding the establishment of a National Institute of Forensic Science (NIFS).

> *As lobbying from the Innocence Project (in favor of NIFS), the National Association of District Attorneys (against it), the American Society of Crime Laboratory Directors (against it), and other organizations continues, the prospects for a well funded, centralized forensic science agency to promote research and regulation seem remote.*

An accurately predicted outcome. Regarding the separation between law enforcement and forensic science provision.

> *The recommendation to move laboratories out from under the administrative control of police agencies also is unlikely to be widely adopted. The International Association of Chiefs of Police already is working to ensure that it never sees the light of day.*

Again, 100% correct and providing evidence that law enforcement agencies rarely, if ever, cede power.

Early US Government Responses

Given the scale of the recommendations, which would, if all were fully implemented, amount to a significant reshaping of the US's forensic science landscape, it took some time for responses to the recommendations to emerge. The early responses were, for the most part, a consideration of how the NAS Report's recommendations might be put into effect, generating further, perhaps more refined, recommendations.

Although supported by many practitioners and academics (Mnookin et al. 2011), the creation of a National Institute of Forensic Science was one of the first recommendations to fall by the wayside. It was probably the very fragmentation of the US justice system, law enforcement and forensic science provision identified in the NAS Report that prevented the creation of a new federal agency. Establishing such an agency would require funding and political will, buy-in and support from politicians across the political divide, which never materialised. Remember, this was just after the global financial crisis struck and the United States was engaged in conflicts in Afghanistan and Iraq. Perhaps vested interest also played a part? NIFS was never seen as a priority by the government, and there was certainly no public pressure to create such an agency.

It was decided that, in the absence of a new agency, existing federal agencies such as the National Institute of Standards and Technology (NIST) and the Department of Justice (DOJ)[10] would be effective in bringing about the reforms needed. As matters progressed, that indeed was the case, the DOJ and NIST jointly tackled the NAS Report's recommendations.

To put it simply, there was no government appetite for the creation of NIFS.

It should be noted that the initial view held internationally was that the NAS Report had exposed issues that were very much for the United States. However, as will be clear from this chapter and others, almost every conversation concerning the reform of forensic science begins with the NAS Report. On reflection, Europe, too, had similar challenges. While it was true that Europe (including the United Kingdom), Australia and New Zealand had introduced quality management systems that addressed and resolved many of the issues raised, there was still a need for reform. There remained one exceptional discipline: fingerprint examination, which is discussed at length in this chapter and mentioned in Chapter 4.

Subcommittee on Forensic Science (SoFS) (2009–2014)

The first response to the NAS Report by the federal government was the National Science & Technology Council (NSTC) forming a Subcommittee on Forensic Science (SoFS) almost immediately after the NAS Report was published. The SoFS report was published in 2014 and claimed to provide a framework for the future.

> [A] *detailed and comprehensive exploration of modern forensic science embarked on by this Subcommittee has broadened the breadth of foundational knowledge and situational awareness in the agencies, informing a meaningful framework for future analysis and coordination.*

The document took its title from the NAS Report 'Strengthening the Forensic Science'. It focused on four of the NAS Report's recommendations for forensic science[11].

- Accreditation of Forensic Science Providers
- Certification of Forensic Scientists
- Proficiency Testing of Forensic Scientists
- A National Code of Ethics for Forensic Science Providers (note – not for individuals)

The SoFS report provided much background information, an analysis of the current situation, described the challenges to implementation, and made some recommendations for further work, which were subsequently taken up by the National Commission of Forensic Sciences (NCFS), of which more later. The SoFS effectively pointed out the difficulties in implementation and handed the baton to the NCFS.

Four approaches to mandating accreditation were considered by SoFS. Of those, two were legislative, and a third was for the DOJ to mandate accreditation of its laboratories and offer incentives for other laboratories, with which it interacts, to do the same. The fourth was to take elements of each of the above, a hybrid approach. No recommendation was made, and no costings were estimated.

The certification of forensic scientists proved to be one of the most challenging as a result of the large number of disciplines and levels within each discipline, including managers, analysts and technicians. It concluded that congressional action might be needed to effect this recommendation. A very similar set of four approaches was suggested, two legislative, one DOJ-led enforcement and a fourth, some combination of the above.

The NAS Report's recommendation for a national code of ethics proved an easy win, as there was a suitable code already published by the Association of Crime Laboratory Directors/Laboratory Accreditation Board (ASCLD/LAB). As there were few cost implications, the SoFS had no hesitation in recommending the adoption of said code.

The report also includes various cost estimates for accreditation and certification, and a list of federal forensic science providers recording their accreditation status.

That report hands over to the NCFS in the following terms.

> *It is the expectation ... that the material collated here will prove useful to policy makers in government as well as forensic scientists, laboratory managers, and other practitioners working together to strengthen the forensic sciences – and to the recently created National Commission on Forensic Science, which is well positioned to consider these and other findings as it prepares to provide policy advice to the U.S. Attorney General.*

Expert Working Group on Human Factors in Latent Prints (2008–2012)

Although the work of this Expert Working Group (EWG) began before the publication of the NAS Report, its work partly overlapped that of the NAS Committee, and its report in 2012 drew significantly on the NAS Report, citing it around 40 times. The subject of the EWG report was the examination of fingerprints as a means of identification (Expert Working Group on Human Factors in Latent Print Analysis 2012).

Human factors include observer effects. As discussed in Chapter 8, those effects are the main result of cognitive biases. For this EWG, human factors also included fatigue and error, as in a mistake. In general terms, human factors might be thought of as any interaction between a forensic scientist and any other part of the forensic science process (ISO 2018), which includes analysis, interpretation and reporting, that might lead to misleading or erroneous evidence. However, in this book, the main human factor considered is cognitive bias.

As explained in Chapter 8, cognitive bias can result in poor decision-making, and to reduce the risk, it must actively be guarded against by shielding the examining scientist from potentially biasing information.

It should be explained that a latent print is the impression of a fingerprint left on the surface of an item. It is latent in the sense that it is invisible to the naked eye and needs to be developed by some means. Once 'visualised', it is in effect the questioned print.

The EWG was convened in December 2008 to conduct a scientific assessment of the effects of cognitive bias/human factors on fingerprint examination. The purpose being to better understand the role of human factors and thereby reduce errors, provide guidance to both practitioners and policymakers and make recommendations. Members of the EWG were broadly based and among the leading experts in their field.

The report is a scholarly, informative, richly detailed and referenced document. It is lengthy, the body of the report being 234 pages. The report makes a total of 34 recommendations. It should be acknowledged that those recommendations relating to the competence of the organisation, its policies and procedures, and the competence of the individual would be implemented by accreditation to and conformance with ISO/IEC 17025, the subject of Chapter 7. Indeed, many of the other recommendations would be covered by a requirement for accreditation to and conformance with ISO/IEC 17025. That leaves validation of methods. Although it is accepted that the steps followed by fingerprint examiners ACE V (Analysis, Comparison, Evaluation and Verification) are not a method, they do provide a framework for examining and assessing the validity of fingerprint examination, which is explored in detail in the EWG report.

Some important points that are revealed are the relationship between the size of a database and the chance of a coincidental 'match'. As the size of a database increases, so does the chance of a coincidental 'match' between a questioned print and one from the database, i.e. a false positive. Given the potential for cognitive bias to infect subsequent steps in the ACE V process, this risk should be recognised and reduced. However, it is hard to see how. The EWG recommends at 3.6.

> *... examiners must recognize the possibility and dangers of incidental similarity. Adjustments such as a higher decision threshold, stricter tolerances for differences in appearance, and explicit feature weighting need to be considered. Modifying quality assurance practices for this scenario also should be considered.*

The report repeats the mandate of the NAS Report regarding the conclusion that a single-source attribution, i.e. to the '*exclusion*' of all others, is not logical or based on science.

It should be noted that the NAS Report extended this prohibition to all feature-comparison disciplines.

The EWG report also proposes a research agenda to identify and develop performance metrics for fingerprint examinations.

It repeats the call in the NAS Report for the ability to exchange fingerprint data across internal borders between local, state and federal agencies, i.e. improve the interoperability of AFISs (Automated Fingerprint Identification Systems).

It specifies the contents of an examiner's report with the aim of transparency and comprehension by the fact-finder, as a non-specialist. Capturing and meeting stakeholder requirements and the contents of reports are requirements of both ISO/IEC 17025 and ISO/IEC 17020, 'Conformity assessment – Requirements for the operation of various types of bodies performing inspection'.[12]

The report repeated the NAS Report's recommendation that all practitioners should be certified as competent and all forensic science providers accredited.

Training, education, competency assessment, continuing professional development and fostering a culture of continuous improvement are very much a theme of the recommendations, all requirements of ISO/IEC 17025 and 17020.

It is the case that the Organisation of Scientific Area Committees for Forensic Science (OSAC) (discussed below), the agency charged with overseeing the development standards, has done little with the recommendations of the EWG in terms of turning them into a standards framework. Even if OSAC had developed standards, there is as yet no enforcement mechanism.

It is unclear what progress is being made to even standardise ACE V, which is highly variable, particularly in the verification phase (Doyle 2019). Drawing on the inquiry into the Brandon Mayfield case from the FBI and the Shirley McKie case for Scottish examiners, verification should be blind to the extent that the reviewing examiner is blind to the conclusion reached and the identity of the initial examiner (Office of the Inspector General 2006; Campbell 2011). In England and Wales, the Regulator's latest codes of practice, which now have statutory force, still permit non-blind verification with its risk of bias and categorical opinions, the most positive implying 'individualisation' (Forensic Science Regulator 2023). As explained in Chapter 6 on 'Interpreting Evidence', categorical opinions (yes/no/inconclusive) are, in logic, a form of posterior probability and therefore must be based on some undeclared prior, the province of the fact-finder or jury. Therefore, by reporting a categorical opinion, the fingerprint examiner usurps the role of the jury. The updating of existing beliefs in the light of new evidence (Bayes' Theorem) is explained in Chapter 6. Figure 9.1 reveals the undeclared prior. It does seem extraordinary that such poor practice is given statutory support.

National Commission on Forensic Science (NCFS 2013–2017)

The next response by the federal government to address the recommendations set out in the NAS Report was the establishment in 2013 of the National Commission on Forensic Science (NCFS) by the US Department of Justice (DOJ). Effectively continuing and building on the work of the Subcommittee on Forensic Science. One of the first acts of the Commission was the creation of 'guidance groups' collectively termed the Organization

Posterior probability	=	Likelihood ratio	x	Prior probability
New knowledge	=	Updating factor	x	Existing knowledge
It's a 'match'	=	?	x	?

Figure 9.1 The undeclared Prior.

of Scientific Area Committees [for Forensic Science] (OSAC). Like NAS, the Commission was established to produce recommendations. However, in this case, recommendations for consideration by the DOJ. It was a federal advisory committee for the DOJ and was initially established for two years to implement as many of the recommendations in the NAS Report as practicable, achievable and politically acceptable.

Its stated purpose was to generate '*non-binding*' recommendations to the Deputy Attorney General aimed at the DOJ agencies only. Therefore, the work of the Commission and any outputs would directly impact the DOJ and the work and practices of its law enforcement agencies, the Federal Bureau of Investigation (FBI), the Bureau of Alcohol, Tobacco, Firearms and Explosives (ATF) and the Drug Enforcement Agency (DEA). However, the OSAC would have greater reach. The Commission's first year's main output was OSAC's creation. Perhaps the major continuing practical impact of the NAS Report is OSAC and its standards-development task. OSAC is discussed next.

The NCFS was broadly based, aiming to cover all forensic science stakeholders, including state prosecutors, defence counsel, judges, and law enforcement agents.

It had three broad and ambitious objectives derived from the NAS Report's recommendations.

Foundational Issues Objective 1, '*strengthening the validity and reliability of forensic evidence*'.

- Strengthening the scientific basis and research standards for forensic science,
- assessing how forensic science is currently used and understood by the community, and
- understanding the community's potential to produce high-quality forensic evidence.

Operational Issues Objective 2, '*enhancing quality assurance and quality control in forensic science laboratories and units*'

- Implementing standards by encouraging[13] the accreditation of forensic science providers and the certification of practitioners;
- implementing quality-control mechanisms[14] to ensure reproducible forensic techniques are used; and
- creating a culture of learning from mistakes with a robust process (root cause analysis and continuous improvement).

Relational Issues Objective 3 for '*identifying and recommend*[ing] *scientific guidance and protocols for evidence seizure, testing, analysis, and reporting by forensic science laboratories and units*'

- Analyse how forensic science is understood and communicated to key stakeholders, including the victims of crime and the general public, and
- Address the language used within the forensic community and expert testimony to discuss forensic findings and recommend practices.

The Commission's charter was extended for another two years but not renewed in 2017 with a change in government. A decision probably made for political reasons, the Commission being a victim of the emerging post-truth society (O'Callaghan 2020). Concern was expressed at the time that 2017 might see the end of the reform period for forensic science in the United States, which began with the 2009 NAS Report (Cole 2018).

It is worth noting that according to Simon Cole, a leading figure.

> *The NCFS, as noted above, was the government's effort towards government regulation of forensic science. It was, of course, not the agency envisioned by the NRC* [NAS]*: it was not permanent, it had no enforcement authority, and it was controlled by law enforcement rather than independent entities. Despite all this,* ***it was the most ambitious effort at government regulation of forensic science in American history****.* [Emphasis added]
>
> *(Cole 2018)*

The Organisation of Scientific Area Committees for Forensic Science OSAC (2014–)

OSAC was initially conceived as a standards development organization (SDO), administered by the National Institute of Standards and Technology (NIST). Its main purposes were seen as standards development and establishing good practice. It was established in 2014 by the NCFS. OSAC was the result of a collaboration between NIST and the DOJ. That collaboration was formalized in a Memorandum of Understanding between the two agencies signed in February 2013 (NIST 2023).

OSAC's stated mission is as follows.

> *... to strengthen the nation's use of forensic science by facilitating the development of technically sound standards, expanding the OSAC Registry with standards that have completed a technical assessment, and promoting the implementation of those standards by OSAC's stakeholders and the forensic science community.*

Its mission was and remains to address a lack of discipline-specific standards; in that sense, its remit is narrow, with many of the NAS Report recommendations being contingent on establishing NIFS and lying beyond the requirement for standards. One of the main recommendations in the NAS Report was separating the functions of forensic science and law enforcement. The reforms now being administered by NIST and the DOJ contradict that recommendation. Others not addressed by NIST/DOJ were a call for more and better research with funding and targeted education programs.

The work of OSAC is really the management of the standards-development process. Its workflow is shown in Figure 9.2.

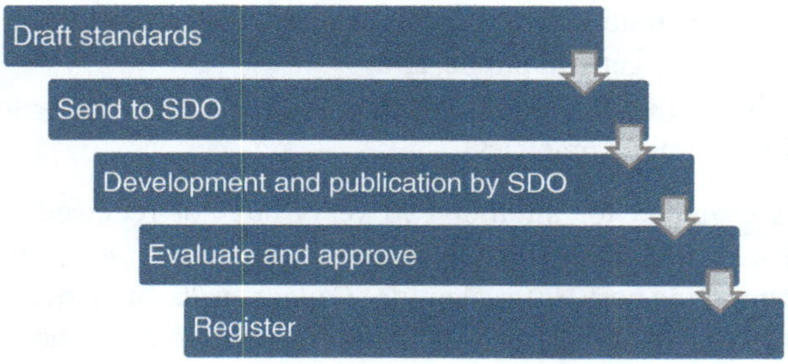

Figure 9.2 OSAC SDO workflow.

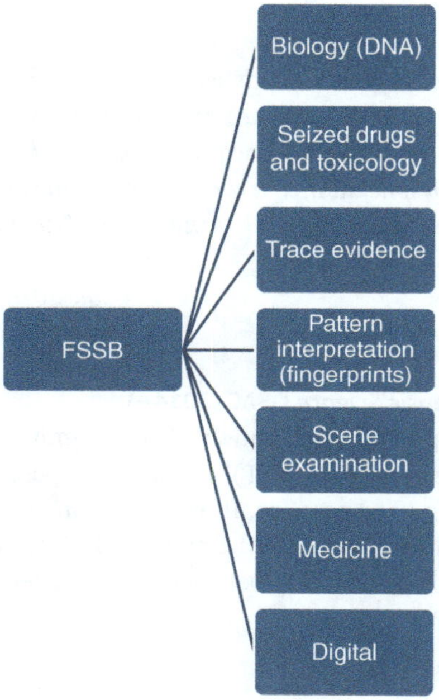

Figure 9.3 FSSB Scientific Area Committees.

OSAC currently comprises 7 Scientific Area Committees (SAC) covering 22 forensic disciplines overseen by the Forensic Science Standards Board (FSSB). The SACs are identified in Figure 9.3.

There is also a human factors committee looking at cognitive bias among other factors that might contribute to errors.

Although it was initially established as an SDO, it essentially farms that out to other organisations such as the American Academy of Forensic Sciences (AAFS) Standards Board (ASB) or adopts existing standards developed by ASTM International (Doyle 2019). So, it exercises a co-ordinating and managing role. Once consensus is reached among practitioners and law enforcement/state stakeholders, the standard is listed on the OSAC Registry, and conformance is encouraged but not mandated.

The relationship between the DOJ and NIST can be represented by the following diagram, Figure 9.4. The FBI retains responsibility for standards in DNA analysis.

OSAC is probably the only major legacy of the NAS Report; NIFS was not created, and the separation of law enforcement and forensic science was not implemented.

Lack of and a Need for a Research Culture

A multi-disciplinary group of leading figures stressed the need to develop a research culture in the '*non-DNA forensic sciences*'.

> *A research culture must be grounded in the values of empiricism, transparency, and a commitment to an ongoing critical perspective. The forensic science disciplines need to substantially increase their commitment to evidence from empirical research as the basis for their conclusions. Sound research, rather than experience, training, and long-standing use, must become the central method by which assertions are justified.*
>
> *(Mnookin et al. 2011)*

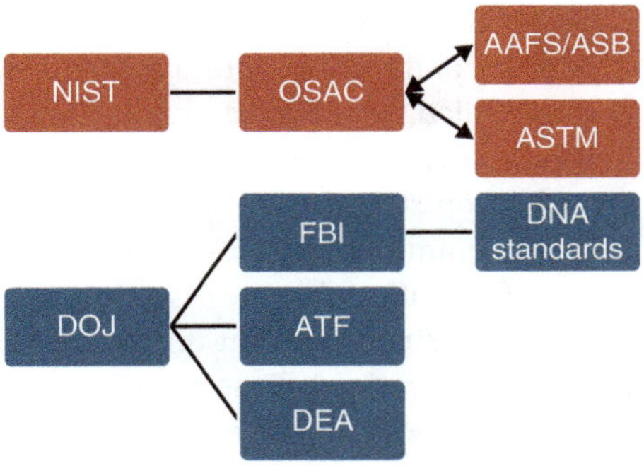

Figure 9.4 The relationship between NIST and the DOJ.

However, a commentary on that publication by Pierre Margot, then Director of the School of Forensic Science at the University of Lausanne, Switzerland, suggested, perhaps unfairly, that the solutions offered by Mnookin et al. might be self-serving. The paper echoes the need for forensic science to move from law enforcement to a scientific culture. A sound scientific structure should be given higher priority than standardisation. The paper recognises the tension between those who advocate the need for shielding the forensic scientist to reduce the risk of bias and the model of the forensic scientist as a researcher with access to all relevant information. While agreeing that a research culture is essential, its focus should be on forensic science questions, building and promoting a singular discipline as an equal of other scientific disciplines. To that end, he calls for the use of the singular as in 'forensic science' rather than the plural 'forensic sciences' (Margot 2011).

However, the authors of both papers agreed that the forensic science community itself should develop, foster and promote a research culture.

Litigation

In the wake of the NAS Report, there was a call for lawyers and judges to strengthen their approach to admissibility.

> *The order[15] provided that in the wake of the NAS Report, the admissibility of trace Evidence 'ought not to be presumed; that it has to be carefully examined in each case, and tested in the light of the NAS concerns, the concerns of Daubert/Kumho case law, and Rule 702 of the Federal Rules of Evidence'.*
>
> *The order also described the procedures governing such a challenge. But the order is not enough. Counsel have to learn that advocacy in cases involving forensic evidence requires familiarity with the kind of issues the NAS Report raised.*
>
> *(Nancy 2011)*

Bias

One immediate reaction was a paper by Michael Risinger (Risinger 2009), one of the authors of the publication, the subject of Chapter 8. Risinger felt that the NAS Report was a victory of sorts after a '*decades-long struggle*' for certain stakeholders to accept and admit the weaknesses in forensic science but regretted the lack of action on bias, the NAS Report calling for more research when Risinger thought none was needed.

The NAS Committee had missed an opportunity to argue for the immediate introduction of masking and sequential unmasking, essential bias-avoidance measures discussed in that chapter which, as recorded, was included in the code of practice of the Forensic Science Regulator in 2010 based on the work of Itiel Dror and colleagues which began in 2005 (Dror and Charlton 2006).

The recommendation in question was number five, calling for more research on the effects of cognitive bias.

Michael Risinger thought this referring of the effects of cognitive bias to more research was the '*worst failure*' of the NAS Report. Recalling that the Report was published in 2009, 'Observer Effects', the subject of Chapter 8, was published in 2002, and Dror's research was first published in 2006.

Impact Today

PCAST (President's Council of Advisors on Science and Technology)

With concern that insufficient progress had been made in the wake of the NAS Report particularly in terms of research to validate subjective feature-comparison methods, and with a change in government looming, with perhaps a different justice agenda (The American Congress of Forensic Science Laboratories 2016), the process of forensic science reform was given extra impetus by the publication in September 2016 of the PCAST Report.

A year earlier, the then US president, Barack Obama, directed the President's Council of Advisors on Science and Technology (PCAST) to address the following question: whether there were any additional '*steps*' beyond those already taken by the Administration in the aftermath of the NAS Report that could help ensure the validity of forensic evidence?

In its report, PCAST identified two requirements:

1. the need for clarity about standards for the validity and reliability of forensic methods in general, i.e. what those standards might be, and
2. the need to evaluate subjective feature-comparison methods to determine whether they have been 'scientifically' established to be valid and reliable.

From this point on, 'subjective feature-comparison' will be abbreviated to 'comparison' or 'comparative'.

PCAST conducted an extensive literature review and consulted representatives of most justice/forensic science stakeholders, including the FBI and NIST, together with a variety of experts.

The PCAST Report was titled 'Forensic Science in Criminal Courts: Ensuring Scientific Validity of Feature-Comparison Methods'. It was essentially a progress report but also highlighted where greater effort was needed, as PCAST saw it, to undertake the necessary research to validate comparison methods. The PCAST Report was strongly worded, perhaps thought necessary to drive home messages in less certain terms.

The PCAST report echoed many of the recommendations made in the NAS Report, such as the need for scientific research to support the claims made by examiners in comparison disciplines and to adopt suitable standards to monitor and improve performance.

In terms of validity, demonstrating the truth of opinions reported, the PCAST report highlighted two concepts: foundational validity of the methods used in those comparison disciplines and validity as used or applied.

Foundational validity was established by determining whether and to what degree a method could produce a reliable result, and validity as applied or used was determining whether and to what degree examiners could produce a reliable result.

Two requirements for foundational validity were as follows:

1. A method for identifying features in both the questioned and reference materials, comparison and, depending on the degree of resemblance found, whether the questioned material 'matched' the reference material. It should be noted that ACE V used by fingerprint examiners would not qualify as a method according to the PCAST criteria, see pages 48 and 49.
2. A number of independent studies were conducted to determine the false positive rate of the method, when examiners declared a 'match' when the questioned and reference materials were from different sources and the false negative rate, when an examiner declares a 'non-match' when in fact the questioned and reference materials have a common source. These rates would also yield true positive and negative rates. It is noteworthy that no mention is made of 'inconclusives'.

The requirement for 'validity as applied' was essentially a test of individual competence,[16]

> *...the examiner must have been shown to be capable of reliably applying the method and must actually have done so.* [emphasis added by PCAST, p56]

According to PCAST, the competence of an examiner is demonstrated through proficiency testing, tests aimed at evaluating and demonstrating competence. PCAST set out several requirements to ensure that the proficiency test was fit for purpose. While the requirements were optimal, they were also ambitious and perhaps idealistic.

PCAST also recommended that the examiner should report relevant statistics, false positive and negative rates and '*where applicable*' random match probability. It was perhaps this recommendation that drew the most ire from the champions of the likelihood ratio approach to evaluation, discussed in Chapter 6. Statistics such as the false positive rate are fundamentally different from the random match probability, which in most circumstances is merely the reciprocal of the likelihood ratio, i.e. $1/LR$. What is being mixed up here are what are known as frequentist and Bayesian statistics, and as the saying goes, 'never the twain shall meet'.

The report sparked much controversy with bodies representing the comparison disciplines forced to defend their discipline vigorously, to reduce the risk of comparison evidence being considered unreliable or even inadmissible.

There was a more nuanced controversy between those who might be described as empiricists, relying on data such as false positive and false negative rates, and those promoting the likelihood ratio approach to the interpretation of evidence.

In this regard, Ian Evett, a pioneering forensic statistician, and others reported the most critical response (Evett et al. 2017).

We suggest that the report has very little emphasis on positive steps and does much to reinforce poor thinking and terminology.

Perhaps the greatest weakness in the PCAST report was the notion that it was for the scientist to consider the probability of the proposition supporting guilt, or at least the probability of guilt given the evidence. The promotion of the prosecutor's fallacy or transposed conditional, discussed in Chapter 5 on logical fallacies.

However, following on from this logical fallacy is a more fundamental issue which comparison examiners have been getting away with forever is that by transposing the conditional and reporting the probability of (the proposition supporting) guilt they are usurping the role of the jury or fact-finder by assuming some undeclared prior probability, as discussed earlier and also in Chapter 6.

It is not for an examiner to report to the court that there is a 1% chance that when a 'match' is claimed, it is wrong, but the probability that the degree of resemblance observed between the questioned and reference material is greater if they are from the same source than not.

As discussed in Chapter 6, this likelihood ratio approach conforms to the principles of balance, considering alternative mutually exclusive propositions; logic, considering the probability of the evidence; transparency and hopefully robustness, in that there exists a body of knowledge supporting the assignment of a likelihood ratio.

The consensus today is that a probabilistic model, even in fingerprints, is to be preferred. Much research in this area has already been reported, with more to come with method development based on the following steps (Robertson et al. 2016).

- Choosing features
- Choosing how to compare them
- Calculating comparison scores based on data gained by experiment
- Assigning likelihood ratios

OSAC and Regulation

As of 2nd of July 2024, OSAC had published 137 standards, covering many aspects of forensic science management practice and delivery.

Regarding regulation, the makeup of SACs and FSSB was questioned by Simon Cole, a leading figure, who thought the balance and representation risked outcomes driven by self-interest. The issue was practitioners populating the SAC and scientists populating the FSSB. Regarding OSAC, he concludes with a series of questions.

Has NIST's OSAC assembled just the right mix of scientific firepower, practitioner buy-in, consumer pressure, government power, cultural change, and persuasive force to be the entity that finally reforms forensic science? We cannot yet know, but the task is daunting.

(Cole 2018)

Noting that OSAC registered standards were regarded by some as mere recommendations, presumably when the standard challenged the status quo, conformance requiring a revision of current practice, several roles for an OSAC 2.0 were floated. One suggestion was that OSAC prepare regulatory legislation requiring conformance with registered standards (NIST 2018). In 2019, OSAC put some meat on the bones of OSAC 2.0. The reforms in the end were quite limited and well short of a regulatory framework with legislative support. They were essentially to make the standards development process more efficient by combining discipline-specific subcommittees (reduced from 25 to 22) or making them smaller, asking for comments and conducting a technical review of standards earlier during the process, i.e. before being sent to an SDO (NIST 2021). There was no further discussion of introducing measures that might mandate conformance to OSAC's registered standards through, for example, legislation.

The United States, founded on free enterprise and low regulation, prefers its standards to be flexible and voluntary, relying on self-regulation for conformance. Therefore, it may be that the United States will never introduce legislation to mandate conformance.

However, there is one major exception, and that is, surprisingly, in DNA Analysis. The passing of the US DNA Identification Act in 1994 requires DNA analysis to meet certain specified standards to populate and interrogate national DNA databases. Again, DNA proves to be an exceptional discipline.

In addition, even if this *laissez-faire* approach is true, it is the case that most US forensic science laboratories, at the local, state and federal level, are now accredited, and a multitude of practitioners are certified, with the DOJ leading by example.

In contrast to the United States, Europe is culturally accepting of a more centralised and prescriptive regulatory approach to standards development and conformance. ISO is headquartered in Geneva, Switzerland, and EU member states are often bound by the same standard. Membership of the European Network of Forensic Science Institutes (ENFSI) requires conformance to international standards. In England & Wales, the Forensic Science Regulator has been given statutory power to enforce conformance (The Forensic Science Regulator Act 2021 (Commencement No. 2) Regulations 2023).

Miscarriages of Justice

In 2019, the Innocence Project hailed the impact of the NAS Report, which concluded that the report had led to changes in the criminal justice system and the 'exoneration' of the innocent (Innocence Project 2019).

According to the Innocence Project report, the NAS Report has resulted in innocent people having their convictions overturned, being freed from prison, and consequently, the people who committed the crimes have been identified.

Handwriting

The subjective feature-comparison discipline of handwriting examination has responded positively to the NAS Report and its call for standards and research to support the claims of this discipline. One of the outcomes was the 'modular' approach, adopting a likelihood ratio approach to evaluation developed by Bryan Found (1962–2016) and Carolyne Bird (Found and Bird 2016). This probabilistic approach, respecting the principles of balance, logic, transparency and robustness, might explain why handwriting was not mentioned in the PCAST report. That reform, a move towards research to provide a greater scientific basis and evaluative reporting based on a likelihood ratio approach, was very much led by Bryan Found, a pioneer of high standards and ethical forensic science (Bryan 2017).

Artificial Intelligence

There is no doubt that artificial intelligence (AI) will revolutionise the comparison disciplines, and even if the opinion before the court is that of a human being, the quality and reliability of that evidence will be significantly improved by AI's contribution, and justice will benefit.

Other Issues

Two major recommendations in the NAS Report have made little, if any, progress: the creation of a National Institute of Forensic Science and greater separation between law enforcement and forensic science provisions.

No NIFS

It was probably the very fragmentation of the US approach to justice, law enforcement and forensic science provision identified by the NAS Report that prevented the creation of a new federal agency. To establish such an agency would require funding and political will. NIFS was never seen as a priority. To put it simply, it was just too difficult.

It was thought that existing agencies such as NIST and the DOJ would be effective in bringing about the change needed rather than creating a new agency. And, as has been discussed earlier, the DOJ and NIST did take on some of the recommendations of the NAS Report. However, it is uncertain that his partnership will deliver the necessary reform in forensic science (Cole 2018).

No Independent Forensic Science

Considering the cognitive biases described in Chapter 8, in particular, confirmation bias and tunnel vision, first recorded by Hans Gross, the risk of infection with such biases must be greater in a law enforcement or prosecution environment than in a purely scientific environment. And with continuing miscarriages of justice, it seems surprising that forensic science in many territories and jurisdictions is still very much residing in a law enforcement environment. Indeed, in many jurisdictions, law enforcement effectively holds the purse strings of forensic science. There is an old saying he who pays the piper calls the tune. However, despite the risks and the importance of an independent body to oversee and regulate forensic science as recommended by the NAS Report, there seems to be little political will to disturb the status quo.

There is a false dichotomy between those who favour Bayesian inference, requiring case details and those concerned about the distorting effect of cognitive bias, which requires shielding the forensic scientist from much case detail. As explained in Chapter 8 and 10, this is managed through CAI and having both a coordinating scientist who can evaluate the scientific evidence in the context of the case and shield the examining scientist from potentially biasing information.

Contribution to Current Practice

One approach to evaluating the contribution to current practice by the NAS Report is to consider each recommendation.

Recommendation 1

The creation of a new federal agency, the National Institute of Forensic Science (NIFS), was not implemented. Although some agencies collaborated to progress some of the recommendations, most notably the creation of OSAC, administered by NIST and its coordination of standards development and its registry of consensus standards. Unfortunately, there is no mechanism for enforcing conformance with those standards.

While inside the United States, the creation of NIFS to implement some or all of the recommendations would have had a significant effect on the management, delivery and practice of forensic science, beyond its borders, the creation would have had little effect other than being a single point of contact for international collaboration. The national and international roles have effectively fallen to NIST.

Although not independent of law enforcement and not a regulatory or oversight body, Australia and New Zealand [oddly] have a 'National' Institute of Forensic Science.

In England and Wales, the Forensic Science Regulator exercises a regulatory and oversight role. The Regulator has recently been given statutory powers requiring specified forensic science activities to be accredited to ISO/IEC 17025 or 17020 (UK Government 2021). Forensic science providers in other parts of the United Kingdom have agreed to conform to the Regulator's many guidance documents.

Recommendation 2: Standardised Terminology and Reporting

As the NAS Report highlights, the variation in terminology is a major issue that has not yet been fully resolved. In the United States, OSAC, in following up on the NAS Report's recommendation, has produced its lexicon and preferred terms (OSAC 2024). In addition, ISO has a technical committee updating its standard for terms and definitions in forensic science, ISO 21043-1. OSAC's preferred terms reference ISO 21043-1. In the United Kingdom, the Regulator has produced guidance on terms and definitions (Forensic Science Regulator 2023). In contrast, ENFSI refers to ISO standards – but not yet ISO 21043 – and International Laboratory Accreditation Cooperation (ILAC) Guides. ENFSI also refers to the OSAC Lexicon. There is evidence of consensus emerging from this enormous international effort on many fronts. However, there seems to be silence on the troubling terms listed in the NAS Report: *'match', 'consistent with', 'identical', 'similar in all respects tested'*, and *'cannot be excluded'*. Perhaps silence should be interpreted as 'not approved for use'?

In 2016, the DOJ began drafting discipline-specific guidance on uniform language and reports. The guidance is regularly reviewed and updated if necessary (Office of Legal Policy US DOJ 2024). The guidance focuses on the conclusions that might be drawn in a particular discipline. These documents included some terms and definitions. Unfortunately, categorical opinions are promoted, and some of the troubling terms listed above are used.

Should these bodies not define the same terms in the same way, then this significant duplication of effort will have been in vain; the effort would be a setback for the standardisation of terminology. So, the NAS Report certainly identified an issue that has resulted in a significant amount of international effort.

On a separate note, the NCFS quickly recommended that use of the phrase '... *to a reasonable degree of scientific [or discipline] certainty*' should cease immediately, which was implemented by the DOJ (Weiss and Laporte 2018), which, in turn, bound its agencies, the FBI, ATF and DEA.

Turning now to standardised reports. As mentioned earlier, the EWG on fingerprints did document the requirements for a fingerprint expert's report. However, it seems that OSAC is yet to reach a consensus and register a standard to cover the contents of reports. Practice directions exist in E&W, New Zealand and Queensland, Australia. The ethical requirement is for complete transparency in demonstrating the quality and reliability of the scientific evidence.

Recommendation 3: More and Better Research

There has certainly been a significant increase in spending on forensic science research in the United States According to the Innocence Project, in the first decade, the US National Institute of Justice (NIJ) funded research recommended in the NAS Report to the tune of $123 million (Innocence Project 2019). For the fiscal year 2024, the NIJ has allocated a total of $12.5 million for research and development in forensic science, spread across approximately 30 awards (National Institute of Justice 2019, 2024).

Additionally, the Bureau of Justice Assistance (BJA) offers over $100 million in forensic science grant opportunities through programs such as the DNA Capacity Enhancement for Backlog Reduction (CEBR) Program, the Paul Coverdell Forensic Science Improvement Grants Program, and others aimed at improving forensic services and capacity (US Department of Justice 2022; Bureau of Justice Assistance 2023).

Forensic science researchers in Europe, including the United Kingdom, have access to the Horizon Europe program, which has an allocated budget for 2021 to 2027 of €95 billion (European Commission 2024).

In addition, there is the European Forensic Science Area 2030 initiative, which aims to enhance collaboration and development in forensic science across Europe. This initiative seeks to improve the quality and coordination of forensic activities, including leveraging new technologies, particularly AI, and data-sharing protocols (Silver 2022).

In Australia, the University of Queensland is leading collaborative projects funded by the Australian Research Council to the tune of $1.3 million (University of Queensland 2018).

This does not include the research conducted 'in-house' by forensic science laboratories.

So, there is certainly much more research being done, as for its quality, well, that assessment lies outside the scope of this book.

It should be noted that in terms of method development and validation there remains a tension between those advocating empirical testing, proficiency testing, and error rate analyses (Koehler et al. 2023) and those advocating a likelihood ratio approach by developing comparison methods based on choosing features, comparing the sets of features, calculating comparison scores for items from known sources and assigning likelihood ratios (Robertson et al. 2016).

Recommendation 4

Remove all public forensic laboratories and facilities from the administrative control of law enforcement agencies or prosecutors' offices.

This separation between law enforcement and forensic science provision in the United States was contingent on the creation of NIFS to drive the recommendation forward. In most jurisdictions, law enforcement agencies are reluctant to cede power and influence once obtained. Therefore, this recommendation faces an uphill struggle and may never come to fruition.

However, as argued earlier, the influence law enforcement has over forensic science introduces a fundamental weakness and risk to justice. Considering the cognitive biases described in Chapter 8, particularly confirmation bias and tunnel vision, first recorded by Hans Gross as introduced in Chapter 1, the risk of infection with such biases must be greater in a law enforcement or prosecution environment than in a purely scientific environment. And with continuing miscarriages of justice, it seems surprising that forensic science in many territories and jurisdictions is still very much residing and operating in a law enforcement environment.

Recommendation 5: More Research on Cognitive Bias

As Michael Risinger pointed out in his paper written almost immediately after the publication of the NAS Report, shielding examiners from potentially biasing information should have been mandated immediately (Risinger 2009). As reported in Chapter 8, awareness of the existence and risks of cognitive bias in forensic science was first raised in 2002, followed by groundbreaking research being conducted by Itiel Dror and colleagues (Dror and Charlton 2006).

However, despite a slow recognition, the risk of cognitive bias is widely recognised today, although bias avoidance measures such as linear sequential unmasking are yet to be universally adopted, for example, in fingerprint examination and the ACE V steps.

Recommendation 6: Development of Tools and Procedures

This was just a hotchpotch of requirements, such as method development and validation studies to facilitate accreditation. Ten US states have mandated accreditation, and around 88% of US forensic science laboratories are accredited (Zarwell et al. 2024). In Europe, Australia and New Zealand, most, if not all, are so accredited. Therefore, this recommendation has been implemented both within the United States and internationally.

Recommendation 7: Accreditation and Certification Mandated

As recorded above, most forensic science laboratories worldwide are now accredited to ISO/IEC 17025. Routine feedback from stakeholders as an instrument of continuous improvement is a requirement of that standard and others that might be adopted, such as ISO/IEC 17020 for inspection activities or ISO 9001 for quality management.

The implementation of the certification of individuals is well underway in the United States, but elsewhere, not so much. It should be noted that any laboratory accredited to ISO/IEC 17025 is effectively certifying its forensic scientists as competent; the weakness is the lack of independence.

The American Board of Criminalistics (ABC) offers examinations in a few disciplines, including 'General Criminalistics'. However, gaining certification seems to be a matter of personal choice. The ABC is accredited to the relevant ISO standard, ISO/IEC 17024 'Conformity assessment – General requirements for bodies operating certification of persons' (American Board of Criminalistics 2024). Again, in the United States, the Forensic Specialties Accreditation Board (FSAB) appears to cover those disciplines that lie outside the scope of the ASB scheme, such as toxicology and document examination. As with the ABC, speciality boards are accredited to ISO/IEC 17024 (Forensic Specialties Accreditation Board 2024). So, in terms of the independent assessment of the competence of an individual forensic scientist in conformance with an international standard, the United States has made far more progress than in other regions. For what it is worth, the United States should be commended for this progress.

In the United Kingdom, the Council for the Registration of Forensic Practitioners (CRFP) briefly appeared (1999–2009) as a body certifying the competence of individuals but failed financially (Doyle 2019).

Insofar as it can be determined, there is no requirement in any common law jurisdiction for forensic scientists to be independently certified as competent before being allowed to give expert testimony.[17] Some European countries operating the civil law system do maintain a register of recognised experts in certain disciplines, for example, the Netherlands Register of Experts (NRGD 2024).

Therefore, while near-universal accreditation is in place, mandatory certification, as a requirement to give expert testimony, seems a long way off and perhaps will never be implemented. In the meantime, as an assurance of individual competence, outside the United States, accreditation to ISO/IEC 17025 will have to suffice, despite the lack of independence.

Recommendation 8: Quality Control, Assurance and Improvement

This recommendation is met through accreditation to ISO/IEC 17025. It should be noted that proficiency tests are a requirement of the standard, and such tests are now part of standard practice.

Recommendation 9: Code of Ethics

As the NAS Report records, several US professional bodies have codes of ethics (however named). Today, most, if not all, professional bodies in most jurisdictions have a code of ethics/practice/behaviour in place, which binds the membership. As recognised earlier in this Chapter, the issues are enforcement and sanction. One means of policing conformance is to include a code in the documented quality management system accredited to ISO/IEC 17025 or 17020. By this measure, the code may be enforced and policed.

As recorded earlier in this chapter, in the United Kingdom, the Regulator has published a code which has statutory support (Forensic Science Regulator 2023).

Many jurisdictions specify legal requirements for expert witnesses and their evidence (Doyle 2019).

Recommendation 10: Education and Training

There has been a significant increase in the number of undergraduate and postgraduate courses in forensic science and related fields. The amount spent on research is set out earlier under Recommendation 3. In many universities, research underpins training and education. Forensic science seems to have been a very popular subject.

One serious issue needs to be highlighted regarding current practice, which can only be remedied by effective training. That is the error of transposing the conditional or the prosecutor's fallacy, discussed at length in Chapters 5 and 6. Despite the consequences of the fallacy and the need to be logically precise when adopting a likelihood ratio approach to interpretation, there is much evidence, both anecdotal and published, that forensic scientists giving expert testimony are transposing the conditional, thereby misleading the court (Koehler et al. 2023). This is a serious training and education issue that needs to be resolved.

In terms of improving the awareness and knowledge of forensic science among lawyers and the judiciary, the picture is patchy. Guides for the judiciary have been produced in the United States and the United Kingdom (National Research Council 2011; The Royal Society 2017). However, lawyers litigating criminal cases may have little contact with forensic science during their career, and so it is a poor investment in time to acquire sufficient knowledge of forensic science. The easiest remedy is for lawyers to confer with scientists at an early stage of proceedings. Lack of knowledge and awareness of forensic science is not an issue in civil law jurisdictions, such as those of continental Europe, as investigations are led by the judiciary, who have experts on tap to advise and guide the investigation and participate in any subsequent legal proceedings.

It is interesting to note that 'Interpreting Evidence' (Chapter 6) is co-authored by a lawyer, and lawyers are among the target audience.

I think it is fair to state that there are many educational and training materials available to judges and lawyers if they wish to get a better grip on forensic science and its role in delivering justice.

Recommendation 12: AFIS interoperability

This is an entirely US Issue.

Fingerprints

There has been much research and other academic activity to move fingerprint examiners from reporting categorical opinions of 'match', non-match and inconclusive to probabilistic opinions based on a likelihood ratio approach. Some continental European examiners have begun to report probabilistically[18], but many in other jurisdictions do not. In addition to the risk of usurping the jury and misleading the court by assuming some unreported prior in arriving at a categorical opinion, there is much useful evidence lost in the discarded 'inconclusive'.

Interestingly, the PCAST report likened the subjective elements in fingerprint examination to those of other comparison tasks such as art authentication. Determining the artist of a painting of uncertain provenance, like fingerprint examination, involves expert judgement and relies on the examiner's experience, expertise and ability to recognise and interpret features. However, the process is inherently subjective.

It seems extraordinary that despite the weakness highlighted in the NAS Report, all the subsequent scholarship, casework failures and the risk of miscarriages of justice, non-blind verification, and categorical reporting are given statutory support by the Forensic Science Regulator of England & Wales (Forensic Science Regulator 2023).

The contents of an examiner's reports were detailed in the EWG report referred to earlier. (Expert Working Group on Human Factors in Latent Print Analysis 2012).

Concluding Remarks

The assembly of the multi-disciplinary committee that produced the 2009 NAS Report was probably the first coming together of most forensic science stakeholders; scientists, lawyers and policymakers in the United States who found a surprising degree of consensus regarding the challenges facing forensic science. It allowed them to determine the strengths and weaknesses in forensic science and suggest a path to reform. It gave the NAS Committee a powerful and authoritative voice.

While the 2009 NAS Report was certainly a milestone or watershed and set an agenda for reform, it essentially captured criticisms of forensic science that had been bubbling under for many years and voiced by many parties. Unsurprisingly, responses to the Report were mixed. Comparison disciplines rushed to defence, concerned that the Report might undermine the credibility of those evidence types; academia welcomed the call for more and better research, and lawyers for greater judicial scrutiny. It certainly increased awareness of the issues and facilitated dialogue between stakeholders.

Overall, the 2009 NAS Report promoted reform, calling for a more robust scientific foundation and the generation of scientific evidence of greater quality and reliability to better serve the criminal justice system.

It also created a NAS Report 'industry', almost two decades later, it remains part of the reform conversation (De Kinder and Pirée 2020).

The outcomes were a bit of a mixed bag. The NAS Report certainly generated a lot of scholarship, reports, papers and conference presentations and is still widely cited today in calls for reform. However, while it did catalogue the problems, it often failed to provide practical solutions. The main recommendation for a National Institute of Forensic Science did not and has not come to fruition, and moving forensic science from a law enforcement environment to one of science seems a long way off, despite the risks to justice. In some jurisdictions, such as England & Wales, the trend is in the opposite direction (Jhalani et al. 2024), putting justice further at risk.

On the positive side, the standardisation of methods and practices with the creation of and continuing work of OSAC is a success, although fingerprint examination remains resistant to change at a fundamental level. Most laboratories in the United States are accredited, and the certification of individuals has made significant progress there. The DOJ agencies publish their quality management systems in the public domain. In addition, research training and education have benefited, and the position has improved.

To a degree, it added to and reinforced the developmental agenda of Paul Kirk recorded in his Ontogeny paper, the subject of Chapter 3. However, the questions of what constitutes forensic science and whether it is a profession remain contested. Perhaps the colloquialism 'you know it when you see it' might apply. For the non-specialist reader, science at the service of justice, or the use of science to help resolve legal disputes, would probably suffice as definitions. These issues are developed in the next chapter.

Key Takeaways

Publication of the NAS Report in 2009 was a watershed moment in the history of forensic science. The report presented a detailed picture of forensic science in the United States.

It was prompted by miscarriages of justice and set an agenda for the reform of forensic science in the United States. It has also been the starting point for many conversations about, and initiatives for reform in, the management, practice and delivery of forensic science in many other jurisdictions. It is still being cited today.

The NAS Report highlighted the need to determine the limitations and scientific validity of many feature-comparison methods, some of which, such as fingerprint examination, had never been challenged and, on examination, fell short of the standard set by DNA analysis. The report called for research to study and establish the scientific foundations and limitations of these comparison methods.

By exposing weaknesses in feature-comparison disciplines, it contributed to overturning wrongful convictions.

In terms of standardisation, the establishment of the Organization of Scientific Area Committees for Forensic Science (OSAC), administered by the National Institute of Standards and Technology (NIST), was an important initiative following the NAS Report's recommendations. OSAC continues to manage the development and promotion of consensus standards to improve the quality and reliability of scientific evidence. It is of note that the European Network of Forensic Science Institutes (ENFSI) in its best practice manuals references standards registered by OSAC.

Two of its most impactful recommendations were not implemented: the establishment of a US National Institute of Forensic Science (NIFS) – #1 and the separation between law enforcement and forensic science provision – #4. Regarding #1, much of the heavy lifting has been provided by NIST. Regarding #4, no progress has been made, putting justice at risk.

The report has been criticised for being somewhat self-serving and not mandating existing bias avoidance measures.

Notes

1 The nucleus of cells is the usual source of DNA for testing. An alternative source is the mitochondria, a component of a cell that provides the energy needed by the cell to function. Nuclear DNA is from mum and dad, while mitochondrial DNA is from mum only.
2 The Innocence Project continues to rely on DNA evidence to challenge convictions supported by feature-comparison evidence.
3 Like 'forensic science' this is broadly defined.
4 The basics of DNA analysis are: sampling, clean-up, quantitation, amplification, analysis and interpretation, see Chapter 4.
5 This is a particular danger with DNA evidence. The DNA of the accused is found at the crime scene. This is technically source-level evidence, which says nothing about the activity that led to the accused's DNA being at the scene. Depending on the case circumstance, there may be more than one 'innocent' explanation for the presence of that DNA. However, in the absence of expert evidence, lawyers might incorrectly interpret the finding of the accused's DNA at the scene as strong evidence of guilt and pressure the accused into a guilty plea. This is an example of the Prosecutor's Fallacy, the subject of Chapter 5.
6 The word 'science' is emphasised in the text with no explanation as to what is meant by the term in this context.
7 At the time of the report, there were many such discipline-specific groups such as SWGDAM, the Scientific Working Group on DNA Analysis Methods.
8 Any probabilistic conclusion would be deemed 'conduct unbecoming ...'.
9 Some fingerprint examiners still use the term 'individualisation' but claim that 'to the exclusion of all others' is not what is meant! (Cole 2014). One wonders what the fact-finder understands by the term?
10 It is important to note that the FBI, ATF and DEA are federal law enforcement agencies and part of the DOJ.
11 There was also consideration of the certification of medicolegal experts but that is outside the scope of this book.
12 A standard applicable to crime scene activities.
13 Note the softening, the NAS Report recommended mandatory accreditation and certification.
14 Again, a low bar, QC is essentially inspection and a responsive mode. QA will provide some assurance but what is required is a quality management system and a culture of continuous improvement.
15 Procedural Order: Trace Evidence at 3, No. 1:08-cr-10104-NG (D. Mass. 8 March 2010).
16 Although by PCAST's definition, it was not competence. However, a discussion on this nuanced distinction is beyond the scope of this book. In this book, ISO's definition is used: 'The ability to apply knowledge and skills to achieve intended results'. ISO9000:2015 3 October 2014.
17 As explained earlier, an ISO/IEC 17025 accredited laboratory is effectively certifying its scientists as competent; however, that process lacks independence.
18 At the world-leading forensic science laboratory, the Netherlands Forensic Institute (NFI) fingerprint examiners are reporting conclusions probabilistically (Forensic Science Regulator 2022).

Bibliography

AAFS. 2009. "Position Statement Response to the National Academy of Sciences' 'Forensic Needs' Report." *AAFS*. 4 September. Accessed July 20, 2024. https://www.aafs.org/article/response-national-academy-sciences-forensic-needs-report.

American Board of Criminalistics. 2024. *American Board of Criminalistics*. Accessed July 18, 2024. https://www.criminalistics.com/.

Association of Firearm and Toolmark Examiners. 2009. "The Response of the Association of Firearm and Toolmark Examiners to the February 2009 National Academy of Science Report 'Strengthening Forensic Science in the United States: A Path Forward'." *ATFE Journal* 41: 204–05.

Baker, Tim. 2024. "Post Office Scandal: £1bn Set Aside to Fund Compensation for Victims – as Govt Vows to Pursue Fujitsu if Fault Found." *Sky News*, 11 January.

Barnes, Jeffery G. 2010. "History." In *The Fingerprint Sourcebook*, edited by Alan McRoberts, 1–17. Washington, DC: National Institute of Justice (US).

Brown University. 2017. "Gatsonis, Constantine." *Resesarch@Brown*. Accessed July 26, 2024. https://vivo.brown.edu/display/cgatsoni#:~:text=Constantine%20Gatsonis%2C%20PhD%2C%20Henry%20Ledyard,Dr.

Bryan, Vale. 2017. "Bryan Found 1962–2016." *Australian Journal of Forensic Sciences* 49 (4): 361–65.

Bureau of Justice Assistance. 2023. "Paul Coverdell Forensic Science Improvement Grants Program." *Bureau of Justice Assistance*. 31 October. Accessed July 18, 2024. https://bja.ojp.gov/program/coverdell/overview.

Caddy, Brian, Graham R. Taylor, and Adrian M.T. Linacre. 2008. *A Review of the Science of Low Template DNA Analysis*. Scientific Review, London: Home Office.

Campbell, Anthony. 2011. *The Fingerprint Inquiry Report*. Inquiry Report, Edinburgh: APS Group.

Cole, Simon A. 2014. "Individualization is Dead, Long Live Individualization! Reforms of Reporting Practices for Fingerprint Analysis in the United States." *Law, Probability and Risk* 13 (2): 117–50.

Cole, Simon A. 2018. "Who Will Regulate American Forensic Science?" *Seton Hall Law Review* 48: 563–81.

De Kinder, Jan and Hugo Pirée. 2020. "The Future of the Forensic Science Providers – Time to Re-think Our Structures?" *Forensic Science International* 316: 1–9.

Doyle, Sean. 2019a. "A Forensic Science Regulator in England and Wales and a Forensic Science Advisory Council." In *Quality Management in Forensic Science*, edited by Sean Doyle, 168–71. London: Academic Press.

Doyle, Sean. 2019b. "Fingerprint Examination." In *Quality Management in Forensic Science*, edited by Sean Doyle, 259–60. London: Elsevier.

Doyle, Sean. 2019c. "Level 3 Standards Development Organizations (SDO)." In *Quality Management in Forensic Science*, edited by Sean Doyle, 31–32. London: Academic Press.

Doyle, Sean. 2019d. "Responses, A United Kingdom Register." In *Quality Management in Forensic Science*, edited by Sean Doyle, 164–167. London: Academic Press.

Doyle, Sean. 2019e. "Standards Applying to the Legal Process." In *Quality Management in Forensic Science*, edited by Sean Doyle, 142–147. London: Academic Press.

Dror, Itiel and David Charlton. 2006. "Why Experts Make Errors." *Journal of Forensic Identification* 56 (4): 600–16.

European Commission. 2024. "Horizon Europe (HORIZON)." *EU F&T Portal*. Accessed July 18, 2024. https://ec.europa.eu/info/funding-tenders/opportunities/portal/screen/programmes/horizon.

Evett, Ian W.V., Charles E.H. Berger, J S Buckleton, Christophe Champod, and Graham Jackson. 2017. "Finding the Way Forward for Forensic Science in the US – A Commentary on the PCAST Report." *Forensic Science International* 278: 16–23.

Expert Working Group on Human Factors in Latent Print Analysis. 2012. *Latent Print Examination and Human Factors: Improving the Practice through a Systems Approach*. Report, US Department of Commerce, National Institute of Science and Technology.

FBI. 2015. "FBI Testimony on Microscopic Hair Analysis Contained Errors in at Least 90 Percent of Cases in Ongoing Review." *FBI*. 20 April. Accessed July 22, 2024. https://www.fbi.gov/news/press-releases/fbi-testimony-on-microscopic-hair-analysis-contained-errors-in-at-least-90-percent-of-cases-in-ongoing-review.

Forensic Science Regulator. 2017. "Codes of Practice and Conduct Friction Ridge Detail (Fingerprint) Comparison." *Forensic Science Regulator*. Accessed July 2024. https://assets.publishing.service.gov.uk/media/64269cba2fa848000cec1096/FSR-C-128__Issue3-archived.pdf.

Forensic Science Regulator. 2022. "FGSSG Fingerprint Interpretation Workshop – Summary." *Forensic Science Regulator*. Accessed July 10, 2024. https://assets.publishing.service.gov.uk/media/61faa3c5e90e0768a5adf2ab/FQSSG_write_up.pdf.

Forensic Science Regulator. 2023. "Code of Practice." *Forensic Science Regulator*. March. Accessed July 17, 2024. https://assets.publishing.service.gov.uk/media/64da431cc8dee4000d7f1c1e/FINAL_2023.1.18_Code_of_Practice.pdf.

Forensic Specialties Accreditation Board. 2024. *Conformity Assessment*. Accessed July 18, 2024. https://thefsab.org/cabs/.

Found, Bryan and Caroline Bird. 2016. "The Modular Forensic Handwriting Method." *Journal of Forensic Document Examination. Special Issue* (Association of Forensic Document Examiners) 26: 7–83.

Hsu, Spencer S. 2017. "Sessions Orders Justice Dept. To End Forensic Science Commission." *The Washington Post*, 10 April.

Innocence Project. 2019. "Ten Years Later: The Lasting Impact of the 2009 NAS Report." *Innocence Project*. 2 February. Accessed July 22, 2024. https://innocenceproject.org/lasting-impact-of-2009-nas-report/.

International Association for Identification. 2010. "IAI Resolution 201–18." *Onin*. 16 July. Accessed July 4, 2024. https://onin.com/fp/IAI_resolution_2010-18.pdf.

ISO. 2018. "ISO 21043-1:2018 Forensic Sciences Terms and Definitions." ISO.

Jhalani, Shrey, Ruth M. Morgan, Amelia Shooter, and John Cassella. 2024. "UK Parliamentary Inquiry Reports in Forensic Science – Plus ça change?" *Forensic Science International: Synergy* 9: 1–13.

Kaye, David H. 2010. "The Good, the Bad, the Ugly: The NAS Report on Strengthening Forensic Science in America." *Science and Justice* 50: 8–11.

Koehler, Jonathan J., Jennifer L. Mnookin, and Michael J. Saks. 2023. "The Scientific Reinvention of Forensic Science." *PNAS: Perspective* 120 (41): 1–10.

Margot, Pierre. 2011. "Commentary on the Need for a Research Culture in the Forensic Sciences." *UCLA Law Review* 58: 795–801.

Mnookin, Jennifer L., Simon A. Cole, Itiel E. Dror, Barry A.J. Fisher, Max Houck, Keith Inman, David H. Kaye, et al. 2011. *The Need for a Research Culture in the Forensic Sciences*. Research Paper, Penn State Law, The Dickenson School of Law.

Nancy, Gertner (Judge). 2011. "Commentary on the Need for a Research Culture in the Forensic Sciences." *UCLA Law Review* 58: 789–93.

National Academy of Sciences. 2009. "Strengthening Forensic Science in the United States: A Path Forward." *Office of Justice Programs*. August. Accessed June 27, 2024. https://www.ojp.gov/pdffiles1/nij/grants/228091.pdf.

National Institute of Justice. 2024. "Funding and Awards." *NIJ National Institute of Justice*. 29 March. Accessed July 18, 2024. https://nij.ojp.gov/funding/opportunities/o-nij-2024-171962.

National Institute of Justice. 2019. "Forensic Sciences." *NIJ National Institute of Justice*. 21 October. Accessed July 18, 2024. https://nij.ojp.gov/topics/forensics/forensic-science-research-and-development.

National Research Council. 2011. *Reference Manual on Scientific Evidence: Third Edition*. Washington, DC: The National Academies Press.

NIST. 2018. "Potential Concepts for OSAC 2.0." *The Organization of Scientific Area Committees for Forensic Science*. 27 July. Accessed July 24, 2024. committees. https://www.nist.gov/topics/organization-scientific-area-committees-forensic-science/potential-concepts-osac-20.

NIST. 2021. "OSAC 2.0: Updating Structure and Streamlining Processes." *NIST*. 22 January. Accessed July 24, 2024. https://www.nist.gov/news-events/news/2019/09/osac-20-updating-structure-and-streamlining-processes.

NIST. 2023. "OSAC About Us." *NIST*. 27 December. Accessed July 4, 2024. https://www.nist.gov/organization-scientific-area-committees-forensic-science/about-us.

NRGD. 2024. *NRGD*. Accessed July 18, 2024. https://english.nrgd.nl/.

NYU School of Law. 2024. "Harry T Edwards Professor of Law." *NYU Law*. Accessed July 26, 2024. https://its.law.nyu.edu/facultyprofiles/index.cfm?fuseaction=profile.biography&personid=19895.

O'Callaghan, Cian. 2020. "Postpolitics and Post-Truth." In *International Encyclopedia of Human Geography (Second Edition)*, edited by Audrey Kobayashi, 339–45. Elsevier.

Office of Legal Policy US DOJ. 2024. "Uniform Language for Testimony and Reports." *Justice*. 6 March. Accessed July 25, 2024. https://www.justice.gov/olp/uniform-language-testimony-and-reports.

Office of the Inspector General. 2006. "A Review of the FBI's Handling of the Brandon Mayfield Case." *US DOJ*. March. Accessed July 12, 2024. https://oig.justice.gov/sites/default/files/archive/special/s0601/final.pdf.

OSAC. 2024. "OSAC Lexicon." *NIST OSAC*. Accessed July 17, 2024. https://www.nist.gov/glossary/osac-lexicon.

R v Hoey. 2007. 49 (NICC, 20 December).

Risinger, Michael D. 2009. "The NAS/NRC Report on Forensic Science: A Glass Nine-Tenths Full (This Is About the Other Tenth)." *Jurimetrics* 50 (1): 21–34.

Roberts, Paul. 1996. "What Price a Free Market in Forensic Science Services?" *British Journal of Criminology* 36 (1): 37–60.

Robertson, Bernard, George A. Vignaux and Charles E.H. Berger. 2016. "Forensic Science Methodology." In *Interpreting Evidence: Evaluating Forensic Science in the Court Room, Second Edition*, 85–98. Chichester: John Wiley & Sons, Ltd.

Silver,, Andrew. 2022. "EU Plans European Forensic Science Area 2030." *Research Professional News*. 17 October. Accessed July 18, 2024. https://www.researchprofessionalnews.com/rr-news-europe-innovation-2022-10-eu-plans-european-forensic-science-area-2030/.

SWGGUN. 2010. "SWGGUN Systemic Requirements/Recommendations for the Forensic Firearm and Toolmark Laboratory." *SWGGUN*. 23 April. Accessed July 21, 2024. https://www.nist.gov/system/files/documents/2016/11/28/swggun_systemic_report.pdf.

The American Congress of Forensic Science Laboratories. 2016. "Position Statement The 2016 PCAST Report." *Crime Scene Investigator*. 21 September. Accessed July 9, 2024. https://www.crime-scene-investigator.net/PDF/american-congress-of-forensic-science-laboratories-response-to-forensic-science-in-federal-criminal-courts-ensuring-scientific-validity-of-pattern-comparison-metho.pdf.

The Innocence Project. 2023. *The Innocence Project*. Accessed October 19, 2023. https://innocenceproject.org/.

The Royal Society. 2017. "Forensic DNA Analysis: A Primer for Courts." *The Royal Society*. November. Accessed July 23, 2024. https://royalsociety.org/-/media/about-us/programmes/science-and-law/royal-society-forensic-dna-analysis-primer-for-courts.pdf.

UK Government. 2021. "Forensic Science Regulator Act 2021." *Legislation*. Accessed July 25, 2024. https://www.legislation.gov.uk/ukpga/2021/14/contents.

Ulery, Bradford T., Austin R. Hicklin, JoAnn Buscaglia, and Maria Antonia Roberts. 2011. "Accuracy and Reliability of Forensic Latent Fingerprint Decisions." *Proceedings of the National Academy of Sciences* 108 (19): 7733–38.

University of Queensland. 2018. "Funding to Create Forensic Expertise." *UQ News*. 15 June. Accessed July 18, 2024. https://www.uq.edu.au/news/article/2018/06/funding-create-forensic-expertise#:~:text=A%20group%20of%20universities%20and,agencies%20interpret%20crime%20scene%20evidence.

US Department of Justice. 2022. "Forensic Grant Opportunities." *Office of Justice Programs*. 24 February. Accessed July 18, 2024. https://www.ojp.gov/events/forensic-grant-opportunities.

Weiss, Danielle and Gerald Laporte. 2018. "Uncertainty Ahead: A Shift in How Federal Scientific Experts Can Testify." *NIJ Journal* (279): 1–8.

Willis, Nick. 2021. *The Great Post Office Scandal: The Fight to Expose a Multimillion Pound IT Disaster Which Put Innocent People in Jail*. Bath: Bath Publishing.

Zarwell, Lucas, John Grassel, and Maya Metni Pilkington. 2024. "Police Crime Lab Accreditation Initiative." *Police Chief Online*, 31 January.

10

The Sydney Declaration

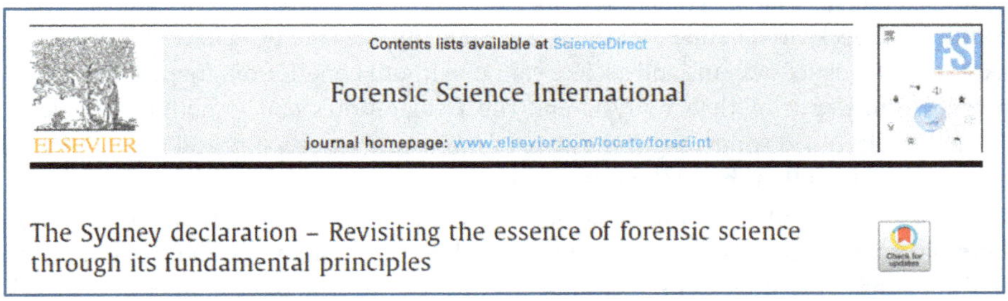
Contents lists available at ScienceDirect

Forensic Science International

journal homepage: www.elsevier.com/locate/forsciint

ELSEVIER

The Sydney declaration – Revisiting the essence of forensic science through its fundamental principles

Image 10.1 Publication header.

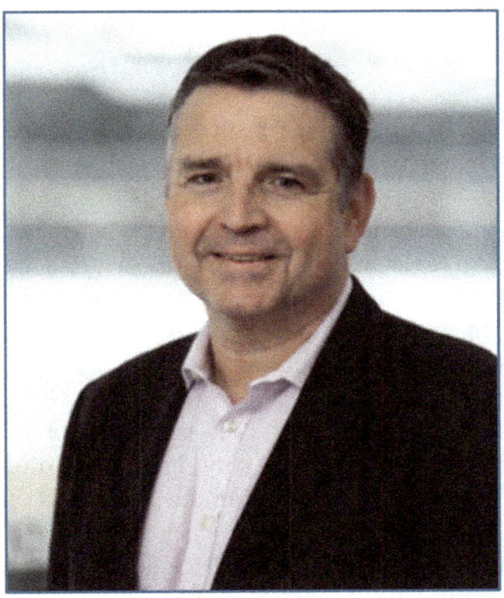

Image 10.2 Claude Roux. Courtesy of Claude Roux.

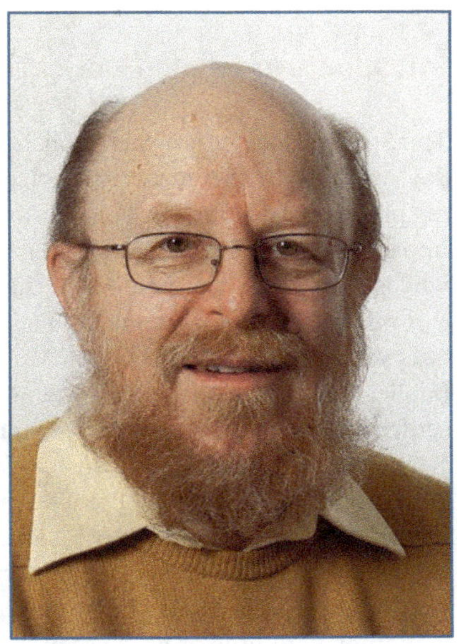

Image 10.3 Pierre Margot. The Double Loop Podcast.

A History of Forensic Science in 10 Publications: How They Established Current Practice, First Edition.
Sean Doyle.

Name of Publication

The publication is titled *The Sydney Declaration – Revisiting the essence of forensic science through its fundamental principles.*

Introduction to the Chapter

The Declaration is the tenth and final publication in the series that contributes to the current practice discussed in this book.

The publication is primarily an analysis of the current state of forensic science as understood by the authors. It seeks to redefine forensic science and affirms core principles that should be adopted to ensure justice systems and society gain maximum benefit from forensic science.

The scope and depth of that analysis and the Declaration's call to action provide an opportunity to discuss at some length the state of forensic science today and potential ways forward, which, given that this is the final publication, seems entirely reasonable.

The publication also promotes forensic science as the science of the trace or traceology and therefore completes a historical arc commenced by Hans Gross and the early pioneers. It, therefore, provides an opportunity to draw together several strands or themes of the book.

For the reasons given above, this chapter is structured somewhat differently from the others in the book.

Introduction to the Publication

The Sydney Declaration was published in 2022. In historical terms, that was only 'yesterday' and far from the 'historical horizon'. That horizon is usually reached when all the leading players have left the stage, so to speak, enabling a detached and objective assessment of impact to be made. So, if it is so recent and its impact on forensic science is yet to be known, why is the publication included in this book? An explanation is required.

It might or might not come as a surprise to the general reader of this history that there is as yet no consensus as to what forensic science actually is (Fraser 2020). Including this publication allows further consideration of this fundamental question, but perhaps not a settlement. The authors of the Declaration present a definition.

One characterisation of forensic science is that it is a collection of disparate disciplines with different principles, approaches and methods, but all with the lofty aim of supporting the law and helping to deliver justice. This is the picture presented in the 2009 NAS (US National Academy of Sciences) Report, the subject of Chapter 9, a fragmented and somewhat disconnected model; fingerprint examiners doing it one way and DNA analysts doing it another, with little or no sense of joint enterprise. The 'it' being 'forensic science'.

The authors of the Declaration seek to advance the counterargument that forensic science is, in fact, one discipline, a science bound by fundamental principles addressing one object: traces resulting from an event under investigation. The purpose of the Declaration is to define forensic science as the science of the 'trace' or traceology and document its underlying principles.

In making the argument that forensic science is a unified discipline, the Declaration draws on much of the history recorded in this book. This includes the forensic criminology[1] of Hans Gross (1847–1915) in Chapter 1, who, instead of identifying the criminal through physical characteristics, used science to detect crime and link the criminal to the crime. The forensic exploitation of dust, a multi-component trace, by Edmond Locard (1877–1966) and his oft-cited but wrongly attributed exchange principle, usually expressed as 'every contact leaves a trace', discussed in Chapter 2. Thirdly, the call for progress on the (unspecified) fundamentals of forensic science and establishing a profession by Paul Kirk in his Ontogeny paper, the subject of Chapter 3.

Therefore, in addition to facilitating further consideration of what forensic science is and what it does, the inclusion of the Declaration also provides an opportunity to reflect on the contributions of Gross, Locard, Kirk and other pioneers from a twenty-first-century perspective.

It should be noted in passing that it is a testimony to the greatness of these early pioneers that their work still has relevance today, over a century later.

This publication, in addition to outlining a possible future for forensic science, also allows for an assessment of the current state of the field. It revisits important issues raised in the book and facilitates consideration of the potential future developments.

Many of the authors are either academics at or have a close association with the École des Sciences Criminelle (ESC) at the University of Lausanne, Switzerland. What is now titled the ESC was established in 1909 by the criminologist Rodolphe Archibald Reiss (1875–1929). As discussed in Chapters 1 and 2, under an earlier title, the ESC is credited with offering the world's first academic training in forensic science, and it and its alumni laid the foundations upon which the Declaration rests. Therefore, Lausanne has an important role in the history and development of forensic science. Including the Declaration in this book will enable some of that history to be recorded and explored.

From a historical perspective, the Sydney Declaration is the latest stage in a concerted campaign led by academics associated with the University of Lausanne, advancing the unifying notion that forensic science is the science of the trace, or traceology; a notion borrowed from history and archaeology. The trace is defined as follows.

> *... the surviving evidence of a former occurrence or action of some event or agent ...*
>
> *(Roux et al. 2015)*

The trace may be thought of as the neutral carrier and transmitter of information; traces available in the present enable the reconstruction of past events. In the context of a criminal investigation, that information can, for example:

- provide leads,
- eliminate and identify suspects,
- reconstruct events and their sequence,
- reveal offences, and
- link crimes.

Examples of traces are fingerprints, fibres, hair, fragments of glass and paint, soil, dust and gunshot residues.

The authors of the Declaration contend that by adopting their definition of forensic science, several benefits follow. In addition to being a unifying concept, it is argued that by their definition, forensic science might have a wider or increased utility in providing forensic intelligence. In addition to its usual role in investigating crime and prosecuting criminals, the provision of forensic intelligence might also contribute to more effective policing, public safety and crime prevention/reduction. Traceologists could also collaborate with criminologists in the broader study of crime for the benefit of society.

Contexts

Historical

The concept of forensic science as the science of the trace can be traced (pun intended) back to Hans Gross and his Handbook, the subject of Chapter 1, which Edmond Locard acknowledges in his treatise on dust (Locard 1929).

> *However, the first author who clearly described cases where this research* [studying dust for the purpose of criminological evidence] *has been made is Hans Gross.*

In this paper, Locard goes on to state.

> *One can hardly speak highly enough of the worth of this magistrate; he was one of the initiators of criminology; and he envisaged not merely a particular phase of the science but its broadest aspects.*
>
> *It is indeed surprising, when reading his volume* [the Handbook] *today to discover that in spite of the progress that has since been made in this field, the ideas, or at least the germ of them, were already found in Gross' works.*

It would be wrong not to also acknowledge the contribution to the origin of traceology to the author Arthur Conan Doyle (1859–1930) and his fictional character Sherlock Holmes. Holmes's ability to solve crimes using abductive and deductive reasoning, proposing explanations and drawing conclusions based on the detection and observation of the merest traces that might be overlooked by others and his almost encyclopaedic knowledge certainly inspired Locard.

It could be argued that this desire to be the scientific generalist, leading and directing the investigation of crime, is borne of a desire to emulate that fictional character. Indeed, Locard was known as the 'French Sherlock Holmes', and Reiss was described by Locard, his friend and colleague, as follows.

> '*... Sherlock Holmes more precisely realised ...*' and '*... had ... the spirit of Sherlock Holmes*'
>
> *(Girod-Frais and Kappler 2022).*

It is interesting to note that there were other 'Sherlocks'. As recorded later in this chapter, Luke May (1892–1965) was 'America's ...' and in Africa, Alfred Lucas[2] (1867–1945), Director of the Government Chemical Laboratory in Cairo, was 'Egypt's ...' (Adams 2016).

Although there seems to be nothing to link Conan Doyle and Hans Gross, perhaps the swirl of ideas highlighted in Chapter 1, of the power of science as demonstrated by Darwin's theory of evolution (1859), which must have influenced Gross, also inspired Conan Doyle. Indeed, Conan Doyle's novel *'The Lost World'*, published in 1912, includes encounters with *'ape-men'; Homo erectus* perhaps, a species of hominid discovered in 1891.

As recorded above, the origins of traceology as a means of reconstructing past events can be linked to Gross, Locard, Reiss and other late nineteenth and early twentieth-century criminologists practising in continental Europe where civil law applied. However, its modern 'father' is Pierre Margot, emeritus professor and former director of the École des Sciences Criminelle (ESC) at the University of Lausanne, a successor of Reiss's Institut de Police Scientifique, founded in 1909.

Margot called for forensic science to be considered a unified body of knowledge in his response to the 2009 NAS Report (Margot 2011a), which was the subject of Chapter 9. At about the same time, he also called for forensic science to be defined as the science of the 'trace', or traceology (Margot 2011b).

In a private communication, Professor Margot reports that the concept of the trace was first included in his teaching at the University of Lausanne in the late 1980s and early 1990s. In 1995, he proposed to the European Network of Forensic Science Institutes (ENFSI) the creation of the European Academy of Forensic Sciences (EAFS) with the idea of focusing on fundamental issues of transfer, persistence and interpretation. Unfortunately, in his view, EAFS was created in 1997 with the silos of 'specialist working groups' in place, effectively focusing on the tools rather than common fundamental issues, on procedures rather than principles.

Following his lead, other similarly minded academics, many former doctoral students of Margot at Lausanne, collaborated in the development and refinement of the arguments advocating for traceology. This process has culminated in the Declaration, the publication of which was perhaps driven by a sense of frustration at the lack of progress towards the model of forensic science advocated for. The consensus among traceologists is that there has been too much focus on the standardisation of methods and practices of individual disciplines, accreditation of forensic science providers and the certification of practitioners as recommended in the 2009 NAS Report. This was at the expense of defining and advancing fundamental principles. In addition, this focus on discipline standardisation further entrenched the fragmentation of forensic science, contrary to a more collaborative, interdisciplinary and inclusive model promoted by the authors of the Declaration.

Science

Echoing Paul Kirk's Ontogeny paper (Chapter 2), the authors of the Declaration, citing the influence of the 2009 NAS report and later PCAST (President's Council of Advisors on Science and Technology) reports (PCAST 2016), both discussed in Chapter 9, contend that the resulting emphasis on quality in forensic science has been misplaced. The organisational/technological framework driven by quality management has not advanced the fundamentals and has therefore contributed to the silos in which the disciplines sink ever more deeply, focusing on the tools rather than the common issues such as transfer, persistence and interpretation.

As recorded in Chapter 9, the US Organization of Scientific Area Committees (OSAC) currently recognises 22 separate forensic science disciplines. The European Network of Forensic Institutes (ENFSI) has 17 discipline-specific Expert Working Groups (ENFSI 2020), and Australia and New Zealand have 13 Specialist Advisory Groups (ANZPAA/NIFS n.d.): further evidence, if any were needed, of the fragmentary condition of forensic science.

The fragmentary nature of forensic science, the resulting reduction in utility and the consequent need to establish forensic science as a single discipline had been recognised many years earlier by, for example, Peter De Forest (De Forest 1998) and the 1995 proposal by Margot to establish EAFS as a body to bridge specialisms.

The authors of the Declaration argue that adopting their definition of forensic science, as the science of the trace, could overcome the fragmentary and disparate nature of forensic science and bring all disciplines under one umbrella with a cohesive set of fundamental principles, as specified in the publication. It should be noted, however, that some of those principles are already in effect, as evidenced in several chapters in this book; for example, the importance of context and the need for logical reasoning in the interpretation of scientific evidence, see Chapter 6 on interpretation.

There is no denying the drift towards greater specialisation and fragmentation, which takes the forensic scientist further and further away from the scene and the trace. All can agree that scientific input at the scene is vital. Mistakes made at the scene, such as overlooking probative evidence, are very hard to rectify later in the forensic science process and may deny investigators and the justice system inculpatory or exculpatory evidence and, as a result, risk a miscarriage of justice (Doyle and Doyle 2011). The question is, how the science is to be delivered at the scene? In many common law jurisdictions, such as those in the United States and Australia, law enforcement or police investigators lead the scene investigation and are responsible for reconstruction, relying on specialist advice and guidance from scientists (and others) who are experts in particular disciplines. However, there is the odd exception where a scientist attends a scene as a matter of routine. One example is ESR in New Zealand (ESR 2024); there may be others[3].

Nevertheless, in common with many authorities, including Gross and the 2009 NAS Report, the Declaration defines crime scene investigation as essentially a scientific endeavour based on the scientific method.

Therefore, in addition to arguing for this universal basis for forensic science being the science of the trace, and affirming a set of fundamental principles, the authors of the Declaration also argue for a generalist role in the scientific investigation of crime scenes – essentially that a scientist should always be at the scene to direct and maximise its scientific exploitation, ensuring that everything that can be gleaned from the scene, is. The purpose is to reveal the history of the scene or the story of the crime – a role exercised by Gross and Locard and defined by Paul Kirk in his textbook 'Criminal Investigation' (Kirk 1953).

The authors strongly argue that the fragmentation of forensic science and increased specialisation has weakened the role of the forensic scientist by encouraging a retreat into the laboratory and an absence from the scene, a trend, they argue, that should be reversed.

The Declaration records another benefit of a scientist being at the scene, and that is the timely sharing of information, which may be relevant in the case of a series of crimes or the investigation of organised crime.

As mentioned earlier, the authors promote expanding the scope of forensic science beyond solving crime to include the support of proactive policing models. Forensic intelligence would contribute to crime prevention and reduction measures, public safety and security. This would be achieved by generating new information, collating it with existing information and exchanging it to better exploit it in identifying trends and patterns, revealing links between crimes and enhancing public safety. In simple terms, in addition to helping to solve crime, forensic science should be used to support more effective policing and identify preventative actions.

Echoing the 2009 NAS Report, the authors of the Declaration call for the development of a scientific research culture, but not as envisaged by NAS. The authors request co-operation between academia and operational forensic science providers to share information to support more effective policing. This is in contrast with the current position where research is focused on particular disciplines, emerging technologies, improving existing technologies and methods and not on the fundamentals.

Terms and Definitions

The Origins of 'Criminology' and 'Criminalistics'

Although there is a section of this book devoted to terms, definitions and explanations, a slight digression to consider more broadly the origin and meaning of some important terms might be of interest to the reader and assist in a broader awareness of terminological issues. Unfortunately, because of the semantic and terminological ambiguity that plagues forensic science, discussed in Chapters 1 and 2 and mentioned throughout this book, it will not bring the clarity some might hope for. Beginning with Hans Gross, most academics would agree that he was a criminologist (Turvey and Petherick 2009; Bachhiesl 2020). Founding the Kriminologisches Universitätsinstitut (Institute of Criminology) at Graz in 1912, Gross studied the entire spectrum of crime, including predisposing/motivating factors, behaviours, crime scene investigation and punishment, together with the broader criminal justice system and its impacts on society at large, see Figure 10.1.

Gross Model of Criminology

Figure 10.1 might help to get a fuller understanding of what Hans Gross considered the 'science' of criminology and the place of forensic science.

Figure 10.1 is part of the branches of criminology according to Gross, page xxvii from the 1904 German edition.

Note to Figure 10.1. Phenomenology is the study of crime, focusing on how it is experienced by those involved or affected by it.

This is only part of Gross's scheme. However, it makes clear that his understanding of criminology was very broad in scope and included all aspects of crime. In addition, what might be thought of as forensic science is in fact a subdiscipline of criminology.

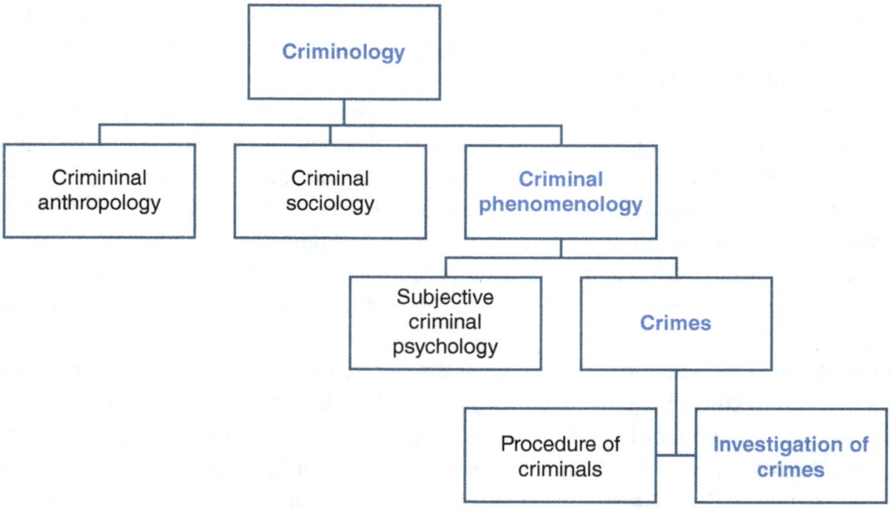

Figure 10.1 Part of the Gross model of criminology.

Criminalistics

Recalling Chapter 1 on the Handbook, it is important to note that the subtitle 'as a system of criminalistics' [as translated] was not part of the original title of the Handbook. While 'as a system for investigating crime' might be a more accurate translation of '*als system der Kriministik*', it seems clear that for Hans Gross, 'Kriminalistiks' was either synonymous with criminology or at least a major part of it. The use of the term 'criminalistics' to mean something that might commonly be understood as 'forensic science' began and has mostly remained in the United States. There are a few strands to the story.

According to Lowell Bradford, as recorded in his paper regarding the origins of the California Association of Criminalists (CAC), which he co-founded in 1954 (Bradford 2007), when he joined the California State Crime Laboratory in 1947, the terms 'criminalistics' and 'criminalist' were not in use. In those days, employees in the state crime lab had the title 'criminologist'. According to Bradford, it was the publication in 1949 of '*An Introduction to Criminalistics*' that first introduced the term 'criminalistics'. Bradford mistakenly names the author as James P. Osterburg. That publication was in fact jointly authored by James W. Osterberg and Chris E. O'Hara and had the defining subtitle '*The Application of the Physical Sciences to the Detection of Crime*' (O'Hara and Osterburg 1949). That book distinguishes criminalistics, '*the science which applies the physical sciences to the investigation of crimes*' from criminology (page x). What may be of significance is that a review of that book reports that this '... *new definition ... provides a word comparable to Kriminalistik ... found in common use in continental Europe*' (Perkins 1950). This may provide the origin of the word 'criminalistics' in the United States, borrowed from the title of Gross's Handbook. The '*Introduction to Criminalistics*' was followed by the publication in 1953 of '*Crime Investigation*' by Paul L. Kirk, the book is subtitled '*Physical Evidence and the Police Laboratory*' (Kirk 1953)[4]. It is noteworthy that in his book, Kirk argues that the criminalist should be a generalist lest some evidence is overlooked, missing the wood for the trees, as might be the case if a specialist is called to the scene. This is a fair point as, for example, a blood stain pattern analyst may not recognise other types of evidence; a point echoed in the Sydney Declaration and the dangers of missing vital clues at the scene highlighted earlier. Kirk argues strongly for a generalist at the scene. For Kirk, the criminalist is *'first and foremost an expert in identification and comparison'*.

Kirk also identifies a limiting factor. In the United States, with its plethora of local 'police labs' or 'crime labs', there would be insufficient resources to support a specialist in multiple disciplines. This can also apply to other territories. However, this does present a risk to justice in that, in the common law system, the status and field of the expert witness are very much part of the evidence, giving it weight. The evidence of a full-time specialist may well be preferred to that of the generalist. This risk has been reduced in common law jurisdictions as the multi-faceted role of the generalist, as exemplified by Gross, is undertaken by different parties, particularly the investigating officer of the police or law enforcement agency (Adam 2016). However, as has been discussed in Chapter 6 and will be further explored in this chapter, there are practical solutions and models of forensic science provision whereby both the scientific generalist and specialist can have a role. In addition, as mentioned earlier, the authors of the Declaration argue strongly that the 'science of the trace' has applications beyond the courtroom, that is, in providing intelligence in support of proactive policing.

Returning to the origins of criminalistics. There is another US strand, Luke S. May (1892–1965), 'America's Sherlock Holmes' (Beck 1992). May published perhaps the first forensic science textbook in the United States, *'Crime's Nemesis'* (May 1936). It was published in 1936 and therefore predates the US publications referred to above. However, concerning terminology, May styles himself a criminologist and president of The Institute of Scientific Criminology. He does not consider himself a criminalist.

Although there appears to be no direct link, many scholars accept that the term 'criminalistics' in English was borrowed in the late 1940s from the work of Hans Gross specifically to distinguish the field from criminology. Criminology today is broadly defined and includes the study of all aspects of crime; its causes, the behaviour and motives of criminals, the scientific methods of their identification, apprehension and prosecution and the broader societal impacts. In contrast, criminalistics, certainly in the United States, became defined as the scientific examination and interpretation of physical evidence with a reliance on the natural sciences, physics, biology, chemistry etc. The purpose is to distinguish those relying on hard science from those relying on medicine.

In Chapter 2, the term 'criminalistique' appears to refer to the scientific investigation of crime.

As will become clear, the boundaries between all the elements of criminology, including forensic science, remain blurred.

Summary of the Publication

Introduction and Definition of Forensic Science

Firstly, it is worth stating that forensic science, however defined, is one of, if not the, most philosophised of subjects. This is because of a lack of consensus on what it is beyond something like 'science in support of the law and justice'. Academic forensic scientists strive to determine what it is they are studying and teaching. This latest attempt, the Sydney Declaration, is perhaps the most intellectually rigorous and certainly the most cohesive attempt to define forensic science. It certainly provides a robust theoretical framework. Whether the fundamental principles of the Declaration (beyond those already adopted) are broadly accepted and can find application in real-world operational forensic science, particularly in common law jurisdictions, is a matter of wait-and-see. Can the theory be turned into practice?

As stated earlier, the Declaration represents the latest stage in a concerted campaign led by a group of academics associated with the University of Lausanne and initiated in 2011 by Professor Pierre Margot (Margot 2011a)[5]. Their purpose is to (re)define forensic science as the science of the trace. For the record, the *'simple definition'* offered is as follows.

> *Forensic science is a case-based (or multi case-based) research-oriented, science-based endeavour to study traces – the remnants of past activities (such as an individual's presence and actions) – through their detection, recognition, recovery, examination and interpretation to understand anomalous events of public interest (e.g., crimes, security incidents).*

The authors argue that the trace is that which links, at the most fundamental level, the fragmentary and disparate disciplines that constitute what is considered to be forensic science.

Four Principles Governing Forensic Scientific Evidence

Buried in what is an extremely dense and wordy text are the important principles of balance, logic, transparency and robustness discussed in Chapter 6.

- Balance – considering alternative propositions; in criminal matters, one supporting the prosecution and the other the defence, but the requirement for the alternatives to be mutually exclusive is omitted.
- Logic – assessing the probability of the evidence, or in this case, the trace, and not the probability of the proposition.
- Transparency – clearly documenting and reporting all the information necessary for demonstrating how the opinion or conclusion was arrived at, including any weaknesses or qualifications.
- Robustness – the opinion/conclusion is based on sound science, research and data.

Case Assessment and Interpretation (CAI), mentioned in Chapter 6 and explained in Chapter 8, is not mentioned in the Declaration, but an earlier paper in the campaign does include it in a proposed model for forensic science (Crispino et al. 2011). This is the model presented in Chapter 6 and the model for forensic science provision presented later in this chapter.

The Seven Principles

The authors of the Declaration specify seven principles that they claim provide a common or unifying framework for the definition of forensic science as the science of the trace. Briefly, these principles are:

1. The trace can provide evidence of source and activity.
2. Crime scene investigation is a scientific activity/endeavour requiring input from a scientific generalist.
3. Forensic science is based on '*scientific knowledge, investigative methodology and logical reasoning*'.
4. The time and distance of the forensic scientist from the crime scene degrades the information the trace might provide.
5. More research is needed to better understand the uncertainties associated with interpretation and communication, e.g. the transfer and persistence of the trace, false positives and negatives.
6. Forensic science isn't just about solving crimes; it also aids proactive policing, reduces and prevents crime, identifies trends, and links crimes through intelligence.
7. Context is vital to interpretation. Therefore, forensic scientists must be impartial and independent to reduce the risk of contextual information-biased outcomes.

Interestingly, the Declaration includes a 'should' and a 'must', terms usually associated with quality standards such as ISO/IEC17025, discussed in Chapter 7. The definition of forensic science given in the Declaration and the seven principles **should** underpin the practice of forensic science. In addition, science **must** be [emphasis added] ...

> *... acknowledged and advocated as the foundation of forensic science and agreement reached on the fundamentality of the 'trace'.*

Summary of Claimed Benefits

In summary, then, traceology will ...

> *... (1) shed light on past events, (2) monitor criminality/security issues and (3) prevent future harms.*
>
> *(Roux et al. 2021)*

Next Steps

The Declaration details the next steps to be taken. They should be *'aspirational'*, the aspiration being a *'globally shared understanding of forensic science and its principles*', as prescribed by the Declaration. These principles should, in turn, be the basis for education, training, research and the provision of forensic science. Furthermore, in contrast with what the authors of the Declaration characterise as a *'technological'* culture, they wish to promote a forensic science culture based on purpose rather than means, as discussed later under motivation, and educate forensic scientists as generalist scientists rather than technicians! That issue will also be discussed later in the Chapter.

The Declaration is in tension between a belief by the authors in the compelling nature of their argument and a realisation that giving practical effect to this 'universal' declaration may be an uphill struggle, particularly in common law jurisdictions. Nevertheless, the Declaration's call to action may be summarised in the following diagram, Figure 10.2.

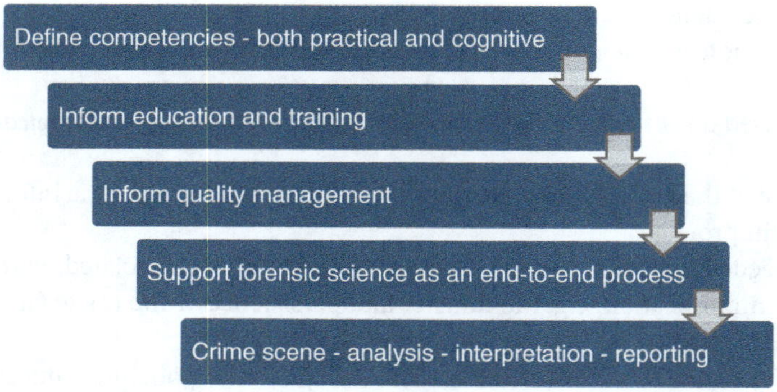

Figure 10.2 The declaration's call to action.

Locard's Traces and Traceology

To get a more practical and broader understanding of the trace and traceology, it might be helpful to return to a source. Unlike the authors of the Declaration, who classify as anything small (microscopic, gunshot residues) or large (a *'megalith'*, a big rock!) when Edmond Locard uses the word trace, he does mean something small; his focus is on the evidential value of dust, a multi-component trace.

Locations for the recovery of dust include clothing, skin, hair, nails (a particularly rich source), ears (the wax being a retentive medium), nostrils, weapons and vehicles. The list of potential components of dust seems endless. Components that might be associated with particular trades or occupations are listed, which are mainly inorganic chemical compounds.

In addition, organic or biological potential components include animal debris, microbes, ova and larvae, feathers, dried blood, dandruff, fish scales, connective tissue, fats, gelatine, muscle fibres, bone, faeces etc.

In terms of identifying the components of dust, Locard provides details of chemical tests for the microscopic amounts of this huge range of substances and materials. Again, the scale and depth of the knowledge held by Locard, as recorded in his publications, are astonishing and on a similar scale to that of Hans Gross.

The following quote reveals Locard's support for traceology, the superiority of the trace as a vestige of a past event over fingerprint evidence of identity. Traceology is not about identity but reconstructing past events (Roux et al. 2015).

> *Fingerprints are wonderful. I would say (...) it is privileged evidence.*
>
> *But, beyond, one can find prints of a variety of species: tooth print, nails, traces from the entire body, hair, dusts. Dust analysis is an infinite, unlimited resource. One can exactly know what the man did.*

Motivation for Writing

The Lausanne School of Thought

As recorded earlier, the University of Lausanne Institute of Police Science was established in 1909 by Rodolphe Archibald Reiss (1875–1929). For a short time, Reiss was a student of Alphonse Bertillon (1835–1914), discussed in Chapter 2, and a friend and colleague of Locard. He was a criminologist like Gross and Locard, but in addition to supporting the justice system, he also prioritised protecting public safety (Girod-Frais and Kappler 2022). Accepting that 'police science' is synonymous with what is commonly understood to be forensic science today, then Lausanne, from the outset, has seen forensic science as having a broader application than just solving crime. According to the Lausanne school, forensic science should also support crime reduction, prevention and enhance public safety. These objectives are very much echoed in the Declaration.

The Institute of Police Science is now titled the School of the Criminal Sciences or École des Sciences Criminelles (ESC), and the subject of research and education remains broadly criminological, an interdisciplinary approach to the study of crime combining science and the law (UNIL University of Lausanne n.d.).

One premise of the authors of the Declaration is that forensic science, as currently practised and as characterised by the 2009 NAS Report, both in its diagnosis and proposed remedies, has isolated forensic science from its broader criminological heritage as practised by Gross and Locard and indeed Kirk (Crispino et al. 2011). As a result, and as mentioned earlier, the current model of forensic science does not fully exploit the value of the trace, particularly in terms of contributing to intelligence and therefore public safety and security.

Lausanne seeks to define forensic science as follows.

> *Forensic science is then, foremost, an interdisciplinary endeavor ... to find out valuable information that may help identify a source or an activity described by their traces (remnants of a presence or an activity).*
>
> *(Crispino et al. 2011)*

Its aim is for forensic science to claim a scientific status in its own right.

Progress has been Misfocussed – One Science to Bind Them All

Echoing the Ontogeny paper, the authors claim that progress has been focused on discipline-specific technology and methods and not on fundamentals. As such, forensic science has been losing status. Accepting forensic science as the science of the trace and adopting the seven principles would realise the Lausanne vision.

> *... of forensic science as a distinctive academic and holistic research-based discipline.*
>
> *(Roux 2018).*

The authors of the Declaration claim that, unlike other more established bodies of scientific knowledge, such as the natural sciences, a shared understanding and broad acceptance of the essence of forensic science, its purpose, and fundamental principles are still misrepresented. This foundation has been overlooked, although recognised by many forensic science pioneers, such as Gross and Locard, and seen as critical to the advancement of forensic science. The Declaration asserts the need for a common understanding of what forensic science is, and it sets out a vision for a unified body of knowledge, forensic science as one discipline.

The Declaration is also borne of a frustration that the disparate disciplines of forensic science seem to be sinking deeper into their silos driven by the requirements of quality management, which is based on methods, or standard operating procedures, and organisations such that forensic scientists become no more than overqualified technicians. A near-contemporary paper by traceologists argues that the focus of forensic science should shift from *'means'* to *'purpose'*. Examples of the purposes are listed.

> *... reconstructing, monitoring and preventing crime and security issues.*
>
> *(Roux et al. 2021)*

The model of forensic science presented by the authors of the Declaration is very much the Lausanne model of a coherent and cohesive unified science based on the 'trace' and being criminological in scope. Whether this will supplant the current fragmentary model of a patchwork of disparate disciplines, we will have to wait and see.

Strengths/Weaknesses/Obstacles/Threats

Strengths

The obvious strength is a unified model of forensic science based on the trace, traceology, applying to all disciplines from fingerprints to DNA analysis and is trans-jurisdictional; it is independent of local political and legal systems that vary, and it works anywhere. According to the Declaration, traceology is described as follows.

> ... [the] *fundamental foundation on which forensic science is built.*

Criticisms and Weaknesses

Comparison with Kirk and the Call for Simplicity

Among the topics discussed in Kirk's Ontogeny paper, the subject of Chapter 3, was the need for fundamental principles, the qualifying elements of a profession and the qualifying aspects of a science.

In his paper, Kirk advances the argument that all sciences are based on simple principles. He then gives examples, for instance, Isaac Newton's laws of motion, such as $F = m \times a$, the laws of thermodynamics and Albert Einstein's equation relating matter and energy $E = m \times c^2$ [6]. All these basic laws are, according to Kirk, *'simple, brief and to the point'* [7].

In his paper, Kirk then goes on to state the following.

> *The true architects of science have always penetrated the superficial to reach the basic design which they could express in brief but truly fundamental terms.*

Kirk's fundamental description of forensic science was the *'science of individualisation'*. As we have learnt throughout this book, individualisation, attributing one source to the exclusion of all others, is an unachievable aim, the pursuit of which has been a barrier to the progress desired by Kirk. However, that definition was *'simple, brief and to the point'*. It could hardly be said that the Declaration meets those criteria. It is an extremely wordy and information-dense document that is at times hard to digest, even for the specialist reader.

As recorded earlier, the Declaration includes the following definition of forensic science.

> *... a case-based (or multi case-based) research-oriented, science-based endeavour to study traces – the remnants of past activities (such as an individual's presence and actions) – through their detection, recognition, recovery, examination and interpretation to understand anomalous events of public interest (e.g., crimes, security incidents).*

Having defined forensic science thus, it goes on to describe that definition as *'simple'*. Perhaps forensic science, as the 'science of the trace', might have been closer to Kirk's criteria and clearer to the reader.

Wordy and Information-Dense

Acknowledging that the Declaration is not intended for a non-specialist readership may explain its style. However, given its radical proposals and aim to win 'converts' and create 'disciples', greater clarity and focus, along with conciseness and brevity, would have helped. This would have avoided unnecessary information and overly complex language.

Science Must Support the Law and Justice

For the general reader, defining forensic science as science used to help resolve legal disputes or in support of law and justice suffices and, reflecting a little more deeply on that definition, it might also satisfy the specialist reader. Forensic science's *raison d'être* is to serve the law by helping to resolve legal disputes and deliver justice. Without the law, there would be no need for forensic science, however defined. Even applied to intelligence-led policing, in that context, forensic science remains supportive of the law and, from a law enforcement perspective, its purpose is to help solve crime. Solving crime brings several benefits, including increased public safety by removing criminals, deterring and therefore reducing the risk of further crimes and, of course, delivering justice for victims and society.

In addition to serving the needs of law enforcement, and perhaps more importantly, forensic science must serve justice. However, in common law justice systems, there are strict rules of evidence, such as the US Federal Rule of Evidence 702 discussed in Chapters 5 and 8. These rules determine the scientific evidence that can and cannot be admitted, the burden being on the science/scientist to satisfy the court of the relevance and reliability of the scientific evidence. These rules are aimed at limiting the evidence placed before the court to that which is strictly relevant so the fact-finder can focus solely on the facts in issue.

Whatever the immediate purpose, forensic science, however defined, will ultimately be used to help resolve legal disputes, such as guilt or not guilt. To do so effectively, the forensic scientist must remain impartial and independent and, when required, provide expert evidence based on observations and findings that are balanced, logical, transparent and robust.

There can be little doubt that, as many authors have claimed, forensic science lies at the science-law interface. As such, it serves the law, and its principal and ultimate purpose in criminal matters is to help solve the crime by identifying the criminal; thus, justice is delivered.

Misunderstood objectives and misaligned incentives, such as rewarding poor behaviours, have contributed to many miscarriages of justice, the recent scandal at the Queensland

Health Forensic Science Service, DNA Laboratory QHFSS, being a good example (Sofronoff 2022). Business-like, key performance indicators were deemed subordinate to the delivery of justice. Forensic scientists must be ever-vigilant; their ultimate role is to help deliver justice.

Too close a relationship with law enforcement puts impartiality and independence at risk. Such a relationship has and will put justice at risk.

A Profession Requires Standards

The authors of the Declaration claim to be the voice of *'a professional community'* but are not focused on organisation and protocols. However, a profession by its very nature is an assembly of individuals with a common principal aim bound by rules, regulations and codes, i.e. protocols. The purpose of those protocols is to distinguish between members and non-members. A profession is a community bound by conformance to standards – it is a standardised organisation.

Forensic Science Supporting the Defence

As described by the Declaration, there seems to be a large defence hole in traceology, its focus being on investigation from a prosecution perspective and supporting more effective policing, including reducing the public fear of crime! The trace is neutral, and findings may support the defence. In any event, any conclusion based on findings remains tentative until tested. Facts are determined by a tribunal, such as a court of law, and not by forensic scientists or law enforcement/prosecuting authorities.

In the inquisitorial or civil law justice system, there is less of a need for a defence expert, and one is rarely instructed. The examining magistrate (or equivalent) is required to seek and obtain all available evidence. In the adversarial or common law justice system, it is for the lawyers representing the parties to the dispute to decide what evidence to place before the court. It is then for the court to decide whether that evidence is admissible and, if admitted, for the fact-finder or jury to attach weight, determine the facts and reach a decision. What might seem to the forensic scientist as compelling scientific evidence of criminal activity, based on observations and findings, could be excluded as inadmissible or not used and therefore not heard by the jury. Even if that evidence is heard by the jury, exculpatory evidence presented by the defence might outweigh that seemingly compelling scientific evidence presented by the prosecution (see the later section on the misleading trace).

It should be recognised that in the common law system, when instructed by the defence and in conducting a review of the relevant evidence, the forensic scientist exercises a role closely resembling that of the generalist in terms of the scope. However, there is an important difference: non-attendance at the crime scene and reliance on findings gleaned at the scene by others. Nevertheless, the defence expert will review procedures and standards for individual evidence types and can also see the wider picture. More importantly, the defence expert is aware of what evidence the prosecution intends to present and the strategy to be adopted. The defence expert will advise and guide accordingly. To be clear, the defence expert, like all expert witnesses, has an overriding duty to the court and must be impartial. The essence of the role is to advise the defence on the strengths and weaknesses of the scientific evidence to be presented by the prosecution. It is perhaps important to stress that in common law justice systems, the burden of proof usually lies with the prosecution, in which case the defence does not have to prove anything or indeed call any witnesses or present any evidence. In terms of the justice system, this makes the role of the defence expert very different to that of the forensic scientist called by the prosecution. The expert called by the prosecution will be expected to support the prosecution's case, otherwise he or she would not be called. Having reported the strengths and weaknesses in the science supporting the prosecution case, the defence expert is unlikely to be called and his or her report not even served on the prosecution.

In passing, it is important to stress that if scientific evidence is to be presented at trial, the instruction of an expert by the defence is essential. As is evident from this book, time and again, an overclaiming prosecution presenting unreliable scientific evidence combined with a lazy defence has contributed to miscarriages of justice.

The apparent absence of consideration of the defence in the traceology model presented in the Declaration might be considered an important omission and may limit its scope.

The Scope Is Not Broad Enough, Forensic Science Is Not Just About Crime

Forensic science might be more broadly defined as the use of science to resolve regulatory disputes. This then brings into scope food forensics, a very active area in which the provenance of foodstuffs and beverages might be in dispute. Included in scope could also be non-criminal environmental forensics, pharmaceutical fraud and human provenance. The use of science in these areas is often to help address questions other than guilt or not guilt.

The focus in the Declaration on the exploitation of the trace in the context of crime/law enforcement/criminology is an example of how forensic science tends to be held in a law enforcement culture from which it needs to escape if it is to flourish.

Scene Activities Are Determined and Managed by Type

The Declaration is about fundamental principles which must be generic to be independent of '*local political and legal structures*' and so be widely applicable. It follows that, according to the Declaration model, the scene must also be a generic concept. While there are indeed general principles of scene management and processing, such as the need to control, preserve, record and collect, scenes can vary from, say, the scene of a suspicious death to a road traffic accident to a post-explosion scene. These scene types require very different skill sets for all those involved. Indeed, many jurisdictions have specialist teams to respond to major scenes. Team members will have been trained in the management and forensic exploitation of such scenes, including having the benefit of knowledge gleaned from related incidents. It is difficult to see how the same generalist might contribute to the investigation of such divergent scenes, and certainly not to the reconstruction of events. It is important to point out that there will be a high degree of collaboration between the specialist law enforcement officers, specialist scientists and others involved in the investigation of major scenes, whether directed by a judge or a law enforcement officer. In addition, there may be political involvement and the need for specialist communicators.

The type of scene will dictate how it is managed, processed and investigated. For a scene involving casualties, the preservation of life may take priority over other scene activities. For a scene involving fatalities, disaster victim identification may take priority.

Whatever the scene, the first and foremost aim is to determine whether a crime has been committed and, secondly, if so, by whom, i.e. identify the criminal(s). There may also be public safety issues.

In conclusion, then, it is difficult to envisage how a generalist might fruitfully contribute to the forensic exploitation of specialist scenes, particularly reconstruction.

Forensic Scientists, Technicians or Scientists

There is a recommendation in the Declaration that forensic scientists should *'first and foremost be educated as scientists and not technicians'*. This seems a harsh judgment on what the authors perceive to be the current situation. Two of the universities that pioneered the teaching of forensic science in the United Kingdom are Strathclyde in 1967 and King's College London (KCL) in 1985, both were and remain master's level courses. Many forensic science laboratories around the world are staffed by graduates of these courses.

The course at KCL is now directed by academics, but certainly in the early days, mostly delivered by practitioners. There was a broad curriculum covering most disciplines in forensic science. That course certainly did not produce technicians (Kings College London 2024).

The course at Strathclyde was mainly delivered by academics and is now complemented by lectures delivered by practitioners (University of Strathclyde 2024).

It is noteworthy that the modern father of traceology, Professor Magot, obtained his doctoral degree in forensic science from the University of Strathclyde, as have many other academic leaders.

A similar story might be told in the United States and countries in continental Europe, such as the Netherlands.

In addition, the university at the heart of the Declaration, Lausanne, certainly does not produce technicians!

While these graduates enter a world of forensic science currently conforming to the 2009 NAS Report model of disparate specialist disciplines, they are nevertheless schooled more as generalists than specialists, but admittedly not to the extent of Gross or Locard. However, it would be hard to make an argument that the extensive knowledge of evidence types and tests held by those pioneers is necessary today. Sadly, the main focus seems to be fingerprints, closed-circuit TV/facial recognition, DNA and digital.

Therefore, the argument that forensic scientists are trained and educated not as scientists but as technicians and are not given a *'foundation in the generalist approach to forensic science'* is not supported by the facts.

A Clash with Common Law

In its criticism of the focus on accreditation and certification, the Declaration appears to clash with some fundamentals of common law. Strictly, a tribunal of fact or court of law is not interested in the opinion of the forensic scientist acting as an expert witness, only in how that opinion was arrived at (Davie v Magistrates of Edinburgh 1953). The idea is to allow the fact-finder or jury to arrive at its own opinion/conclusion, which, having access to all the evidence provided by both parties, may well be an entirely different conclusion, as discussed in the section on the misleading trace. Therefore, to present findings that might be relied on by the fact-finder, the expert witness must conform to recognised standards and be subject to the independent oversight afforded by accreditation and certification.

The Development and Refinement of Traceology

As mentioned earlier, the contention that forensic science is the science of the trace was first mooted by Margot at Lausanne in the late 1980s and early 1990s. Traceology has subsequently been developed and refined in a series of publications, which are listed in the Biography, culminating in the Declaration.

An example of that development is that in earlier traceology publications, the trace was thought of as something small, as did Locard. Indeed, the trace was so small as to need a microscope for its recognition. According to the Declaration, a trace may now be as large as a *'megalith'*, a large rock. The Declaration's suggestion that a trace as something small was an incorrect assertion by reactionary *'chemists'* is somewhat disingenuous, as some of the authors of this publication have also held that view, as evidenced by earlier papers advancing the notion of traceology (Roux et al. 2015).

Increasing Complexity Means Increased Specialisation

Science used in support of the law and justice is becoming increasingly complex. Examples include the use of probabilistic genotyping, forensic genealogy and next-generation sequencing[8].

There is an adage attributed to several individuals, including the physicists Albert Einstein and Ernst Rutherford, that if you can't explain something simply, then you don't fully understand it. Explaining these complex technologies and the results produced simply is a challenge, a challenge that might only be met by specialists. Effective communication is a key competence in forensic science. In addition to increasingly complex analytical tools, there are also complex investigational tools such as Case Assessment and Interpretation (CAI), explained in Chapter 8 and discussed later in this chapter.

At some point, complexity will exceed the knowledge and understanding of a 'generalist', and the generalist must then give way to the specialist who should be better able to communicate in terms comprehensible to a lay fact-finder. Indeed, in both common and civil law systems, it is the role of the forensic scientist to aid the inquiry by providing knowledge and expertise beyond that of other parties.

It is difficult to see how increasing complexity can be accommodated in the traceology model of forensic science.

One of the Main Purposes of Forensic Science Is to Help Avoid a Miscarriage of Justice – Culture and Education Need Improvement

According to traceologists, the purpose of forensic science as a distinct discipline includes reconstructing, monitoring and preventing crime, together with addressing security issues.

The continuing miscarriages of justice will not slow the calls for improvements in quality and operational procedures, aims which the authors of the Declaration take issue with. As mentioned earlier, they contend that the emphasis on quality has not advanced the fundamentals of forensic science.

Cultural and educational weaknesses that risk miscarriages of justice remain high priorities for improvement. Much anecdotal evidence and many trial transcripts demonstrate that forensic scientists giving expert evidence often transpose the conditional. As discussed in Chapter 5, transposing the conditional risks unfairly strengthening the prosecution's case and is the logical equivalent of arguing that my sheep is a cow because it has four legs! In addition, as mentioned later, misunderstood objectives may persist, and poor-quality forensic science – however defined – continues to contribute to miscarriages of justice. Those responsible for educating and training forensic scientists must accept some responsibility for these weaknesses.

Before moving forward, these issues need to be addressed. Whatever forensic science is or is not, scientists will continue to give expert evidence to courts of law, and that evidence must be of sufficient quality to be relied upon by the fact-finder or jury to reach a safe decision by a fair process. Unless and until that objective is met, making philosophical claims about the epistemological basis of forensic science may seem a luxury to some.

It could be argued that one of the purposes of forensic science, however defined, is to prevent or at least reduce the risk of a miscarriage of justice.

Obstacles

The Challenge of Silos

There can be no doubt of the fragmentary nature of forensic science with discipline-specific approaches, categorical reporting here, likelihood ratios there, etc. This is not helped by fragmentary forensic science provision and law enforcement. The Netherlands perhaps offers a good model where there is a single police force and a single forensic science provider, the Netherlands Forensic Institute[9], housed at one location, facilitating an interdisciplinary and collaborative approach.

A less-than-ideal model would be federal Germany with its 16 states, most with their own forensic science laboratory or England and Wales (E&W), a single jurisdiction with 43 (yes, that's correct!) different police forces. E&W additionally and uniquely has a forensic science market that requires the protection of commercial advantage and intellectual property with tight regulatory oversight to ensure a level-playing field (UK Government 2024). One consequence of the market is that it introduces an additional layer of fragmentation, i.e. several different providers supporting one investigation (Gallop and Brown 2014).

There are nine police forces across Australia and New Zealand. Each state and territory police force in Australia has its own forensic division, and each state and territory has its own forensic science agency. As for the United States, the 2009 NAS Report (Chapter 9) highlighted the fragmentation and disconnects there, and one in particular, the barriers to the useful exchange of fingerprint data.

It does seem that, in many jurisdictions, the current fragmentation is so entrenched that a coherent and cohesive interdisciplinary approach to forensic science provision is an unlikely prospect, certainly in the near future.

Fragmentary Forensic Intelligence

While not supported by traceologists, as they accept but argue against the fragmentary status quo, there is movement regarding the exchange of forensic information for both investigation and intelligence. OSAC, ISO and the EU[10] have all individually taken steps to standardise procedures and terminology. As mentioned throughout the book, terminological ambiguity in forensic science is a major issue. These initiatives aim to ensure that forensic scientific evidence can be exchanged across borders, useful databases established and populated with valid data.

Regarding drug-related crime, the United Nations Office on Drugs and Crime (UNODC) has a long history of gathering intelligence. The UNODC conducts impurity profiling of drugs and gathers data to monitor the variation of production methods in cannabis (UNODC 2001, 2009).

These initiatives do not necessarily facilitate the timely provision of forensic intelligence advocated in the Declaration. However, they do provide intelligence which, in due course, will help to prevent and solve crimes.

Can Traceology Be Adequately Resourced? Terrorism Is

If the fundamental principles set out in the Declaration do become broadly accepted, then the degree to which they might be applied in practice will depend, to some extent, on the priority crime is given by society.

The resources required to implement the recommendations in the Declaration would essentially be knowledge and money. The generalist, undertaking a role similar to that of Gross or Locard, would need to acquire their extensive knowledge, or close to it. Society would need to provide the funds to educate such generalists to effectively examine a scene, recognise, recover and interrogate the trace in detail, for both evidential and intelligence purposes. The necessary resources might be hard to justify in low-level repetitive crime such as burglary or vehicle theft. However, the authors of the Declaration make a case for such resourcing to enable the gathering and exploitation of information for intelligence purposes.

For crimes that are a threat to society itself, such as terrorism, adequate resources are already in place. Natural scientists are recruited at the postgraduate level and then serve a multi-year apprenticeship in the specialism. Those scientists often visit the scene (e.g. post-explosion, cache or bomb factory and any other related scene) and perform the role of the scientific generalist as part of a multidisciplinary team (Broome and Todd 2012). In terms of trace (as in very low levels) detection and analysis, much is invested in research and development to answer the key questions, as much to enhance public safety as to identify the criminal(s) and solve the crime. For an idea of that investment, see 'The Forensic Investigation of Explosions' (Beveridge 2012).

Major law enforcement agencies across the 'western' world populate and maintain various shared databases for intelligence purposes, such as profiling terrorists and analysing criminal networks. Teams of highly trained and experienced investigators and scientists are on standby to respond to terrorist incidents. In addition, for counter-terrorism, a more complete criminological approach is used, e.g. (HMG 2011). So, for some major crimes, particularly those against society, the model detailed in the Declaration is largely in place.

Society allocates resources according to the type of crime, those that are a threat to society itself having the highest priority. The question is, would society be persuaded to adequately resource traceology and fully exploit the trace for low-level repetitive crime?

The Current Roles of Police, Investigators and Forensic Scientists Are a Barrier to Implementation

As mentioned earlier, in common law jurisdictions, the many roles undertaken by Gross and Locard are now divided among several other professions (Adam 2016). The principal role is that of the investigating officer, a police or law enforcement officer who leads and directs the investigation, relying on a multi-disciplinary team including specialist police officers, scientists and crime scene examiners to address the key questions: who, what, when, etc.

The senior investigating officer (SIO) will have been schooled in extracting information from the scene and will have much experience of general crime scene investigation or, for major crime scenes, specialist knowledge. As reported in Chapter 1, English versions of Gross's Handbook were used as manuals for detectives in London's New Scotland Yard until the 1970s. The SIO would direct crime scene investigation in the full sense of the term, i.e. reconstruction and solving crime and not just crime scene management, examination and processing – control, preserve, record, recognise and recover.

In civil law jurisdictions, such as those in continental Europe, the investigation is often led by an examining magistrate, an officer of the court, with experts such as scientists asked to assist the investigation as and when required, very much the model employed by Gross.

It is also important to note that, as far as the police/law enforcement in common law jurisdictions are concerned, once a person has been charged with an offence and sent for trial, that is pretty much the end of the matter. Whereas, for the forensic scientist, his or her most onerous task is just about to begin, providing impartial testimony that is balanced, logical, transparent and robust. Thereby assisting the fact-finder or jury to better understand the scientific evidence presented and reach a safe decision by a fair process. In contrast, police witnesses will be partisan, convinced of the defendant's guilt and accordingly biased in the evidence presented, as is their duty.

Standards for Intelligence and Evidence

The Declaration argues that for intelligence purposes, findings and observations gleaned from the trace might be put to early and non-judicial use, i.e. not necessarily placed before a court of law and tested. There is an argument made by some of the authors that if used for intelligence, for example, to link crimes, rather than as evidence before a court of law, that information need not be subjected to the checks and balances afforded by quality management (Bruenisholz et al. 2016). However, that intelligence may at some stage become evidence or at least be supportive of evidence and, because of its poorer quality, may misdirect an investigation. Recalling Chapter 8 on tunnel vision and Hans Gross' caveat about the preconceived theory, feeding an incorrect line of inquiry risks a course of action that would, and on many occasions has, resulted in a miscarriage of justice. It is worth considering for a moment the high standards required of DNA evidence from its earliest days (USA DNA Identification Act 1994) as discussed in Chapter 4. The key point is that information held on databases must be of sufficient quality to be reliable[11].

In many jurisdictions, laboratories that produce DNA information to be placed onto a database must be accredited to the international standard ISO/IEC 17025, the subject of Chapter 7, for that activity.

If the purpose of non-judicial use is to define possible explanations based on abductive reasoning (making educated guesses) as intelligence in support of the early stages of an investigation, then there is no quality issue.

Threats

Forensic Scientist, Criminologist or Criminalist

The Declaration strays into areas that might be properly termed forensic criminology[12]. Some forensic criminologists, listing the 'failures' catalogued in the 2009 NAS Report, for example, claim that they are better placed to undertake the traditional role of the forensic scientist, as understood by the authors of the Declaration (Gotham and Kennedy 2019). Furthermore, as forensic criminologists, they are better qualified to do so (Petherick et al. 2009).

It may be that criminologists, as social scientists, are better at exploiting traceology than natural scientists. This also seems to be the position of many of the authors of the Declaration, as expressed in 'The Routledge International Handbook of Forensic Intelligence and Criminology' (Rossy et al. 2018).

In which case, it might be time to consider resurrecting the term 'criminalistics' and 'criminalists' for those engaged in applying the natural sciences to the forensic exploitation of physical evidence, the investigation of crime and the resolution of legal disputes. Criminalistics is then a subdiscipline of forensic science, as forensic science is a subdiscipline of criminology.

It may become the role of the forensic scientist or criminalist (natural scientists) to generate the data, and for that data to be processed and analysed by criminologists (social scientists). Who knows what the future might hold?

To be fair, there is no doubt that closer cooperation between forensic scientists, as producers of forensic intelligence, and criminologists would be of benefit to society, as argued by Rossy et al. (Rossy et al. 2018).

The Misleading Trace

Unfortunately, because of the uncertainties of transfer, particularly secondary transfer[13] and persistence[14], these factors may confound any attempt at reconstruction. If recognised and recovered, the trace may be a remnant of an irrelevant event several times removed from the crime or crime scene. Because of the possibilities afforded by transfer and persistence, finding a person's DNA at a crime scene may not be evidence of their presence. Furthermore, the finding of an alleged perpetrator's DNA on the clothing of the alleged victim might be evidence of innocent social contact, or even presence at a common location, rather than criminal sexual contact.

In fairness, persistence and secondary transfer confounding the notion of the informative trace would be addressed by further research, which is acknowledged in the Declaration among the uncertainties. However, given the dropping of some trace evidence types, as discussed later in this section, obtaining funding for studying the transfer and persistence of 'retired' evidence types might be difficult, particularly for low-level repetitive crime.

As highlighted in the Declaration, the major uncertainty is that there is no way of knowing what actually happened in the past.

In common law justice systems, there will always be (at least) two editions of 'the truth' presented. Parties will select and focus on that part of 'the truth' that supports their case and ignore that part of 'the truth' that does not. The truth is in inverted commas because in all justice systems it is the fact-finder or jury that decides what 'the truth' is.

The trial of O.J. Simpson, as discussed in Chapter 5 on logical fallacies, is an example of how, in the adversarial or common law system, a 'truth' can be advanced that is not supported by the scientific evidence, in this case, blood groups. That 'truth', unsupported by the scientific evidence, but presented by a skilled advocate, was the one that seemed to be accepted by the jury in reaching its verdict. In essence, it is the lawyers who, for strategic or tactical reasons, decide what and how scientific evidence will be presented and what will be contested.

It is of interest to recall a case well known to forensic scientists, and that is *R v T* (R v T 2010). In appealing the trial court verdict, the defence had discovered that the expert who gave footwear evidence in support of the prosecution case had employed a likelihood ratio (LR) approach in evaluating the evidence and had not disclosed that fact at trial. The Court of Appeal reviewing the case took a dim view of the evaluative process based on what it considered flimsy data and effectively ruled that, outside the field of DNA analysis, where hard data is available, the LR approach should not be employed. The judgment of the Court of Appeal was roundly criticised by most of the forensic science community (Aitken et al. 2011; Thompson 2012). However, it is important to note that under the adversarial system the same lawyer who exposed the non-disclosure of the use of the LR in *R v T*, in his next case, might need to rely on the LR to help prove his client's innocence, which of course he would have a duty to do. As stated earlier, in common-law justice jurisdictions, it is lawyers who decide what evidence is to be presented and how it is to be presented, and courts decide what is to be admitted. This case helps emphasise the point that science is, to some extent, the servant of the law, and perhaps a definition of forensic science beyond that may be untenable.

Furthermore, if the trace can mislead to the extent that its absence cannot be taken as proof that it was never present and that its presence is not supportive of an alleged activity, then the question might arise: what is the point of looking for that trace? In other words, its presence may be a false positive and its absence a false negative. This evidential ambiguity has contributed to a decline in the search for certain traces[15]. Take gunshot residues (GSR), positive findings are often qualified by the caveat that the presence of GSR is not proof of firearms involvement, and contamination may be the source. On the other hand, the absence of GSR does not exclude firearms involvement. While the FBI denies it, the suspicion is that this lack of probative value through evidential ambiguity led the FBI to drop GSR in 2006 (Bykowicz 2006). Another example is the microscopic examination of hair, which has been discontinued after misleading evidence given by FBI examiners was revealed to have contributed to numerous miscarriages of justice (FBI 2015). Again, hair from different people has been declared to have the same source and hair from the same head has been declared to have different sources. The microscopic examination of hair is now only used to select candidate hairs for subsequent mitochondrial DNA analysis. Further, in 2005, following a critical report, the FBI 'retired' bullet lead analysis (National Research Council 2004; FBI 2005). A recent study by the US National Institute of Standards and Technology (NIST) has pretty much done for bite mark analysis (NIST 2023).

To be fair to the authors of the Declaration, they highlight the uncertainties and the need for research to gain a better understanding of those uncertainties, particularly of persistence and transfer, as stated earlier. Research is also required to determine the most probative features of the trace and the variance of those features that could affect probative value. However, to repeat the point, obtaining funding for that research might be difficult for 'retired' evidence types.

Biography of the Publication

The modern biography of the Declaration begins with Pierre Margot's lectures at the University of Lausanne in the late 1980s and early 1990s. However, in this book, the development of the Declaration is recorded as beginning in 2011.

2011 Commentary on the need for a research culture in the forensic sciences
(Margot 2011a)
2011 Forensic science on trial – What is the law of the land?
(Margot 2011b)
2011 Forensic science – A true science?
(Crispino et al. 2011)
2012 From forensics to forensic science
(Roux et al. 2012)
2014 Traceology: The trace as the fundamental vector of police science/forensic science
(Margot 2014)
2015 The end of the (forensic science) world as we know it? The example of trace evidence
(Roux et al. 2015)
2017 Traceology, the bedrock of forensic science and its associated semantics
(Margot 2014)
2021 A different perspective on the forensic science crisis
(Weyermann and Roux 2021)
2021 Shifting forensic science focus from means to purpose: A path forward for the discipline?
(Roux et al. 2021)
2022 Traceology, criminalistics, and forensic science
(Ristenbatt et al. 2022)
2022 The Sydney Declaration – Revisiting the essence of forensic science through its fundamental principles
(Roux et al. 2022)

The publication of the Declaration in 2022 has been followed by a special edition of Forensic Science International, 'The Sydney Declaration and the Status of Forensic Science', July 2023, which records several responses to the Declaration.

Professional Biography of the Authors

The principal author is Claude Roux, a former doctoral student of Pierre Margot at the University of Lausanne and now Professor of Forensic Science and Director of the Centre for Forensic Science at the University of Technology, Sydney. According to one biography, *'his professional motivation has been largely driven by his vision of forensic science as a distinctive academic and holistic research-based discipline'*. This explains his role in promoting traceology.

Another of the co-authors is Pierre Margot, already identified in this chapter as the modern father of traceology. He is a graduate of the University of Lausanne and obtained a doctoral degree in forensic science from the University of Strathclyde, Scotland. After post-doctoral positions in the United States, Switzerland and Australia, he was appointed professor at the ESC, University of Lausanne. He was the fourth to occupy what is the first academic chair of 'forensic science', created in 1909 at the University of Lausanne by Rudolphe Archibald Reiss, one of the pioneers of forensic science mentioned earlier in this chapter and discussed in Chapter 2. As of 2018, Margot had supervised over 30 PhD theses, and his research group had published over 220 peer-reviewed papers in the previous decade. In recognition of his contribution to forensic science over those decades, Margot has received many accolades.

Under his leadership, the Institute of Police Science and Criminology (IPSC and now ESC) of the University of Lausanne was a rich source of research and scholarship producing forensic scientists who have gone on to be leaders in their own right, for example, Claude Roux, Christophe Champod, the current Director of the ESC and others such as Olivier Ribaux, Professor Margot's immediate successor, Frank Crispino and Chris Lennard who are among the authors of the Declaration.

Impact Today

There has been an almost evangelical promotion of the Declaration at conferences, in social media and, as mentioned earlier, a special edition of the journal Forensic Science International responding to the Declaration; the Swiss having a deserved reputation for zealously fostering and promoting reformation!

As this chapter has emphasised, defining forensic science as the science of the trace at a fundamental, or even philosophical level, might be broadly accepted, for example, by both fingerprint examiners and DNA analysts. However, given the barriers and challenges detailed in this chapter, such as fragmentation and separation from the crime scene, it is difficult to see how this definition could overcome the deeply entrenched current model and lead to the common approach to operational practices, training, education, and research desired by the authors.

Contribution to Current Practice

The academics, graduates and students at the ESC remain true to the unified model of forensic science; narrow in definition, inclusive in scope and a subdivision of criminology, established at the University of Lausanne by Reiss in 1909. The question is, can Lausanne reconfigure forensic science to conform to its model? Success is claimed in the Cantons of Switzerland and Liechtenstein. However, we shall have to wait and see if success comes in common law jurisdictions such as Australia, but it won't be for want of trying!

The Way Ahead

Separation from a Law Enforcement Culture

One of the recommendations made in the 2009 NAS Report, the subject of Chapter 9, was greater separation between forensic science and law enforcement. Science, it argued, was better conducted in a science environment rather than one of law enforcement. The model presented in the Declaration, with its emphasis on knowledge creation for more effective policing, would more closely integrate forensic science and law enforcement. As recorded earlier, placing forensic science more firmly in the law enforcement camp could put at risk the impartiality and independence of the forensic scientist when acting as an expert witness. However, a separation between an examining scientist who may give expert evidence of opinion and a coordinating scientist, either non-testifying or giving factual expert evidence, as advocated in Chapters 6 and 8 and the model presented later in this chapter, might address this issue somewhat.

Another concern is that closer integration of forensic science and law enforcement may strengthen the misplaced belief by some forensic scientists that they are 'soldiers' in the 'war' against terrorism, drugs or crime in general, again endangering impartiality and independence. The forensic scientist's belief that they are on the prosecution team has contributed to many miscarriages of justice; examples are discussed in Chapter 7, the wrongful conviction of those accused of carrying out bombings in Britain in the 1970s being a good example of these misunderstood objectives (R v McIlkenny & Ors 1991). There is also the risk of contamination with the many cognitive biases that can infect an investigation, as discussed in Chapter 8.

All can agree that to achieve the aim of establishing a scientific research culture, forensic science must have a strong scientific foundation. However, to achieve that aim, it could be argued that there needs to be a move away from the pervasive law enforcement culture. The most direct way of doing this is to make forensic science provision and all that supports it, training, education and research, independent of law enforcement and strengthen relationships between forensic science laboratories/providers, universities and professional bodies.

It is often said that to fully understand who holds the power in any system, one should *'follow the money'*[16]. If forensic science is directly or indirectly funded by law enforcement, then law enforcement and not science will effectively set the research agenda or at least prepare the first draft. While conducting research in support of more effective policing is essential, it is questionable whether such research will improve forensic science and, as stated earlier, calls into question the impartiality of forensic scientists.

Research in a law enforcement culture will tend to focus on the propositions favourable to the prosecution; the probability of the trace given the prosecution proposition (supporting guilt), rather than the probability of the trace given the defence proposition (supporting innocence). In terms of logic, the focus of the research needs to be as much on scenarios producing likelihood ratios (LR) of less than one as those producing LRs of greater than one, more simply, focus on false positives. To give a specific example, research on circumstances in which the presence of gunshot residue is not the result of firearms involvement is unlikely to be supported.

The history of the implementation of Case Assessment and Interpretation (CAI), discussed in Chapter 8, does not bode well. While the use of the LR approach has gained ground in interpreting scientific evidence, discussed in Chapters 5, 6 and 8, a collaboration between the scientist and law enforcement to use the LR approach at the earliest stages of an investigation to identify traces with the highest probative potential has made little progress (Gallop and Brown 2014). The experience in E&W is revealed by the following quotes.

> *... re-positioning of forensic scientists within the decision-making hierarchy was out of keeping with traditional police views. CAI was found to conflict with the increased pressure on police forces to prosecute suspects:*
>
> *We had another group of officers who kind of misinterpreted really ... we had to do a bit of work re-assuring them that we weren't out to ... how shall I put it? Help the defendant ...* interviewee.
>
> *(Lawless and Williams 2010)*

It is worth repeating the important point made in Chapters 4 (DNA) and 9 (2009 NAS Report); the evidence type that has had the greatest impact on the management, delivery and practice of forensic science and on justice itself is DNA analysis. DNA 'fingerprinting', as it was, originated in an entirely scientific culture and not law enforcement. In contrast, those comparison disciplines that emerged from a police/law enforcement culture have been the most heavily criticised and were/are often of questionable reliability, see the chapter on the 2009 NAS Report.

As mentioned earlier, the focus in the Declaration on crime to the exclusion of exploiting the trace for resolving non-criminal disputes supports the contention that forensic science is overly influenced by law enforcement.

Several of the authors, including the lead author, are based in Australia, a territory in which the police have a significant influence on forensic science research, management, delivery and practice through the Australia New Zealand Policing Advisory Agency (ANZPAA NIFS 2024). Australia could then be a good place to start moving away from a law enforcement culture. However, David H. Kaye[17] in his review of the 2009 NAS Report indicates the uphill struggle that might be (Kaye 2010). Which, given the lack of progress on the recommendation, which was made in 2009, is evidence of its unlikely success.

Greater separation between forensic science research and provision from law enforcement would not only allow science to take the lead in setting the research and development agenda but would aid the delivery of justice by removing the potentially biasing influence of law enforcement. Of course, as part of the justice system, forensic science would remain a partner of law enforcement, but a more equal partner.

Police Unlikely to Cede Power

Given the influence and indeed control exercised by the police and law enforcement over forensic science in common law jurisdictions, it is unlikely they will cede that power easily. Ironically, those best placed to lobby for moving forensic science from a law enforcement culture to a science culture are the authors of the Declaration, doing so by exercising their academic freedom.

The current fragmented model means that it may be that only when all the constituent parts and disparate disciplines have conformed separately to the traceology model will traceology be accepted as the fundamental model of forensic science, as the authors of the Declaration campaign for.

However, the current 'silo' model is so deeply entrenched that the alternative model advanced by the Declaration might never emerge in common law systems. In the meantime, the authors could begin by lobbying for independence from law enforcement.

The fundamental challenge is to rest power from the current holders, and the way to do this is to strengthen relationships between universities, forensic science providers and professional bodies to rebalance the relationship between science and law enforcement.

Organic Development of Specialisms

While there is no doubt forensic science is fragmented, the operational models presented by the traceologist do not always ring true. From personal experience, laboratories' capabilities develop organically and often around a particular type of threat or crime, for example, document examination and fraud. At the questioned documents section of the UK's Laboratory of the Government Chemist (LGC), scientists, who are mostly chemists, examine handwriting, test papers, inks and toners, examine and compare photographs, visualise indented impressions and look for physical matches. The Forensic Explosives Laboratory of the UK's Ministry of Defence was established in the 1880s to combat terrorism and has developed and maintains a range of analytical techniques (spectroscopic, spectrometric, and chromatographic). It provides a holistic service from the crime scene to court and feeds into several intelligence capabilities. It also has a team dedicated to research (Dstl 2021). On a different scale, the agencies of the US Department of Justice had a similar organic development in response to particular crimes/threats (FBI: major/organised crime, ATF: prohibition and DEA: drugs). These agencies again offer a holistic service and contribute to many databases for intelligence purposes.

In summary, many current forensic science laboratories were established and are maintained to respond to particular threats to society. They provide a holistic crime-scene-to-court service, contribute to intelligence-led policing and invest heavily in relevant research based on identified capability gaps. However, it is conceded that they are not typical 'crime labs'.

Budgets

As recorded earlier, in many jurisdictions, budgets are allocated according to the type of crime. The investigation of a possible murder or terrorist incident will have a larger budget than, say, burglary, usually classified as volume crime. These budgets translate into the allocation of resources. For low-level crime, the likely response is a cursory scene visit from a uniformed police officer and the provision of a crime number for an insurance claim. This response provides little or no opportunity to exploit the trace for intelligence purposes. Given the call on the public purse in many jurisdictions, such low-level repetitive crime is unlikely to see an increase in funding and will therefore fall outside the scope of traceology.

The Future

What the future holds for traceology is unclear. The decades-long campaign with an almost evangelical zeal to promote the main themes – forensic science as the science of the trace, that crime scene investigation is a scientific endeavour, that the traceology model will benefit more effective policing through generating, exploiting intelligence and the benefits of a generalist at the crime scene – has yet to have a discernible effect or impact beyond those that advocate for it and in some civil law systems. Traceology probably won't have much of an impact until the stakeholders holding the purse strings are convinced of its practical merits and the advantages of having a scientific generalist at the scene, as promoted by the Declaration. Until that time, forensic science will continue to be reactive, responding to miscarriages of justice which demand political action. The response is often a very costly inquiry, which typically finds 'missed opportunities' and concludes that 'human failings' rather than 'systemic failures' are at fault. Recommendations are made, often for tighter regulation, but implementation depends on politics; some quick fixes may be applied, and the world moves on. Unfortunately, most developed societies do not see justice, beyond 'banging up the bad guys', as a high priority; therefore, it is often the case that there are few votes in improving criminal justice systems.

This reveals the fundamental challenge. All criminal justice stakeholders should promote an effective criminal justice system as the hallmark of a civilised society, and, as such, it should be adequately resourced, perhaps on an equal footing with health and education. Defining 'justice' as people getting what they deserve, a criminal justice system must deliver justice for all: suspects, offenders, victims and society.

Responsibility for the Next Steps

According to the Declaration, responsibility for the next steps lies with any party but the universities. However, universities are surely in the best position, possessing the power and independence (one would hope!) to lobby for change.

The Declaration looks in part to practising forensic scientists to spread the word. However, most forensic scientists are either directly employed by law enforcement agencies, particularly in the United States, or indirectly by government labs relying on the work provided by law enforcement for their income and economic survival. Even in E&W, where the market has led to the establishment of 'independent' forensic science providers, their income is derived from work commissioned by the police. As the commissioning authority, the police have a great deal of influence, and forensic science providers tend to be treated as little more than test houses (Gallop 2020).

Drawing Strands Together, A Model Forensic Science Provider

Building on the 'ideal' forensic science laboratory described in Chapter 8, a model comprising the following elements is suggested.

1. Separation from law enforcement
2. Case assessment and interpretation (CAI)

3. A coordinating scientist
    a. A generalist who participates in the CAI process
    b. Allocates tasks to examining scientists and shields them from potentially biasing information
    c. Testifies only on matters of fact
    d. Acts as the generalist directing forensic activities at the scene, as promoted in the Sydney Declaration and leads on forensic intelligence
4. An examining scientist, a specialist shielded from potentially biasing information
5. Blind verification in comparison procedures
6. Accreditation of organisations
7. Independent certification of individual competence
8. A policed and enforced code of ethics
9. Quality management system in the public domain, including SOPs
10. Evidence conforming to the principles of
    a. Balance – always considering alternative mutually exclusive propositions,
    b. Logic – always considering the likelihood of the evidence and not the proposition
    c. Transparency – clearly setting out the link between the evidence and any conclusion drawn and highlighting any weaknesses
    d. Robustness – a sound basis of evidence (research and data) in support of the interpretation process
11. Independent peer review of reports
12. Reports conforming to the practice directions of the jurisdiction

Key Takeaways

The Sydney Declaration was published in 2022. It is the latest stage in a concerted campaign by a group mainly comprised of academics, many with links to the University of Lausanne, Switzerland. The purpose of the campaign is to (re)define forensic science as the science of the trace. The trace is the remains of an (unlawful) activity and the neutral carrier and transmitter of information, essentially regarding source, activity and enabling the reconstruction of past events. By such a definition, the authors seek to unify the many and varied disciplines that constitute forensic science. The definition provides a sound theoretical framework and answers the call of Paul Kirk in his Ontogeny paper for progress on fundamental principles. The challenge is for the (re)definition to find general acceptance and turn theory into practice. The campaign continues.

The trace is certainly a concept that can link forensic science disciplines and provide coherence and cohesion to the study of forensic science and the education of forensic scientists. Whether traceology will have an operational impact beyond a few civil law jurisdictions is open to question; only time will tell.

The term 'trace' is related to the 'exchange principle' wrongly attributed to Edmond Locard and often paraphrased as 'every contact leaves a trace', the subject of Chapter 2. Although it seems reasonable, the principle can never be proved, and one exception would undermine it.

To fully exploit the information the trace can provide, the authors argue that a scientific generalist should be at the scene of the crime as a matter of course. The role described is like that of the early criminologists Hans Gross and Edmond Locard. However, the role envisioned in the Declaration is somewhat narrower in scope.

The authors go on to argue that by being at the scene, the scientific generalist can pass on information promptly for intelligence as well as evidential purposes, for example, to link to other crimes. They also contend that information used for intelligence purposes can be of a lesser quality than information used for evidential purposes; this is problematic.

The authors reasonably assert that intelligence gathered and processed by traceologists can aid the investigation of future crimes and support more effective policing. However, supporting more effective policing through a closer relationship with law enforcement might put impartiality at risk.

The role of the generalist, as described by the authors, more easily applies to repetitive volume crime such as burglary and the like. It is unclear how it might apply to major crimes such as murder or terrorism, which are usually investigated by a multi-disciplinary team of specialists.

The analysis of the current situation presented in the Declaration is generally true, but there are exceptions. In some jurisdictions and for some major crimes, forensic scientists regularly attend scenes, participate in multi-disciplinary teams and provide a crime scene-to-court service. Furthermore, databases are maintained and populated with valid data for intelligence purposes.

The main challenge faced is that the current forensic science model in many jurisdictions supports law enforcement, which is only one element of the criminal justice system, but the model is deeply embedded. Furthermore, forensic science is fragmented, as is the environment in which it operates. Disparate disciplines lie deep within their silos, and crime scene management, processing and investigation rest very much with other parties. In common law jurisdictions, such as those in the United States, law enforcement takes the lead, and in civil law jurisdictions, such as in continental Europe, the examining magistrate (or equivalent) does. Forensic scientists, usually specialists, are 'on tap' and not 'on top'. In addition, the trend is towards greater specialisation driven by increasing complexity, such as the application of forensic genealogy and familial searching.

In part, the Declaration seems to blur the distinction between forensic science and criminology, given the Declaration's Lausanne origins, perhaps intentionally. Much of what the Declaration advocates for is criminological. So much so that even if the authors succeeded in establishing the science of the trace as a holistic discipline, it would remain a subdiscipline of criminology and perhaps forensic scientists would become subordinate to, and therefore under the direction of, criminologists!

In addition to blurring the distinction between forensic science and criminology, the publication has some other weaknesses. It is, in parts, a hard read. Significantly, it pays little or no attention to the impact of miscarriages of justice, which will continue the pressure for quality improvements and greater regulation. In addition, continuing miscarriages of justice call into question the training and education of forensic scientists whose actions contribute to some miscarriages. It also fails to recognise that too close a relationship with law enforcement will put impartiality at risk.

It should be borne in mind that the trace can be misleading through variable and uncertain persistence and secondary transfer, such that the absence of evidence may actually be evidence of absence!

The Declaration also calls for forensic science to adopt a scientific research culture. One example given is that information held within forensic science laboratories might be made available for interdisciplinary study between practitioners and academics. This might be best achieved by requiring forensic science providers to place in the public domain their quality management system, including standard operating procedures, and perhaps one day even case files.

Another step towards a scientific culture would be separating law enforcement from forensic science provision, as recommended by the 2009 NAS Report. Much of this book has highlighted the influence on the development of forensic science of molecular biology (DNA analysis, Chapter 4), mathematics (the likelihood ratio approach to interpretation, Chapter 6), philosophy (logical fallacies, Chapter 5) and psychology (cognitive bias, Chapter 8). None of these contributors to current practice had their origin in law enforcement.

The role of Arthur Conan Doyle's fictional character Sherlock Holmes in the promotion of traceology, and more broadly forensic science, cannot be underestimated. His name and behaviour are applied to many of the key players.

Finally, it is generally accepted that forensic science, however defined, lies at the interface of science and the law, the aim being to aid the delivery of justice. The authors of the Declaration argue for a greater role for forensic science in the criminal justice system. However, forensic science is and will remain subservient to the law and that must be accepted as a fundamental principle. The law will determine the success or otherwise of the Declaration.

Notes

1. A concise definition of criminology is the study of all aspects of crime. A fuller definition is given in the chapter on Terms, Definitions and Explanations. Other definitions are given in this chapter. According to some, forensic criminology is the scientific study of crime and criminals for the purposes of addressing investigative and legal issues; it is a subdiscipline of criminology (Turvey and Petherick 2010).
2. Author of 'Forensic Chemistry and Scientific Criminal Investigation', which cited Gross' Handbook.
3. In a private communication, Professor Margot reports that after 25 years, there are now many Lausanne ESC graduates exercising crime scene examination roles in the police forces of Switzerland and Liechtenstein.
4. This publication is probably the closest to Gross' Handbook in the English language but only very occasionally references Gross and that is to a 1934 English edition edited by N Kendal. For any student of forensic science Kirk's 'Crime Investigation' is a must read.
5. Professor Margot would be the first to acknowledge that he is following in the footsteps of his predecessor, Reiss.
6. Force = mass times acceleration. Energy = mass times the speed of light squared.
7. It is worth pointing out that these laws make a prediction or are predictive, whereas the nature of forensic science, as emphasised in the Declaration, is retrodictive, that is the reconstruction of past events from traces available in the present.

8 Probabilistic genotyping involves mathematically generating virtual full DNA profiles based on limited information; it is discussed in Chapter 4. Forensic genealogy involves using genetic information, usually from consumer DNA testing companies, and combining it with traditional genealogical methods, like tracing family trees, to establish relationships and identify individuals. Its most famous use to date was in identifying the 'Golden Gate Killer' (St. John 2020). Next-generation sequencing or massive parallel sequencing provides far more information than normal DNA STR profiling and can produce useful profiles from highly degraded DNA.

9 Arguably one of the best forensic science laboratories in the world. A national facility housed under one roof!

10 Organization of Scientific Area Committees – register of standards and lexicon. ISO Technical Committee 272 – ISO 20143. European Union – Council Decision 2008/615/JHA.

11 Of sufficient quality to enable a tribunal of fact (jury) to reach a safe decision by a fair process.

12 The scientific study of crime and criminals for the purpose of addressing investigative and legal issues, a subdiscipline of criminology (Petherick et al. 2009).

13 Secondary transfer is any transfer of the trace beyond primary or direct transfer.

14 How long a trace may remain in place after deposition.

15 The advent of fast and/or powerful evidence types, DNA, CCTV, FP and digital have also contributed.

16 Made popular by the 1976 docudrama 'All the President's Men'.

17 Distinguished professor of law emeritus at Penn State Law and frequent commentator on forensic science, see Forensic Science Statistics and the Law https://for-sci-law.blogspot.com/.

Bibliography

Adam, Alison. 2016. "Hans Gross and Criminalistics." In *A History of Forensic Science – British Beginnings in the Twentieth Century*, edited by Alison Adam, 63–66. London & New York: Routledge.

Adams, Alison. 2016. "The Influence of Scientific Criminology and Criminalistics." In *A History of Forensic Science: British Beginnings* Crispino, Frank, Olivier Ribaux, Max Houck, and Pierre Margot. 2011. "Forensic Science – A True Science?" *Australian Journal of Forensic Sciences* 43 (2): 157–76.

Davie v Magistrates of Edinburgh. 1953. SC 34 (Court of Session (Scotland)).

De Forest, Peter R. 1998. "Proactive Forensic Science." *Science & Justice* 38 (1): 1–2.

Doyle, Sean and Dianne Doyle. 2011. "The AFSP Standard – A Lesson for Law Enforcement Agencies." *Science and Justice* 52: 17–19.

Dstl. 2021. *Dstl Marks 150 Year History of Its Forensic Explosives Laboratory*. GOV.UK. 11 August. Accessed September 4, 2024. https://www.gov.uk/government/news/dstl-marks-150-year-history-of-its-forensic-explosives-laboratory.

ENFSI. 2020. *Working Groups*. Accessed August 16, 2024. https://enfsi.eu/about-enfsi/structure/working-groups/.

ESR. 2024. *Forensic Scene Investigation*. Accessed September 11, 2024. https://www.esr.cri.nz/expertise/forensic-science/forensic-scene-investigations/.

FBI. 2005. "FBI Laboratory Announces Discontinuation of Bullet Lead Examinations." *The FBI Federal Bureau of Investigation*. FBI National Press Office. 1 September. Accessed September 9, 2024. https://archives.fbi.gov/archives/news/pressrel/press-releases/fbi-laboratory-announces-discontinuation-of-bullet-lead-examinations.

FBI. 2015. "FBI Testimony on Microscopic Hair Analysis Contained Errors in at Least 90 Percent of Cases in Ongoing Review." *FBI News Press Release*. 20 April. Accessed August 2023. https://www.fbi.gov/news/press-releases/fbi-testimony-on-microscopic-hair-analysis-contained-errors-in-at-least-90-percent-of-cases-in-ongoing-review#:~:text=%E2%80%9CThese%20findings%20confirm%20that%20FBI,Project%2C%20which%20is%20affiliated%20with.

Fraser, Jim. 2020. "Preface and acknowledgements to second edition." In *Forensic Science: A Very Short Introduction*, written by Jim Fraser, xviii. Oxford: Oxford University Press.

Gallop, Angela. 2020. "Unnatural Selection – Forensic Science on the Endangered List." *The Barrister* Easter: 26–27.

Gallop, Angela and Jennifer Brown. 2014. "The Market Future for Forensic Science Services in England and Wales." *Policing* 29 (June): 254–64.

Girod-Frais, Aline and Julia Anna Kappler. 2022. "Rudolf Archibald Reiss and the Importance of Forensic Science." *SIAK International Edition* 19 (5): 4–17.

Gotham, Kevin Fox and Daniel Bruce Kennedy. 2019. "Introduction to the Practice of Forensic Criminology." In *Practicing Forensic Criminology*, edited by Kevin Fox Gotham and Daniel Bruce Kennedy, 1–21. London: Academic Press.

HMG. 2011. *CONTEST The United Kingdom's Strategy for Countering Terrorism*. London: The Stationery Office Limited.

Jackson, Graham and Alex Biedermann. 2019. "'Source' or 'Activity' What is the Level of Issue in a Criminal Trial?" *Significance* 16 (2): 36–39.

Kaye, David H. 2010. "The Good, the Bad, the Ugly: The NAS Report on Strengthening Forensic Science in America." *Science and Justice* 50: 8–11.

Kings College London. 2024. *Forensic Science MSc/MRes*. Accessed August 24, 2024. https://www.kcl.ac.uk/study/postgraduate-taught/courses/forensic-science-msc-mres.

Kirk, Paul Leland. 1953. *Crime Investigation: Physical Evidence and the Police Laboratory*. New York: Interscience.

Lawless, Christopher and Robin Williams. 2010. "Helping with Inquiries or Helping with Profits? The Trials and Tribulations of a Technology of Forensic Reasoning." *Social Studies of Science* 40 (5): 731–55.

Locard, Edmond. 1929. "The Analysis of Dust Traces." *Revue Internationale de Criminalistique* 1 (Nos. 4-5): 176–249.

Margot, Pierre. 2011a. "Commentary on The Need for a Research Culture in The Forensic Sciences." *UCLA Law Review* 58: 795–801.

Margot, Pierre. 2011b. "Forensic Science on Trial – What is the Law of the Land?" *Australian Journal of Forensic Sciences* 43: 89–103.

Margot, Pierre. 2017. "Traceology, the Bedrock of Forensic Science and Its Associated Semantics." In *The Routledge International Handbook of Forensic Intelligence and*

Criminology, edited by Quentin Rossy, David Décary-Hétu, Olivier Delémont, and Massimiliano Mulone. London: Routledge.

Margot, Pierre. 2014. "Traceology: The Trace as the Fundamental Vector of Police Science/ Forensic Science." *Revue Internationale de Criminologie et de Police Technique et Scientifique* 67 (1): 72–97.

May, Luke S. 1936. *Crime's Nemesis*. New York: The Macmillan Company.

Mulone, Massimiliano, Quentin Rossy, David Décary-Hétu, and Olivier Delémont. 2018. "Introduction." In *The Routledge International Handbook of Forensic Intelligence and Criminology*, 1–3. London: Routledge.

National Research Council. 2004. *Forensic Analysis: Weighing Bullet Lead Evidence*, 226. Washington, DC: The National Academies Press.

NIST. 2023. "Special Programs Office. Forensic Science Program." *NIST*. 13 March. Accessed August 14, 2024. https://www.nist.gov/spo/forensic-science-program/bitemark-analysis-nist-scientific-foundation-review.

O'Hara, Chris E. and James W. Osterburg. 1949. *An Introduction to Criminalistics: The Application of the Physical Sciences to the Detection of Crime*. New York: The Macmillan Company.

PCAST. 2016. *Forensic Science in Criminal Courts: Ensuring Scientific Validity of Feature-Comparison Methods*. Report, Washington, DC: President's Council of Advisors on Science and Technology.

Perkins, Robert M. 1950. "Book Review, Introduction to Criminalistics." *University of Miami Law Review* 3 (2): 257–60.

Petherick, Wayne A., Brent E. Turvey, and Caire E. Ferguson. 2009. *Forensic Criminology*. London: Academic Press.

R v McIlkenny & Ors. 1991. 287 (Cr.App.R.).

R v T. 2010. 2439 (EWCA).

Ristenbatt, Ralph R., Jack Hietpas, Peter R. De Forest, and Pierre A. Margot. 2022. "Traceology, Criminalistics, and Forensic Science." *Journal of Forensic Science* 67 (1): 28–32.

Rossy, Quentin, David Décary-Hétu, Olivier Delémont, and Massimiliano Mulone. 2018. *The Routledge International Handbook of Forensic Intelligence and Criminology*. Abingdon, Oxon: Routledge.

Roux, Claude. 2018. "Contributors." In *The Routledge International Handbook of Forensic Intelligence and Criminology*, edited by Quentin Rossy, David Décary-Hétu, Olivier Delémont, and Massimiliano Mulone, xx. London: Routledge.

Roux, Claude, Benjamin Talbot-Wright, James Robertson, Frank Crispino, and Olivier Ribaux. 2015. "The End of the (Forensic Science) World as We Know It? The Example of Trace Evidence." *Philosophical Transactions of the Royal Society B* 370: 1–8.

Roux, Claude, Frank Crispino, and Olivier Ribaux. 2012. "From Forensics to Forensic Science." *Current Issues in Criminal Justice* 24 (1): 7–24.

Roux, Claude, Rebecca Bucht, Frank Crispino, Peter De Forest, Chris Lennard, Pierre Margot, Michelle D. Miranda, et al. 2022. "The Sydney Declaration – Revisiting the Essence of Forensic Science Through Its Fundamental Principles." *Forensic Science International* 332: 1–10.

Roux, Claude, Sheila Willis, and Celine Weyermann. 2021. "Shifting Forensic Science Focus from Means to Purpose: A Path Forward for the Discipline?" *Science and Justice* 61: 678–86.

Sofronoff, Walter. 2022. "Final Report Commission of Inquiry into Forensic DNA Testing in Queensland." Commission of Inquiry.

St. John, Paige. 2020. "The Untold Story of How the Golden State Killer was Found: A Covert Operation and Private DNA." *Los Angeles Times*, 8 December.

Thompson, William C. 2012. "Discussion Paper: Hard Cases Make Bad Law – Reactions to R v T." *Law, Probability and Risk* 11 (4): 347–59.

Turvey, Brent E. and Petherick A. Petherick. 2009. "Preface: The Origins of Forensic Criminology." In *Forensic Criminology*, edited by Wayne A. Petherick, Brent E. Turvey, and Claire E. Ferguson, 24. London: Academic Press.

Turvey, Brent E. and Wayne A. Petherick. 2010. "Preface: The Origins of Forensic Criminology." In *Forensic Criminology*, edited by Wayne A. Petherick, Brent E. Turvey and Claire F. Ferguson, 21. Burlington, MA: Academic Press.

UK Government. 2024. *Forensic Science Regulator*. Accessed September 12, 2024. https://www.gov.uk/government/organisations/forensic-science-regulator.

UNIL University of Lausanne. n.d. *School of Criminal Sciences*. Accessed August 26, 2024. https://www.unil.ch/esc/fr/home/menuinst/lecole.html.

University of Strathclyde. 2024. *MSc Forensic Science*. Accessed August 22, 2024. https://www.strath.ac.uk/courses/postgraduatetaught/forensicscience/.

UNODC. 2001. *Drug Characterization/Impurity Profiling – Background and Concepts*. Guidance, New York: United Nations.

UNODC. 2009. *Recommended Methods for the Identification and Analysis of Cannabis and Cannabis Products*. Guidance, New York: United Nations.

Weyermann, Céline and Claude Roux. 2021. "A Different Perspective on the Forensic Science Crisis." *Forensic Science International* 323: 1–7.

Index

A History of Forensic Science in 10 Publications: How They Established Current Practice, First Edition.
Sean Doyle.

g

h

www.ingramcontent.com/pod-product-compliance
Lightning Source LLC
LaVergne TN
LVHW062200200926
848484LV00006B/1291

* 9 7 8 1 3 9 4 1 7 0 7 6 0 *